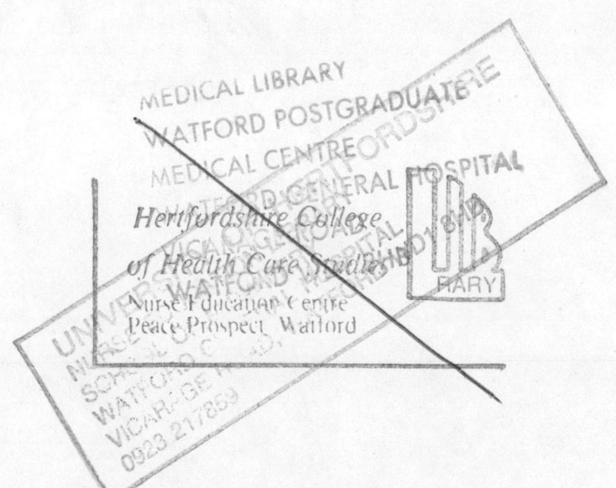
MEDICAL LIBRARY
WATFORD POSTGRADUATE
MEDICAL CENTRE
WATFORD GENERAL HOSPITAL
VICARAGE ROAD
WATFORD WD1 8HB
Hertfordshire College
of Health Care Studies
Nurse Education Centre
Peace Prospect, Watford
0923 217859

COUNSELLING IN REHABILITATION

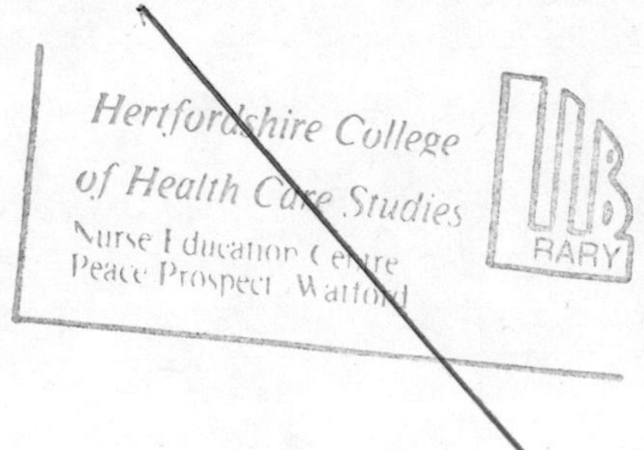

COUNSELLING IN REHABILITATION

William Stewart
BA, RGN, RMN, Dip. Soc. Studies

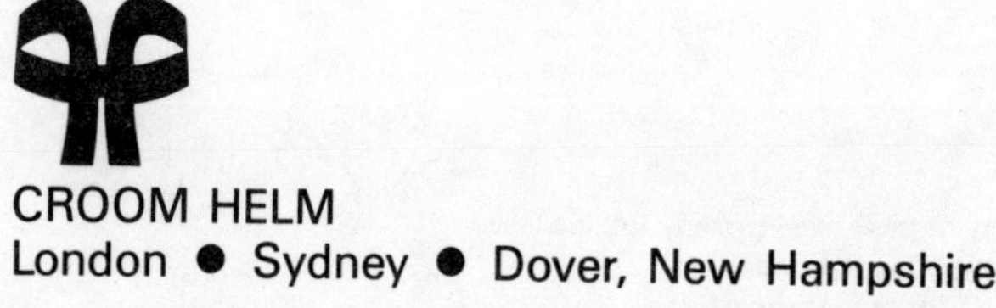

CROOM HELM
London • Sydney • Dover, New Hampshire

Croom Helm Ltd, Provident House, Burrell Row,
Beckenham, Kent BR3 1AT

Croom Helm Australia Pty Ltd, Suite 4, 6th Floor, 64–76 Kippax Street,
Surry Hills, NSW 2010, Australia

British Library Cataloguing in Publication Data

Stewart, William, 1927—
Counselling in rehabilitation.
1. Counselling
I. Title
362.1'04256 RM735

ISBN 0-7099-4310-5

Croom Helm, 51 Washington Street, Dover,
New Hampshire 03820, USA

Library of Congress Cataloging-in-Publication Data

Stewart, William, 1927-
Counselling in rehabilitation.
Includes index.
1. Health counseling. 2. Rehabilitation
counseling. 3. Sick—Psychology. I. Title.
[DNLM: 1. Counseling. 2. Rehabilitation.
WB 320 S852c]
R727.4.S74 1985 362.4'0486 85-18992

ISBN 0-7099-4310-5 (pbk.)

Filmset by Mayhew Typesetting, Bristol, England
Printed and bound in Great Britain
by Billing & Sons Limited, Worcester.

CONTENTS

To

Ron Tebay

a constant inspiration and
support over many months of writing

PREFACE

'Counselling In Rehabilitation' is written for all people — professionals (of whatever discipline) and lay — who are, in any way, involved with others who, by reason of crippling disease or accident, need rehabilitation in order to prevent, minimise or alleviate disability.

The spur to write this book was a challenge issued by a group of students on the 'Rehabilitation Studies' (Diploma/MSc) course at Southampton University, to which course I have the privilege to be a contributor. This is a unique, multidisciplinary course which draws students from every health care discipline worldwide.

Not until I was challenged to write a book devoted to counselling in rehabilitation did I realise how scarce such publications are. I was not asked to write for professional rehabilitation counsellors (there are already a number of such books) but for therapists using counselling as one of their repertoire of skills. It has been my firm belief, over many years, that all health-care workers have a counselling component as an integral part of their work. Yet very few of them receive counselling training. The workshops I run, and this book, attempt to remedy this deficiency.

The emphasis throughout the book is on the personal, emotional and social aspects of disease and disability, rather than on practical rehabilitation. I hope that you, the reader, will gain fresh insights from this approach to help you in your own counselling.

Two basic premises form the basis of 'Counselling In Rehabilitation':

1. Every therapist uses counselling skills, and wants to improve them.
2. Every illness and disability imposes its own stresses which influence every part of the person's life.

Counselling, as an integral part of therapy, may help to relieve such stresses and so assist recovery.

All references to therapists and patients in this book have been made under fictitious names.

ACKNOWLEDGEMENTS

There are many people to whom I owe thanks and without whom this book would not have been written. There are the students who provided the initial impetus; the people who talked so readily to me about their various illnesses and disabilities; the care staff who talked about their 'problem patients'; the librarians at Southampton Medical Library, particularly Jacquie Welch, the 'computer on-line wizard'; and the librarians at Knowle Hospital and Tachbury Mount Hospital. You were all so patient and helpful, thank you.

FOREWORD

The medical model of illness is a powerful one. At its centre is physical pathology, to which diagnosis and physical intervention are directed. Advances in knowledge have given us the ability to alleviate many of the diseases from which previous generations suffered. Yet with these advances, skills that previously constituted medical treatment have been neglected, not only by the medical profession but also by increasingly technologically minded nurses and therapists. Our considerably improved state of health and life expectancy has relieved many of us of the experience, in our formative years, of illness and disability — experience which previously was shared and intuitively understood. Most of us first meet serious illness and disability in a novel or in poetry, television, or perhaps in religious writings. The reality when it comes is strange and frightening and our reactions often delay or divert us from taking full advantage of medical treatment.

Rehabilitation is becoming increasingly recognised as an intellectually respectable part of the process of recovery and adjustment after an illness. It is a part which needs to be taken seriously by all those who are caring for the patient even in the acute stage of a disease. To ensure that rehabilitation occurs successfully, health care staff need to develop a perceptive and imaginative approach to their patients. People generally have come to realise that they do not have to choose between a physically effective cure for their pathology and humane guidance as to how to cope with it. They quite rightly want both.

In practice these responsibilities fall particularly to nurses and therapists because they have so much more time in personal contact with the patient. But the issues set out in this admirable book are of fundamental importance to all of us who are involved with the process of recovery from disease and adjustment to its effects. Doctors are respected for their wide knowledge of the complexities of disease, yet many seem to understand little about the psychological and emotional impact of an illness on a person and on his family. In failing to take advantage of their position to help the patient through these experiences, they fail also in their aim of alleviating suffering. A glance at any standard medical textbook will make clear how little emphasis current training places on these subtle, important and fascinating aspects of disease.

This book, by an experienced counsellor and teacher, explores these issues and the strategies necessary to help those whose rehabilitation is faltering because of a lack of understanding or failure of satisfactory adjustment. It exemplifies the approach of the successful counsellor in its clear and unpedantic style, leaving valuable signposts that can be returned to as occasion demands.

The early part of the book explores the goals of rehabilitation and how its aims are identified for an individual patient. It charts the process of counselling and how counselling differs from giving advice, being sympathetic, or psychoanalysis. It is certainly possible to counsel effectively using only intuition and imagination. But the true professional accepts that this can take one only so far, and that to provide effective help to all one's different patients requires a more structured understanding of the issues and also of what is taking place between the patient and the therapist.

We all have a personal philosophy that explains our relationship with other people, and one such philosophy is suggested in this book with characteristic deference and humour, drawing attention to the wisdom of retaining a healthy scepticism that any one such theory has 'the answer'. But whatever one's personal philosophy, the need for a clear map of the process of rehabilitation is self-evident. It will be found in the account that follows of the experience of disabling illness, coming to terms with disability, and the nature of anxiety, stress, pain and sensory deprivation. A particularly welcome emphasis in this book is the patient's family, whose role is so crucial and whose own needs and difficulties must be kept permanently in focus.

At times like ours when health resources provided by the state are restricted by lack of money, it is particularly important to use those that we have to the best effect. Faced with the bewildering complexity of human nature and experience, is it reasonable to expect a doctor, nurse or therapist — especially a young one at the start of his or her career — to handle all these issues? Who has not experienced the impulse to restrict one's goals, to keep one's head down and to move on rapidly to the next patient? With the help of this book the anxieties, the fears, the irrational behaviour, and the unhappiness that sometimes has to be worked through in rehabilitation will no longer be a source of consternation and confusion, but will be recognised as familiar signposts on the road to recovery.

D.L. McLellan,
Europe Professor of Rehabilitation,
University of Southampton

1 THE PHILOSOPHY OF REHABILITATION

Towards a Definition

> If we could bequeath one precious gift to posterity, I would choose a society in which there is a genuine compassion for the very sick and the disabled, where understanding is unostentatious and sincere, where, if years cannot be added to the lives of the chronically sick, at least life can be added to their years; where the mobility of disabled people is restricted only by the bounds of technical progress and discovery; where the handicapped have the fundamental right to participate in industry and society according to their ability; where socially preventable disease is unknown and where no man has cause to be ill at ease because of his disability.
>
> Mr Alfred Morris, during the second reading of his 'Chronically Sick and Disabled Persons Bill', House of Commons, London, 1970.

'Rehabilitation is the process of restoring a person's ability to live and work as normally as possible after a disabling injury or illness. It aims to help the patient achieve maximum possible physical and psychologic fitness and regain the ability to care for himself. It offers assistance with the learning or relearning of skills needed in every day activities, with occupational training and guidance and with psychologic readjustment.'[1]

This definition, by using the word 'restoring', assumes that at some time in his life the patient has lived and worked 'normally', and within the strict dictionary definition 'to restore to a previous condition', this is accurate. But rehabilitation is concerned with many people who would not fall within the definition. They would include those physically disabled from birth and those with mental handicaps. While it may not be possible to 'restore' these people to any former state of 'wholeness', rehabilitation workers are active in working with them. If it is not possible to 'rehabilitate' it is very possible to 'habilitate'; to enable such people to strive toward that which they and other people would accept, without prejudice.

An idea contained in the definition is that rehabilitation is geared only to work. While the definition does say 'live and work', it would appear to overlook certain categories of people for whom work — earning a living — is not a prime concern. It could be argued — quite cogently — that school children, housewives and the elderly, for example, while not earning their living, do work. This apart, if, for the purpose of this book, rehabilitation is to include 'habilitation' of those people who have been mentioned above, the emphasis needs to be placed on 'living' rather than on work, always bearing in mind that work may be or may become an essential feature of living.

I make no pretence of dealing with the physical aspects of rehabilitation, nor with the various topics generally covered by books on rehabilitative medicine, though to separate the psychologic (hereafter referred to as 'psychological') from the physical may prove to be totally impossible. As Professor Glanville says, 'Rehabilitation implies the restoration of patients to their fullest physical, mental and social capability.'[2] He adds, '. . . and one might add, 'in the shortest possible time.'' Thus, two new ideas have been presented for consideration, 'social' and 'shortest possible time'. These two additions both broaden and deepen the scope of rehabilitation. Without the word 'social', one could assume that concern was only for 'getting the patient better'; 'fit to get back to work'. If this were the case, all of the rehabilitation could take place within the hospital with the person either as an in-patient or attending as an out-patient. By including the social aspects, recognition is given of the undeniable fact that the person is on the one hand a patient but on the other a member of society. His social needs and his rehabilitation needs impinge upon and influence each other. The therapist* who concentrates on the physical and mental aspects of the treatment and ignores the social, treats only part of the problem and does not meet fully the patient's needs.

It could be argued that even the definition quoted from the Mair Report (note 2 above) omits one vital factor and underplays another. If one is treating a 'whole person' (and this is implied in the two definitions quoted) then one must recognise that that person has a spiritual side to his nature which may or may not be associated with religious expression. This would not be the place to enter into a discussion of the validity of the statement just made, nor of the merits of considering the 'spirit' as the intellect or the emotions. The reader may reject this, or any other part of the book, as inappropriate. So be it. I write from a personal belief that deep within man is a part of his personality which responds to 'deep calling unto deep'. In a later chapter this theme will reappear as we consider the subject of

---

* Within the context of this book, whenever 'therapist' is mentioned, it refers to anyone involved in the treatment of the patient.

'self-knowledge'. The part of the Mair definition which has been underplayed is the 'emotional'. The difference between 'mental' and 'emotional' is more than just a play on words. 'Mental' refers to activities of the mind; there would be little argument against that. It would be more difficult to state with any degree of accuracy where the seat of emotions is located. What is irrefutable is that people do have emotions or feelings. The feelings a person experiences strongly influence the way he co-operates with the therapist in the rehabilitation programme. To ignore his feelings is tantamount to telling him that they are of no significance. Patients who give only mental assent to their rehabilitation are not fully committed to it. Full commitment demands intellectual and emotional understanding and acceptance.

The phrase in the first definition, 'regain the ability to care for himself' also requires qualification. Some people, even following intensive rehabilitation, may never be able to care for themselves in quite the way they did before the accident or illness that resulted in their need for it. That is where the Mair Report definition applies. Rehabilitation should aim at the fullest possible restoration or maintenance of living. Many people require continual support for the remainder of their lives *in some specific activity of daily living* and may yet be quite independent in all others. If the patient, as a result of rehabilitation, achieves a degree of independence, more than was present before, it has been a success.

The final part of the definition to be considered is 'psychological readjustment'. Perhaps it is worth saying again; those who suffer from crippling disease, injury, accident or surgical intervention need different psychological help from those with congenital or chronic disability, whether of a physical, mental or emotional nature. This distinction has already been stated but in drawing this section to a close it was felt necessary to restate it. For in no sense can these two broad groups of people be lumped together and offered the same psychological help.

To summarise the foregoing argument, this definition is offered as the philosophy upon which this book is based:

> Rehabilitation implies the restoration or maintenance of, or the improvement in, the physical, mental and emotional states of a person, of any age, suffering from the effects of congenital mishap, crippling disease, injury, accident or surgical intervention. The social needs of the individual, his family and the society of which the person is a part, are crucial factors in the rehabilitation process which is concerned as much with preventing further deterioration of the condition as it is with alleviating the effects of the condition by appropriate treatment.

When Should Rehabilitation Commence?

'Rehabilitation is "creative convalescence" and as such, represents that active contribution made by medical, paramedical staff and patient to the restoration of health during the recovery phase which follows intensive definitive treatment.'[3] P.J.R. Nichols, from whose book the above definition is taken, writing several years later, drew attention to the

> relative lack of interest among the medical professions in the problems of convalescence. Publications on the subject are scanty, little research has been undertaken, and little attention has been devoted to the medical aspects of recovery. The main interests of clinicians often lie only in diagnosis and acute definitive treatment. The doctor's role in the convalescent period is often considered of minimal importance, and the patient's attitude during the period is traditionally passive.[4]

The Tunbridge Committee in the opening paragraph of its Report says,

> Insufficient attention is paid to the rehabilitation of the sick and injured. We believe that the restoration of normal to near normal capacities will become increasingly important during the next decade so that the need for rehabilitation is urgent.[5]

From these quotations the conclusion could be drawn that rehabilitation may not figure prominently in the thinking of some doctors. Rehabilitation for their patients is likely to be a neglected part of treatment. If it is started at all its effectiveness could be seriously impaired by being both inadequate and inappropriately timed. This begs the question, 'what is the appropriate time?'

Mattingly writes,[6]

> It has been said that rehabilitation should begin in the ambulance. This is perhaps an exaggeration, but it should certainly start soon after admission to hospital. It is essential to prevent complications of bed-rest such as bed-sores, urinary infections, venous thrombosis, muscle-wasting and contractures by good nursing, physiotherapy and early mobilisation.

While the preventative aspect of rehabilitation should not be overlooked, the note of caution sounded by Mattingly must be heeded. This caution is emphasised in,

> It is often stated that doctors should take into account the problems of rehabilitation on first contact with the patient. This is clearly untenable for many patients either because of the severity of their condition and the urgent need for immediate treatment or because the existence of multiple pathologies, particularly in persons over the age of 60, often makes immediate assessment difficult.[7]

These are warnings against rushing in, in the belief that it is never too early to start rehabilitation. On the other hand the therapist should start to establish a relationship with the person so that long-term rehabilitation will be built on a firm foundation. While it is true that too early attention to rehabilitation — other than preventative — may be inappropriate, it is never too early for the therapist to think about it, so that when the time is right, some sort of plan has been tentatively formulated. Thinking about rehabilitation may also influence the choice and direction of treatment, although this does not imply that the responsibility for assessment and prescribing treatment is taken over by any person other than the doctor. In establishing a relationship with the patient, the relatives should not be excluded, for it is crucial that their commitment and co-operation is secured before active — and possibly long-term — rehabilitation is contemplated.

For rehabilitation to succeed, the person must be an active partner and not a passive recipient of a programme designed exclusively for him by the therapist. Brechin puts forward the idea that rehabilitation be considered as an educational process where the therapist becomes a teacher, helping people to develop ways to '. . . cope with and control their disability and to utilise available rehabilitation resources and personnel, whenever such aid is needed.'[8] The shift from an authoritarian, 'telling' approach toward a relationship of equality is significant. Counselling, within the context of this book, is founded upon a relationship in which the person being counselled is encouraged to work toward solving his own problems. Within this relationship the therapist is a facilitator and, at times, a teacher. But for the client, counselling demands active participation which is directly opposed to the traditional expectations of the patient's role. Therapists may very well discover that much more is expected of them by patients who demand an active say in their own rehabilitation.

The preceding paragraphs open the question, 'when should rehabilitation commence?'. It might be too simplistic to say, 'when the patient is ready', but in a sense that is correct. 'Ready' not just physically — in that he has reached a certain stage of treatment — there must be an emotional readiness; a willingness and a preparedness to start to look at, and plan for, the future. Indeed it would probably be right to say that for some patients (particularly those undergoing planned surgery) the seeds of rehabilitation are sown before rehabilitation itself is possible. A patient, receiving treatment, and well prepared for what is to take place and the possible effects, is more likely to accept the principles of rehabilitation because it has already been clearly indicated to him that he is an active partner in his treatment and recovery. He becomes the client of the therapist counselling him. This section opened with a quote from the late Philip Nichols, 'Rehabilitation is creative convalescence'. For certain people, those who can look forward to a return to normality or near normality, this phrase speaks volumes. For others, because of the severity of their disability, this period of 'creative convalescence' may stretch far into the future. Indeed for some, the process of rehabilitation may, or should, never stop.

Who Needs Rehabilitation?

An examination of the Proceedings Review of the Twelfth World Congress of Rehabilitation International, held in Sydney in 1972, reveals that there is no section of patient care where rehabilitation is inappropriate. In considering the question, 'who needs rehabilitation?', one could become overwhelmed by the task and how to tackle it. One could answer it by looking at the various conditions which are most frequently presented; but whole books have been devoted to single conditions. Another possibility would be to relate the answer to conditions which affect various bodily systems — neurological, respiratory, cardio-thoracic, abdominal. Both of these approaches would be more than adequate but the approach in this book is to consider rehabilitation in relation to the various parts of the definition on page 3. It is not only people who suffer major disasters who need a period of creative convalvescence; anyone whose normal functioning has been disrupted by illness or injury, for even a short period, requires some degree of rehabilitation, some period of readjustment. There are several groups of patients for whom rehabilitation may not be considered vital, if too narrow a definition is considered. Children, married women, the aged and those suffering from incurable disease all pose special problems, if return to work is the major consideration. An active programme of rehabilitation for a young man, the victim of a severe accident, causing brain damage and physical disability, could make all the difference between a semi-dependent life at home and a totally dependent existence in an institution. The housewife, severely burned by boiling fat, may need to be rehabilitated if she is to pick up the threads of housework again. The old lady who falls and breaks her hip needs more than the provision of a walking frame. The middle aged woman with progressive cancer needs more than a prosthesis to compensate for her lost breast. Is there any person who is, or has been, a patient, who would not benefit from rehabilitation? This ideal may not be easily attainable, and any rehabilitation programme brings with it certain moral and ethical considerations which will now be considered.

Moral and Ethical Considerations

Some moral and ethical points have already been touched on by the broadening of the definition to include people other than those suffering from the effects of injury or disease. Some other moral questions are: should rehabilitation be started at all? If there are limited resources (people, finance, time) which patients should take priority? Having started, can rehabilitation be maintained? If it cannot, what does this do for the person, his relatives and society? The Tunbridge Report[5] states, 'Psychiatric and geriatric patients make the greatest demands on the rehabilitation services . . .. Rehabilitation for these patients may be to concentrate on minimising the effects of institutionalisation.' If this is still an accurate picture of services today, is it justified that these two groups of patients should be allocated more resources than other groups? Should a young disabled man deserve more consideration than emotionally ill or aged people? Should limited resources be channelled toward disabled people who will eventually make a significant contribution to the rapidly shrinking group of workers who have to support a rapidly increasing ageing population? These questions are similar to those asked by NHS members as they plan Regional and District patient services. At some stage someone, or some group of people, lays down priorities, influenced by the available resources and community needs. The decisions the planners make may not please or satisfy everyone: decisions rarely do! Just so in rehabilitation. Resources are limited, governed mainly, but not solely, by finance. Even if unlimited money were available, it is possible that there might never be enough therapists to treat all who need their services. It is more likely that the pit is bottomless, just as provision of any health care service appears to be. Demand for rehabilitation will always outstrip supply.

As Regional and District decisions have to be made about providing services, so local decisions have to be made about who receives rehabilitation. There may well be some patients who would benefit greatly but who receive only perfunctory rehabilitation because the therapists are already working at full stretch. It is very possible that in some instances decisions as to who receives rehabilitation are never consciously taken. A doctor who does not place rehabilitation high among his priorities may seldom refer other than severely injured patients for rehabilitation. Those not referred may be the ones who would benefit greatly from an active, albeit short, rehabilitation programme. Some doctors may not refer all who need rehabilitation, knowing that limited resources are already stretched to their limits.

Another point to consider relates to the expectations of the patient, his family and society. A person who has suffered extensive injuries, involving, for example, the head and spinal cord, would seem an obvious candidate for rehabilitation. A programme started at the optimum time and carried through with dedication by all care staff could very well produce results that promise a good recovery. The expectations of the patient and his relatives, however, may not be fully realised. Through nobody's fault, the patient may not be able to progress further. The person who has been brought so far along the road toward independence but is then forced to settle for something less, may well spend the rest of his life in an emotional strait-jacket, held prisoner by his frustration. This raises the question, should rehabilitation only be started if there is a guarantee of success? While this may appear to be an absurd question, not worthy of consideration, it is one which some patients, or their relatives, in times of stress and disappointment, may ask. It is similar to that which is often asked about treatment that has failed and the patient dies. Andrew, aged 4, had leukaemia and was treated for a year with all the modern treatments. They were to no avail: he died a protracted death. His shattered parents, in their anguish, berated the doctor thus, 'You should never have started treatment. You've been experimenting on our son.' Their words were bitter, but no words could express the loss they felt of their only child. For them, 'Hope deferred maketh the heart sick'[9] was a nightmare reality. But was it wrong of the doctor to start treatment? Can one not commence rehabilitation because of the fear that recovery may be less than total? Is progress measured only by total success, or should it be measured by achievement, however small?

In this section more questions have been asked than answers given. But to many of these questions there is no one answer. In a sense this is paving the way for later chapters of the book which deal explicitly with counselling. Counselling demands a high tolerance of ambiguity and the ability to work with questions which do not have definitive answers. 'The main attributes of counselling lie in an exchange of feelings and attitudes, rather than in an exchange of information, answering questions, offering solutions or giving advice.'[10]

Constraints and Conflicts

Some constraints and conflicts were briefly discussed in the previous section. This emphasises the impossibility of keeping topics in watertight compartments. In this section some of those issues will be raised again, in different contexts. One such issue was that of finance; and finance can seldom be considered without making it a political issue. Without labouring the point, finance for health care is limited, and it is possible that the allocation of monies to rehabilitation services is given a low priority by many health authorities. How money is allocated should always be governed by need but political issues often constrain the decision-makers in their choice of options.

> 'It's always best on these occasions to do what the mob do.'
> 'But suppose there are two mobs?' suggested Mr Snodgrass.
> 'Shout with the largest', replied Mr Pickwick.[11]

This quotation gives some indication of one political point. Some branches of medicine, traditionally, have always had louder and more persuasive voices than some others. This has a great deal to do with prestige within the medical professions but also how they are regarded by the general public. To save the life of a person who has been badly mangled in an horrific car accident, by hours of intense surgery, will normally attract more publicity than months, or years, spent by therapists in helping that same patient to become independent and to cope with the after-effects of the accident. The paraphernalia and the prevailing air of mystery of the Intensive Care Unit are more terrifyingly impressive to the relative than the pulleys and weights and parallel bars that the patient may use under the instruction of the therapist. If patients or their relative were asked, 'Where would you allocate money: to a larger ICU or for a better equipped gymnasium?' they would, in all probability, answer in favour of the former. But what price a life saved if the rehabilitation services are inadequate? Is a life saved, but doomed to living at less than optimum, worthwhile? Would relatives who voted money to the ICU have a different opinion when caught up in endless years of total and unremitting care, simply because there were not sufficient resources available for effective rehabilitation? Patients and their relatives are not likely to be involved in deciding which services are allotted money (though it might improve the health care services if they were!) but someone, some group must be their advocate.

One of the phenomena of the British way of life (though it could apply elsewhere) is the voluntary movement. Voluntary organisations will raise thousands of pounds for what they, and others, regard as worthy projects. Diagnostic equipment, appliances for specialised treatment and many social and recreational machines are provided in this way. Specialised units have been built by donations from appeals. When equipment is installed, or buildings erected, the care and maintenance and the funding of the staff to run these units is generally handed over to the health authority. Could any health authority reject the gift of a new terminal care unit, for example? An expensive piece of equipment, such as a whole body scanner, which requires a special building to house it, may incur very costly running and maintenance overheads. Such a useful machine should, of course, be used to its maximum, but eventually it will need to be replaced. Then the authority is likely to be faced with the difficult decision of whether or not to allocate money in this direction. If they do, some other service may be deprived: if they do not, society may well accuse them of mismanagement.

Pressure groups are able to influence health authorities in two ways. There have been many instances where hospitals, threatened by the axe, have been saved by the efforts of pressure groups. The health authority has capitulated to public opinion. The other side of the picture is that pressure groups can very often act against the best interests of people requiring care. Many instances should be quoted where people have campaigned against hostels for the mentally handicapped, or the emotionally ill, being sited in a particular town, estate or street. The campaigners are probably quite caring people, but their fears of plummeting house prices and noisy or embarrassing indicidents are, to them, real. How can one reassure the mother of a tiny infant who comes out of a shop to discover Brian, a mentally handicapped man, peering into the pram and making strange noises? The mother is not to know that Brian is harmless and he loves babies. Brian looks odd and behaves strangely. Recently she read in the newspaper of an incident where a mentally handicapped man (or was he mentally ill, or both? she is not certain) was accused of murder. She joined a pressure group to fight against having a house in her street taken over as a home for six mentally handicapped people. They won the fight and six people have to live many more months in an outdated hospital. Their rehabilitation programmes, started in the hospital are curtailed until a house can be found for them. Society may thus be both friend and enemy to those people who need rehabilitation. If society can constrain rehabilitation, so may relatives. Let us consider an example. Janice was an eight-year-old, suffering from cerebral palsy and was cared for, during term time, in a special residential school. At the end of the second term, the physiotherapist had succeeded in getting her to walk. But when she returned, she was back in her wheelchair.

'Why are you not walking, Janice?' the physiotherapist asked, 'Mummy says it's easier for her if I'm in the chair', was her reply.

So the process was started again, and again Janice returned from the next holiday unable to walk. Just why Janice's mother wanted her daughter kept in a wheelchair would be difficult to determine. But what is fairly certain is, inconvenient as it was or however much of a tie it was or however much of a burden (and would become increasingly so), the mother — and possibly Janice — gained something from what was happening. While it may have been true when the mother said that it was easier for her to have Janice in the wheelchair, that may not have been the whole truth. Her words to the physiotherapist are revealing, 'I've got her where I want her'. The whole truth was psychologically hidden from her. If counselling had been available (the physiotherapist moved from the locality soon afterward) the mother might have gained some insight into what was happening between herself and Janice and between them and the physiotherapist. These insights might have helped her to work toward Janice being where she wanted to be, rather than being where her mother wanted her to be.

Much of what will be discussed in later chapters centres around the relationship that exists between the therapist and the client, but it also focuses on the relatives as part of the total working relationship. To involve the patient in a programme of rehabilitation and ignore the relatives would place rehabilitation on a shaky foundation. An intensive programme produces physical and emotional strains on the patient. Difficulties experienced in the Department will often spill over into the home environment. The patient who experiences disappointment over slow progress, or total inability to perform, is likely to take his frustration home with him. There he may take it out on his relatives by being aggressive, angry, sullen, argumentative and so on. On the other hand he may attack himself and become depressed and withdrawn and cast an air of gloom over everyone. During times of discouragement, his relatives need to be able to support him; they will do this far more easily if they understand what is happening. If they have been involved, they themselves will feel supported within the relationship that exists between therapist and patient.

Willing relatives can be encouraged to become able assistants in the rehabilitation process rather than passive appendages.

Another constraint is the patient himself. Just as Janice's mother received some psychological gain from keeping Janice dependent in a wheelchair, so also may patients gain something from prolonging the period of creative convalescence. People who are involved in insurance claims may have vested interests in delaying full recovery. But even that motive may not be on a conscious level. Those who are not involved in litigation, or awaiting compensation may also have something to gain from prolonging the period of treatment. Being at home may be more congenial than being at work. While sick benefit may not fully compensate, the patient and his family are unlikely to starve. One could ask, 'Does this hinder or assist speedy recovery?' The relationship which the patient has established between the therapists and his fellow rehabilitees may be more satisfying than any others he knows. Some people thrive on sympathy and on being dependent on other people. The examples of how the patient views the relationship between himself and his disability are legion, but perhaps enough has been said at this stage to alert the reader to take a closer look at this particular aspect of rehabilitation.

> In all distresses of our friends
> We first consult our private ends;
> While nature, kindly bent to ease us,
> Points out some circumstance to please us.[12]

Well-meaning friends can play havoc with the patient's recovery by well-intentioned, but misplaced advice. How surprising it is that so often other people know so much better than we what we should do! Or as Swift, in the above stanza, so aptly says; we always tend to gain from our friends' troubles. In chapter 8, Elizabeth tells her story of her feelings following major abdominal surgery. But a little of what she says is pertinent here.

> I had been home two weeks [from the convalescent home] and not feeling too bright, in fact at times quite tearful. Rosemary came to see me and said, "I know what you should do; go on retreat." [Elizabeth is a devout Roman Catholic.] "I'll come in tomorrow, first thing, and expect you to have reached a decision."
>
> This went on for a whole week. I couldn't make up my mind. I was so confused. Spiritually it was probably right; but physically it was quite beyond me.

Elizabeth made light of what had obviously been a trying experience. She continued,

> and in the end I was so wound up that although I'd been tearful when it all started, now I couldn't control my floods of tears. In desperation I 'phoned my priest who, when he came, was astonished that I should even be thinking about a retreat. He confirmed that the rigours of the spartan retreat would probably send me to an early grave. Rosemary was very put out that I'd even consulted the priest, let alone taken his advice. She hasn't been near since.

What Rosemary stood to gain from this, is difficult to judge; but what is obvious, is how much of a burden she had oppressed Elizabeth with. This advice, had it been acted upon, might well have resulted in a serious relapse and prolonged the period of convalescence. Friends who say, 'I know what you should do'. Or, 'This will do you good', or some such similar comment, should be listened to very carefully, yes, but watched — carefully.

The final point to be considered is, how care staff themselves may constrain active rehabilitation. This may seem contradictory, but mention has already been made of how some doctors appear not to be orientated toward rehabilitation, or if they are, they do not think about it soon enough. Nichols[13] says,

> The Piercy Committee (1956) clearly spelt out the philosophy that rehabilitation must be a single continuous process, beginning with the onset of sickness or injury and continuing throughout the treatment until final resettlement is achieved, fully acknowledging that rehabilitation is not to be regarded as the application of special techniques but is an integral part of total patient care.

In the section, 'when should rehabilitation commence?' attention was drawn to the inappropriateness of introducing the idea of rehabilitation too soon. How can this be reconciled with the above quotation? If, at the onset of illness or injury, or soon after a diagnosis of congenital handicap has been made, it is recognised that rehabilitation must be 'an integral part of the total patient care', then it could be justifiably said that rehabilitation has commenced. If this recognition is backed up by establishing a bond with the patient and the relatives, within which an in-depth assessment of them is carried out, the process is already well-developed before special techniques need to be introduced. The physiotherapist who ensures that the patient learns to breathe properly, following an abdominal operation, is laying the foundation stone for future rehabilitation. The nurse who assesses that the patient is now able to do something for himself which has previously been done for him, is ensuring that rehabilitation is continued. Yet nurses — who of all professionals have the most sustained contact with the patient — may hinder rehabilitation, in the same way as did Janice's mother, by not perceiving the patient's need to be independent as quickly as possible. It may not be easy for a nurse to stand back and watch an old lady struggling to get into her stockings while one hand lies helpless by her side, paralysed by a disabling stroke. Yet nurses who are rehabilitation orientated know that the patient must struggle toward independence. Any short-circuiting of this process will prolong the period of dependence. Janice's mother never learned this important lesson.

The final section of this chapter returns to society, of which we are all a part. In many ways, people who require rehabilitation could be regarded as a minority group in society.

> Disabled people can be conceptualised as a disadvantaged or minority group because they have a great deal in common with the old, blacks, women, the poor and other minorities in that they are treated and reacted to as a category of people.[14]

Here the writer is referring to those whose disability is permanent, but there is some justification in considering even those suffering from transitory disability as belonging to a minority group. The writer goes on to say, '. . . the disabled person is often considered to be less intelligent, less able to make the 'right' decisions, less 'realistic', less logical and less able to determine his own life than a nondisabled person.' If people adopt this attitude, the disabled gradually come to accept this as their role in society, as if they had no other part to play. They then retreat into their disabled ghettos. It is as if society needs to classify people into two distinct groups, 'them' and 'us': the disabled and the able. But, 'We need to see the disabled in a pattern or grid involved with the rest of society. None of us stays in one place in this grid.'[15] This message is timely. For even though we may not experience crippling injury or disease, few of us will escape the effects of the ageing process. So, by comparison, a man of 60 could be said to be disabled when engaged in a race with a man 40 years his junior!

If the attitude of society toward the disabled is to regulate them to the status of second class citizens, by implication it also suggests that valuable resources and facilities should be reserved for the first class citizens — the able. Hand in hand with this attitude goes its twin sister — the disabled should be grateful for what they are given. The following quote demonstrates this.

> Unfortunately, those people whose task it was to rehabilitate me also made certain assumptions about me and the world I was to inhabit after I left the home. The assumption about me was simple. I should be grateful for whatever existence I could scrape together . . . whatever it [society] meted out to the cripple, the cripple accepted. The way of the world was not to be challenged.[16]

It is sad that many people in the 'caring professions' adopt a similar attitude toward those in need of rehabilitation. The professional — of whichever discipline — who plans a rehabilitation programme, based solely on clinical experience and not in consultation with the patient or his relatives, is treating the patient as if he had no rights. Many professionals give the impression that they know what is best for the patient. They should know what *may* be appropriate to treat a certain clinical condition, but that is only part of the programme. The patient is not a clinical condition. If a relationship is not established in which the patient feels an equal partner, the therapist will be perceived as being dominant. If the patient accepts this *status quo* he will comply but in complying he will do only what he is told. There will be no creative commitment to rehabilitation. That has been surrendered to the therapist. Prolonged compliance leads to apathy: apathy generates failure. The patient who kicks against compliance and dependency is often labelled 'difficult' or 'non-co-operative'. A consequence of this is that the therapist withdraws and distances herself, emotionally, from the patient, thus making effective rehabilitation even less likely.

This chapter will be drawn to a close with a quote from Professor Aitken, 'The main thing is, of course, that the various professionals should be aware of the patient's many emotional and practical needs, rather than remaining blinkered and concerned only with the task in hand.'[17]

Summary

This chapter has been concerned with exploring the philosophy of rehabilitation upon which the remaining chapters are founded. Some of the issues raised are likely to be controversial and may not be accepted by every reader. The definition was broadened to include as wide a range of people as possible, with disparate conditions, giving rise to different rehabilitation needs. A note of caution was sounded about attempting to introduce active rehabilitation too soon; at the same time it was felt that it was never too early to start to think about it.

The view was put forward that rehabilitation is an educational process wherein the therapist is a teacher, helping the person devise strategies to cope with and control his disability. It was suggested that not only those suffering the effects of crippling disease or injury need rehabilitation; people who have been temporarily disabled by minor illness or accident, or those recovering from planned surgery, also need a period of 'creative convalescence'.

The whole topic of rehabilitation raises many moral and ethical questions, some of which are discussed in this chapter. It was pointed out that not many answers are given but it was felt to be right that they should be asked. One of the major issues raised was who, or what group of people, should be given priority in the allocation of scarce resources. Pressure groups very often influence these decisions.

The final section dealt with the various constraints to rehabilitation. The patient cannot be considered in isolation from the society in which he lives. That society, by its attitude toward disability, can assist or hinder rehabilitation. It can be exceptionally caring towards one group of people and at the same time, incredibly callous toward another. Care-givers, relatives, well-meaning friends and the patient himself all influence the success or failure of rehabilitation. Success is more likely if the patient and his relatives are fully committed to what is happening by being encouraged to be active partners and not passive recipients of a programme designed to meet clinical needs but which ignores all others.

Notes

1. Miller, B.F. and Keane, C.B. (1978), *Encyclopaedia and Dictionary of Medicine, Nursing and Allied Health*, W.B. Saunders, Philadelphia.
2. Professor H.J. Glanville, quoting from the Mair Report (1972) in *Rehabilitation of the Neurological Patient*, L.S. Illis, E.M. Sedgwick and H.J. Glanville (eds). Blackwell Scientific Publications, Oxford, 1982.
3. Nichols, P.J.R. (1982) *Rehabilitation Medicine*, Butterworths, London.
4. Nichols, P.J.R., ibid.
5. Rehabilitation. Report of a Sub-Committee of the Standing Medical Advisory Committee, 1972. The Tunbridge Report.
6. Mattingly, S. (1977) *Rehabilitation Today*, Update Books, London.
7. Tunbridge, Sir R.E. Twelfth World Congress of Rehabilitation International Sydney 1972, Proceedings Review.
8. Brechin, A., Liddiard, P. and Swain, J. (eds) (1981) *Handicap in a Social World*, Open University Press, Milton Keynes.
9. Proverbs 13 verse 12.
10. Stewart, W. (1977) *A Guide to Counselling*, Wessex Regional Training Guide.

11. Dickens, Charles, *Pickwick Papers*, Chapter 13.
12. 'Verses on the death of Dr Swift' by Jonathan Swift, 1731.
13. Nichols, P.J.R. (1979) Newsletter. 'Demonstration Centres in Rehabilitation', April.
14. Brechin, A.G. *et al*, *Handicap in a Social World*.
15. Wilke, Harold, Twelfth World Congress of Rehabilitation.
16. Kriegel, L. 'Uncle Tom and Tiny Tim; some reflections on the cripple as negro.' *The American Scholar, 38*, pp. 412–30 quoted in '*Handicap in a Social World*'.
17. Burningham, Sally (1982) Report of a conference, *Remedial Therapist* 'A Team Approach to Counselling, Vol. 5 issue 5, 29 October.

2 THE PHILOSOPHY OF COUNSELLING

This chapter covers the basic concepts and principles of counselling. They are presented in alphabetical form for easy reference.

Acceptance

> By acceptance I mean a warm regard for him as a person of unconditional self-worth — of value no matter what his condition, his behaviour or his feelings. It means a respect and liking for him as a separate person, a willingness to possess his own feelings in his own way. It means an acceptance of and a regard for his attitudes of the moment, no matter how negative or positive, no matter how much they may contradict other attitudes he has held in the past.[1]

This definition by Carl Rogers introduces acceptance as an emotional process — how the counsellor feels. Inherent in the idea of acceptance is that the counsellor does not judge the client by some set of rules or standards. This means that counsellors have to be able to suspend their own judgements. 'They assign no condition to be met before extending help. They do not attach "if" clauses — if you study, if you behave, if you apologise, then I will consider you a worthwhile person.'[2]

Acceptance springs from the well of compassion and is demonstrated in a desire to help, not to control, criticise or condemn. Acceptance, in the sense in which it is used in counselling, is akin to the Christian ideal 'loving the sinner not the sin'. This ideal may seem too high for many of us to reach, but the fact that we may feel to be a long way from it should not prevent us from counselling, provided we are open to receive new insights to help us along the road to that ideal. How does the client feel who is accepted in this way? Harry and Margaret Dean tell us, 'He feels warm inside, safe, free to be himself, prepared to let down his guard, willing to share. The door to his inner healing appears to be not too far away.'[3] No discussion of acceptance would be complete (and the discussion here is brief) without stating the obvious; that in order to accept the client, the counsellor must accept himself — warts and all! This theme will be taken up again in Chapter 5 on self-awareness.

Hamilton says, 'It [acceptance] is translated through courtesy, patience, willingness to listen and not being critical of whatever the client may reveal about himself.'[4] This 'non-judgemental' attitude is crucial in counselling. Davison suggests that acceptance is similar to mother-love that loves and supports her child through bad times as well as good. 'In it he feels a sense of security, because of it he is encouraged to go on trying, his self-esteem is enhanced and he comes to feel that after all he can face life with confidence.'[5] Susan Gilmore adds something very important; that acceptance does something for both client and counsellor. 'Extending acceptance to a client is a very active and emotion-laden experience for both the client and the counsellor.'[6] This suggests that when the counsellor accepts the client, the client in return accepts the counsellor. Reciprocity is rewarding.

People who engage themselves in counselling, either as clients or counsellors, open themselves to be more accepting of themselves and other people.

Advice

People frequently open conversations with, 'Can you give me some advice?' One answer would be, 'Yes', and having listened to the story, an opinion is given which may or may not be accepted and acted upon. There are many times in life when advice asked for could quite readily be given.

> Where advice can be given safely is in practical issues but not where emotions are involved. Many simple issues, however, have wider implications. The stronger the emotional content or the more serious the implications, the less is advice appropriate. Where emotions are involved advice, even if asked for, is frequently ignored if it does not match up with what the person feels is 'right'. Advice not asked for is certain to be ignored.[7]
>
> The dictionary defines counsel as advice.
>
> In its widest sense, and certainly as a lawyer would use it, it is not 'do this' but rather, 'this is what is possible', an opening up of alternatives and possibilities. In this sense the dictionary definition could be correctly applied to counselling.[8]

Thus we see that there is room for advice, particularly if the request relates to some professional activity, for example, some aspect of clinical treatment. Refusal to offer advice may give the impression that the counsellor is not interested. But the counsellor who answers the question, 'What would you advise me to do?' with, 'What ideas have you had?' is helping the client to realise that he, himself, has a part to play in seeking an answer.

That there is a place for advice-giving is not disputed. The Citizens' Advice Bureau Service exists solely for the purpose of giving advice, and does it successfully. Advice is often appropriate in crises; at times when the client's thoughts and feelings seem stunned by the event. At times like these the adviser must exercise greater caution than when the person is fully responsive and responsible. Advice offered and accepted in such circumstances and then acted upon could prove to be, if not 'bad advice', not totally appropriate to meet the needs of the person receiving it. People under stress are vulnerable.

Advice is a form of persuasion. Hollis classifies advice as 'direct influence' and discusses three main safeguards for its use:

1. The worker must be reasonably sure that he knows enough about what is best for the client.
2. . . . be quite sure that the need for advice rests in the client and not in the worker. This is a matter for self-examination for the worker.
3. . . . induce the client, whenever possible, to think things through for himself. Clients often seduce the worker into thinking advice is necessary when it is not.[9]

Hollis also draws attention to what may be called 'advocating',

> the putting of a certain urgency behind the advice that is offered . . . .. When there is a possibility of severe consequences of an impulsive, ill-considered action, or when sufficient time is not available before action is threatened . . . the technique of advocating may be worth trying.

The therapist who says to a patient who has just recovered from a coronary, 'I would certainly advise you not to drive your car', is advocating, as is the nurse who says to the mother, 'You really ought to take your child to see the doctor.' In both these instances, the consequences of not heeding the advice warrant the additional urgency of advocating.

Advice is not generally a popular word in counselling circles, mainly because of the way its meaning has become restricted to, 'This is what I think you should do', or 'If I were you I would do . . . . ' Advice put over in that way is likely to backfire or, as we saw with Elizabeth (p. 12), actual emotional harm may result.

Confidentiality

'The preservation of confidential information is a basic right of the client and an ethical obligation upon the counsellor.'[5] A slightly different view is put forward in, 'The counsellor has to decide when silence about confidential information is too great a price for society to pay.'[2] This view is supported by, 'Learning to discriminate between "confidential" and "secret" material. Everything said in a counselling interview is confidential but not everything is secret.'[7]

If clients were asked what is their understanding of 'confidentiality' they would probably say that they didn't want the details of what they disclosed gossiped about or discussed with people who didn't have to be involved. They would, in all probability, agree that the counsellor, where necessary, would be free to discuss broad details with professional colleagues, but only after their prior consent had been obtained.

Case conferences are a common feature of many professional groups, and the therapist — as counsellor — may be so involved. It is quite conceivable that during the course of counselling, certain details will emerge that will be too intimate, painful or embarrassing to be revealed and discussed even among trusted colleagues. That is one time when the therapist has to make a conscious decision between what is merely confidential and what is secret. Another time would be when making notes to which other people may have access. If the therapist asks herself the question, 'If this detail is withheld, will it seriously affect someone else's understanding of the client's case?' If the answer to this is 'no', then, quite safely and legitimately, it may be left out.

None the less, the wise therapist will be alert not to give an unconditional guarantee of confidence before hearing the facts. The person who opens with, 'Now I want to tell you something in strict confidence' should be guided into an exploration of precisely what he means by 'confidence'. For, as will emerge later, the therapist may be forced to consult with a more experienced counsellor if what the client reveals requires skills and insight which at this stage the therapist does not possess. Most counsellors at some time in their careers have been faced with the painful decision of whether or not to respect confidence or, for the good of society, or to prevent something disastrous happening, to break it. But whatever is decided, no action should be taken without discussion with the client.

An example of this conflict may suffice.

Staff Nurse Harmsworth came to the hospital counsellor in a distressed state. This was the first time she had visited a counsellor. She expressed many worries about her work on a medical ward where she had been since she qualified a year previously. The counsellor (who was also a nurse) thought that some aspects of her behaviour were a bit odd. She was jumpy and suspicious and seemed very tired although it was only mid morning. The girl suddenly burst out crying and between her tears said, 'I've been stealing drugs from the drug cupboard.' It transpired that prescribed drugs had not been given to patients even though they had been signed for and checked. The counsellor was on the horns of a dilemma. On the one side was her loyalty to her client and on the other, her loyalty to the hospital, the nursing profession and society. She discussed this conflict with the nurse and the result was that she accompanied the nurse and helped her tell the sad tale to the appropriate nurse manager. That was not the end. The nurse became a regular client of the counsellor who supported her through a very difficult time of disciplinary hearings which finally lead to a severe warning but not dismissal. The counsellor would have been in a very difficult position had not the nurse gone to her manager. To safeguard society she might well have had to break this confidence. If she had kept confidence, and something disastrous happened, could she have been accused of negligence and disloyalty?

This raises an important ethical consideration. Counselling at work is different from counselling in a private setting. There the counsellor owes no allegiance to the organisation with which the client may be in conflict. Thus, in some respects, the therapist may be forced to resolve conflicts of which private counsellors have no direct knowledge. Not that conflicts never come their way. As Shertzer says,[2] counsellors must always consider the welfare of the wider society; so they too may have to make difficult and painful decisions about confidentiality different from the therapists' decisions.

Common Elements

Most counselling theories and models include the following elements.

1. Counselling is a 'high level *communication*' activity.
2. Clients have the right to choose the *direction* of their own lives. (This will be discussed in the section, 'Self-responsibility'.)
3. Counsellors must be *flexible* to adapt their styles to the needs of

their clients.

4. Clients *learn* more about themselves and are thus more able to cope realistically with the world in which they live.
5. Clients who are *motivated* to seek counselling are more likely to benefit from it than those who are pressed into it.
6. The *purpose* of counselling is to help the client become or remain the person he feels he wants to be.
7. The central feature of most counselling approaches is *relationship*. (This will be covered in a later section.)
8. The counsellor has *respect* for the unique individuality of the client.
9. Both client and counsellor receive *rewards* from counselling.
10. The richness of the counsellor's inner world and his life experience are seen as crucial elements in *supporting* the client.

Definitions

> People are engaged in counselling when a person, occupying regularly or temporarily the role of 'counsellor' offers or agrees explicitly to give time, attention, and respect to another person or persons temporarily in the role of client. The task of counselling is to give the 'client' an opportunity to explore, define and discover ways of living more satisfyingly and resourcefully within the social grouping with which he identifies.[10]

On first reading this definition may appear rather long and complex. To some people it may give the impression of a legal function rather than one concerned with exploring feelings within a trusting relationship, as the next definition shows.

'Counselling or psychotherapy is defined as the helping process in which the relationship is necessary and sufficient.'[11]

A very simple definition of counselling is, '. . . a process of helping people with their problems'.[12]

One of the difficulties already inferred in this section is that a definition which seeks to be all-encompassing tends to become unwieldy and loses something of its impact. A short, pithy statement may be more acceptable but may be criticised for not saying enough. Two such statements are:

'. . . to help an individual to achieve some adjustment either within himself or within his environment.'[7]

'Patient counselling is helping the patient to cope with his condition and the treatment involved.'[13]

This second definition could be expanded to read '. . . helping the patient and his relatives to understand and cope . . ..' For the patient to cope adequately with his treatment he needs to understand. And as was discussed in chapter 1, the relatives may also need help to understand, if they are to cope with the condition and resultant treatment.

This definition is the one probably most relevant for therapists, but a great deal is implied rather than made explicit. No mention is made, for instance, of the qualities of the counsellor nor of the quality of the counselling relationship. Therapists will appreciate that the words 'understand' and 'cope' mean more than an intellectual exercise or a physical adjustment. An undiscerning person reading this definition, without hearing the deeper emotional undertones, may conclude that this is all these words do mean.

The final definition to be considered is,

> A way of relating and responding to another person so that that person is helped to explore his thoughts, feelings and behaviour; to reach clearer self-understanding and thus is helped to find and use his strengths so that he copes more effectively with his life by making appropriate decisions, or by taking relevant action.
>
> Essentially then, counselling is a purposeful relationship in which one person helps another to help himself.[14]

Therapists should have no difficulty in relating this definition to rehabilitation. One comment must suffice to bring this section to a close. The word 'cope' in this and the previous definition implies that all conditions may not be resolved nor cured. Many patients who attend for rehabilitation suffer disabilities that will remain with them for life. Therapy without counselling will help with the physical task of coping; counselling, as a vital and integral part of the rehabilitation process, will provide opportunity for them to explore the emotional aspects of coping.

Defence Mechanisms

Defence (or mental) mechanisms were formulated by Freud in his treatment of neuroses. Defence mechanisms operate to protect the ego by keeping the state of things as they are. The principal mental mechanisms to study in relation to interaction are:

1. PROJECTION — 'A bad workman always blames his tools.'
2. RATIONALISATION — 'I failed my driving test because I had a rotten headache.' In other words this is a more acceptable reason than the plain, unvarnished truth.
3. DISPLACEMENT — Kicking the dog when in reality the person would like to kick the boss (or someone else).
4. SUBLIMATION — Usually referred to in a sexual context. Finding an outlet more acceptable for inner drives.
5. DENIAL — Complete denial is seldom encountered. An example would be the person who refuses to accept that his leg has been amputated.
6. REPRESSION — Where an emotion is shut out of the conscious. As the therapist is unlikely to be working directly with the unconscious, she will seldom work with repressed material. It is possible, however, that some repressed material may be triggered off as other things are dealt with and cleared out of the conscious.
7. REACTION FORMATION — An example would be the heavy drinker who gives up alcohol and becomes an ardent 'ban the drink' campaigner.
8. REGRESSION — A person who returns, even momentarily, to a previous stage of development and exhibits the behaviour appropriate to that stage is regressing.
9. COMPENSATION — The man who is a cripple and becomes a mountaineer is compensating.

While it is true that Freud formulated the idea of mental mechanisms, they are not confined to pathological states. We all (unconsciously) use them to allay anxiety. Defence mechanisms that are too rigid often conceal or disguise the real problem. If, as a result of counselling, the client realises that some particular way of behaving is inappropriate and he expressly seeks counselling help to modify his behaviour, so be it. But direct work with defence mechanisms is best left to those qualified to do so — psychoanalysts.

Defence mechanisms operate in the unconscious; counselling seldom focuses on unconscious material. That is one of the principal differences between counselling and psychoanalysis.

> The principal difference between psychoanalysis and counselling is that psychoanalysis deals more, but not exclusively, with the unconscious and the past, while counselling deals more, but not

> exclusively with the conscious and the present, the here-and-now and the very recent past.[15]

People who work in the field of rehabilitation will often be acutely conscious of the particular mechanisms a specific patient is using to defend himself. While the therapist should acknowledge and recognise them, it would be unwise to attempt to break them down. To do so may expose the client's ego thus leaving him vulnerable to internal and external influences.

Empathy

One way of looking at empathy is, '. . . the ability to feel oneself in the shoes of the other person and thus obtain a knowledge that is almost first hand.'[16] This is the ability to walk in the world of the other person. It may seem that this is slightly presumptuous. Can we ever walk totally in the world of another person? There is the danger that if we do, we shall lose that degree of objectivity that is essential in counselling. But if we can see what the other person is seeing, and hear what he is hearing, and to a degree feel what he is feeling, then we have achieved empathy.

Katz[16], speaking of Harry Stack Sullivan says, '[he] believes that empathy is a form of communication on a non-verbal level which can be traced back to the relationship of the infant to its mother.'

Reik[17] points out that an essential element in empathy is being able to vibrate unconsciously in the rhythm of the other person's impulse and yet be capable of grasping it as something outside oneself and comprehending it psychologically, sharing the other's experience and yet remaining above the struggle.

It is this quality of objectivity that distinguishes empathy from sympathy. It could be said that empathy is objective compassion and sympathy, subjective compassion where one person has over-identified with the feelings of the other. Mrs Dale, an elderly lady, was grief-stricken when her only grandson was involved in a motor cycle accident. She said to someone who had enquired about her loss of weight,

> It's David. He's only twenty one and he's going to be paralysed for the rest of his life. I can't get over it. I feel what he feels. I cry his tears of rage. I feel the anger he feels. I feel the pain and frustration and despair.

Mrs Dale had become immersed in David's feelings. She was David. She was walking totally in his world; it wasn't something outside herself; she could not remain above the struggle.

Sympathy often leads to an inability to take action or to action which is inappropriate. An example of the difference between empathy and sympathy is where a traveller falls into a storm ditch and lies there with a broken leg. A passer-by looks in and says, 'Poor fellow, let me help you' and he jumps in with him and comforts him but cannot get him out because he is not strong enough. A second person comes along, puts one foot into the ditch, reaches down to grasp hold of the injured man and pulls him out. Empathy needs one foot in reality.

Thus, for counselling to be effective, the counsellor relies on empathic understanding rather than on sympathy. But there is no such thing as a permanent or absolute state of empathy. It is not a quality which can be acquired once and for all. It is never static. It fluctuates according to the situation and the person with whom one is involved. Sometimes our empathy is 'spot on'; at others it would appear to be overshadowed or off-centre.

If empathy is important, so also is being able to convey that we understand or that we are attempting to. Gilmore[6] suggests several ways of increasing understanding of the client and of conveying this understanding. One such aid is the 'ballet analogy'. The counsellor is watching a ballet in which each dancer, in turn, is the client. He is also the orchestra, the lights and the story. If the counseller immerses himself in this he will understand, by watching, listening and moving in the inner world of the client. He will thus be able to convey this understanding to a more responsive client who does not have to be told that empathy exists; he will feel it.

Insight

Insight in counselling refers to the extent to which the client is aware of his problem, its origin or origins and the influence his problem exerts on him. Insight may be sudden — like the flash of inspiration; the 'eureka experience'. More usually it develops stage-by-stage as the client develops psychological strength to deal with what is revealed. Very often the last bit of the jigsaw drops into place after counselling has ceased, when the individual has time to think over what has taken place and when he is removed from the pressures of what can be a fairly intense experience. Insight cannot be given by one person to another; neither can it be forced on him. The counsellor may see the problem and its solution very clearly but until the client perceives it for himself the counsellor can only stay with him and guide him until he can. If he is rushed he will, in all probability, retreat and any gains may well be lost. He is guided towards insight by building up the relationship and fostering his ability to take steps toward self revelation.

Dean[3] sounds a warning note.

> Leaving a person with insight for which he has found no practical application is not at all satisfactory. A person's awareness may have been heightened but that is all. The old thought patterns and behaviour patterns remain. So insight may be followed by a high degree of frustration.

It is important, therefore, that the client is helped to see how he can put his insights to practical use.

Mentor Consultation

For counselling to be productive the counsellor must be continually moving forward toward increased understanding of himself in relation to other people. Time and again he will be brought into contact with clients whose problems will awaken within him something which will create resistance or conflict *within that relationship and specific to it*. The client's difficulty will not be adequately resolved until the counsellor's own resistance or conflict is resolved. It is true that the client may seek help from other sources, but if so the counsellor's personal development may be retarded. When faced with a situation where his own emotions are thrown into turmoil, or where counselling appearing to have reached stalemate, there are three courses of action the counsellor may take. He can pull the blanket over his head and hope that the problem will go away, he can work at it on his own, or he can seek help.

In counselling we hope that the client will achieve a degree of insight in order to see his problem more realistically. If insight is essential for the client, how much more is it essential for the counsellor? If it is necessary for the client to seek help from someone to work through his problem (if he been able to work it out for himself, surely he would), it is equally important for the counsellor. There is an element of truth in what people say: that one must have experienced something before one can really help others. This does not mean that the counsellor must have passed through an *identical* experience, but it is important that every person who engages in counselling has been the recipient in a helping relationship. Many people who counsel have personal experience of what it is like to be a client, and it has been this experience that has prompted them to become counsellors. Not everyone has had this first-hand experience and yet it is possible to experience similar feelings when it becomes necessary to seek the help of someone else during counselling.

The person in need of counselling has probably put off seeking help and has tried to work it out for himself, but to no avail — the problem is still there. He is bound to feel inadequate; that he should have been able to manage. He may think, 'Can this other person really help?' The counsellor may experience similar feelings when it is obvious that the counselling relationship has turned sour; that the client is being difficult, resistant, hostile or whatever. It is easier for the counsellor in this position to go to someone else for help than it was for the client to approach the counsellor in the first instance. At that stage the counsellor, in his heart, knows how the client feels. He may resist it, and rebel against it, but only if he submits to this experience, when it becomes necessary, will his counselling once more assume accurate empathy.

The mentor assumes an important role in counselling. He will assist the counsellor to resolve the difficulty that has arisen between himself and his client, mainly because he can stand outside and explore with the counsellor what is happening within the client, the counsellor and the relationship between counsellor and client. The mentor will be able to use what happens between himself and the counsellor — the relationship — to point to what may be happening between the counsellor and the client. This is similar to how the counsellor may be able to point out to the client that what happens between them may be similar to what happens between the client and other people. For the counsellor who has such a mentor relationship the potential for personal awareness is infinite. The counsellor who chooses to disregard such a relationship will lose out and runs the risk of eventually becoming ineffective in his counselling.

In some circles this aspect of counsellor development is called 'supervision'. A dictionary definition of 'supervisor' is, 'A person who exercises general direction or control . . .. One who inspects and directs the work of others.'

A 'mentor' is 'A guide, a wise and faithful counsellor; so called from Mentor, a friend of Ulysses, whose form Minerva assumed when she accompanied Telemachos in his search for his father.'[18]

The fact that 'supervision' is the generally accepted term should not detract from the generally accepted meaning in counselling. Marteau points out,

> The function of the supervisor is to help the student increase his skills and develop in the understanding of his own and his client's feeling in such a manner as to increase his sensitivity to and awareness of both. While this relationship is concerned with the emotional development of the student it is not meant to become predominantly therapeutic. Thus the task of the supervisor differs from that of the counsellor, falling between the polarities of counselling and tutoring.[19]

Presenting Problem

The problem which the client chooses to bring to the agency, or the 'presenting problem' as it is sometimes called, is of considerable significance. Sometimes it is in the nature of a trial balloon, the client quite deliberately choosing to bring up something which is not of primary importance in order to test out the agency, but more often it represents that aspect of the client's problem which, at this present time, is giving him the *most* anxiety.[5]

The implication of this is that we need to be aware that the client does often present something as a 'lead in' to what is of greater significance. Perhaps it is to test the counsellor; to see if he can get on the same wavelength. But he may also do this to ease himself in. Perhaps it would be too emotionally demanding to talk about the significant problem before the counselling relationship had been firmly established. Whatever the reasons, it is always wise to sit back and wait for the client to develop the theme. To take the analogy of the ballet (p. 27), the presenting problem could be thought of as the overture. The audience does not judge the performance only on hearing the overture; they wait for the action. Just so in counselling. Precipitate action, based on the presenting problem, may well prove to be unhelpful and time wasting.

Problem-solving

Not all counselling is concerned with problem-solving but a great deal of it is. Some people want to increase their self-awareness, to understand a bit better how they interact with others, or to develop more insight of the helping relationship by first-hand experience. All of these may apply to counselling in rehabilitation but it is more likely that the therapist will be involved with patients and their relatives who have definite problems with which they need help. Very often the client presents the 'problem' to the counsellor in a jumbled and unclear way. In the early stages, therefore, it is useful to have a plan which counsellor and client can work on together to bring order out of chaos. The model presented here may help. As patient and therapist work through this together, step by step, it will let the patient see that there is a logical way of tackling his problem. It will also help the therapist by relieving some of the anxiety of not knowing where to start.

A Problem-solving Model

Identify the Problem

1. Is there a problem? If so, what is it precisely?
2. Who says there is a problem?
3. Who has the problem?
4. What other people are involved? How are they involved?
5. What is my role to be in helping . . . resolve this problem? (Name the person or persons.)
6. What are my impressions of . . .?
7. Why do I think and feel this way about them?
8. Any other points relevant to this stage?

Explore the Problem

9. What areas does . . . need help to explore?
10. How long has the problem existed?
11. What steps have been or could have been taken to resolve the problem?
12. Would (a) doing nothing (b) making changes create risks?
13. What changes are possible?
14. Which of (a) or (b) involves the greater risk?
15. What does . . . have to (a) gain (b) lose?
16. What is the goal I think . . . could work toward?
17. Any points relevant to this stage?

Action Plan

18. What action plan could I help . . . draw up?
19. What steps could . . . take to reach the goal set in 16?
20. Are there any changes I would (a) advise (b) advise against?
21. If any of the changes involve other people, what strategies can be

devised to facilitate change?

22. What is my role in the action plan?
23. How will I know if change has taken place?
24. Are there any external factors which could work in favour of . . . achieving his goal?
25. Are there any external factors which could work against . . . achieving his goal?
26. Are there any internal factors which could work in favour of . . . achieving his goal?
27. Are there any internal factors which could work against . . . achieving his goal?

Evaluation

28. What questions do I need to ask in an attempt to evaluate the problem-solving process?

Source: Appendix 'F' in William Stewart, *Counselling in Nursing: A Problem Solving Approach*, Harper and Row, London, 1983.

Rapport

> Rapport is a word used a great deal in any discussion on relationships. It would appear to derive from the special relationship that exists between hypnotist and subject. But in a more general sense it is a relationship based on a high degree of community of thought, interest and sentiment.[20]

Rapport may be considered from three standpoints: harmony, compatibility and affinity.

An analogy may be taken from nature in which there is a strong striving for balance and harmony. But harmony is seldom achieved, or if at all it does not persist. In counselling, harmony is often — to borrow from Matthew Arnold — an 'elusive shadow', but a shadow that we must try to convert into substance.

Compatibility between people depends upon such factors as personality, looks, intelligence, emotional stability, understanding, kindness, tenderness and common interest. In friendship we can pick and choose but in rehabilitation neither therapist nor client is able to be quite so selective. This means that therapists, in order to be effective counsellors, must strive hard to 'make themselves *as compatible as possible* with as wide a range of people as possible. If this sounds a formidable task, it is, but not a superhuman one.'[8]

Affinity has to do with the quality of the relationship. Another analogy may be drawn from chemistry and physics where specific elements are attracted to each other to form a compound, or where iron is attracted to a magnet. The two elements have formed a unique bond, just as two people do who come together in marriage. Counselling is a significant and unique bond between counsellor and client, or between therapist and patient in rehabilitation. They have been bonded together for a specific purpose and when that purpose has been fulfilled, the relationship will be dissolved. The bond of affinity will be severed.

> The more one invests in a relationship, the stronger the bond grows; and the breaking of it may bring pain. But to compensate, both client and [therapist] nurse take with them something of the investment of the other person to enrich their respective experiences.[8]

Relationship

> The excellency of every art is its intensity, capable of making all disagreeables evaporate, from their being in close relationship with beauty and truth. John Keats

Many writers on the subject of counselling emphasise the relationship aspect. It would be foolhardy and possibly arrogant to imply that this subject could be covered in a section of one chapter when others have devoted whole volumes to the counselling relationship. This chapter, therefore, will concentrate only on certain aspects of this important topic.

The reader could be forgiven for thinking that the counselling relationship is something special and different from any other relationship. The only sense in which it may be different is that it is not an end in itself; it is a means to an end.

Certain characteristics can be identified which are common to any positive relationship.

Gilmore[6] lists the following characteristics:

Respecting	Being genuinely interested in
Valuing	Appreciating
Liking	Wanting to share the experience of
Prizing	Receiving a person as he presently is

Being delighted with Being concerned about Caring for	Having a deep regard for the basic worth of this human being.

Although Gilmore was speaking of a particular aspect of acceptance, her list applies equally to the total counselling relationship.

The counselling relationship is more than a collection of attributes and attitudes. It will only be significant to the client when it is translated into action which touches him. Various writers speak of 'genuineness', 'congruity', 'openness', 'warmth' and many other desirable qualities. But one word sums them all up, 'caring'. Caring is not slushy and sentimental. It is based on sincerity and is characterised by warmth and vitality. It is not smothering or cloying, nor does it encourage dependence; but it permits the client to work toward independence. An analogy may be drawn from the relationship of a child to its parents. When the child is young, caring is almost total and includes all aspects of care. As the child grows, he takes over some of the functions previously undertaken for him by his parents. Eventually he assumes complete independence and lives his own life. It is a wise parent who has prepared the child well for eventual independence, by gradually relinquishing control.

In the early stages of counselling, the client may be more dependent on the counselling relationship than the counsellor would wish. But as the client develops insight, and as he is encouraged to develop strategies to cope with his difficulties, he should become increasingly independent. Parents are aware that the time and energy they devote to caring for their child may not always bring joy and pleasure to them. Many parents are overburdened with guilt when their child, whom they have reared to the best of their ability, rejects all their efforts and brings them nothing but heartache and trouble. When the counsellor offers himself in relationship with clients he, too, is vulnerable. And sometimes pain and disappointment takes the place of joy and pleasure when, for example, clients terminate the relationship prematurely. But both pain and sorrow, as well as joy and pleasure, are necessary for the deepening of the counsellor's ability to relate to a wide range of people.

Resistance

Resistance is likely to be present in any counselling. Many people who require counselling also experience resistance to it. This paradox is something which every counsellor must recognise and accept. As a general rule the resistance is not personal. The client experiences resistance, in the first instance, because of what is happening within him. Conflict of any kind creates its own resistance. Another reason for resistance is linked with the feeling of not being master of his own ship. Personal disappointment, fear, resentment, frustration and anger are feelings which are all liable to be present. He may realise that his personal life is in chaos and his inner world in turmoil. He may feel guilty that his disability should make him so dependent on others, including the therapist. Guilt causes us to anticipate censure which leads to a build-up of resistance.

Anticipated change may also cause resistance. The person with the problem is put in the position of having to change some aspect of his behaviour. (There is of course the possibility that in fact it is not he, the client, who needs to change his behaviour but other people who have somehow managed to manipulate him into the situation of believing that he is the one who should change.) He may agree that change is required, indeed is desirable, but paradoxically he resists the change. In a sense this is related to his perception of the counsellor. If he sees him as someone who can enforce change (and many people have some strange ideas of what counselling actually is!), he may show more resistance than if he regards him as a person who will enable him to make his own changes. If the person does not accept that he has a problem he will almost certainly be resistant. If therapists remember that all patients may experience resistance, not only to counselling but to therapy itself, they will be prepared for it when it shows itself, possibly in antagonism, rudeness, anger or any other negative feeling.

If the counsellor attempts to push the client ahead too fast, or talks too much, or adopts a negative approach, resistance is likely to result. The client in rehabilitation is most likely to be labouring under strong emotions — feelings of rejection, for example — and it would be reasonable to assume that it could be difficult for him to concentrate on a constructive appraisal of the situation until he has been allowed to ventilate such feelings. The prudent therapist will discern the early-warning signs of heightened emotions and permit, and indeed encourage, the client to give vent to them. Just as effective ventilation will rid a room of stale odours, so ventilation of negative feelings will reduce resistance.

Resistance may manifest itself at any time during counselling. It may become apparent in the way the client blocks what the counsellor is putting forward. Instead of considering what is being said, he objects to it and argues against it without consideration. This may be due to the fact that the counsellor has touched a trigger spot, a tender area, a hidden something he does not want to discuss. If the counsellor says something like, 'I seem to have touched on a tender spot, perhaps you would rather not discuss it at this stage', he is telling the client quite clearly that he has recognised his feelings, that he is still alongside him. But he is also leaving the way open in his 'at this stage' for the client to discuss it when he is ready and if he so desires.

Resistance does not emanate exclusively from the client; this would put the relationship on an unequal basis. In every counselling interview the therapist's own emotions, attitudes, opinions and beliefs are brought sharply into focus and at any given moment he may discover that some sacrosanct attitude or belief has been brought into conflict with an opposite attitude or belief of the client. When that happens, the way may be cleared by a frank admission from the therapist that this has happened. But at the same time, the focus must not be removed from the client. The session should not turn into one where the therapist and patient reverse roles. This does not imply that 'co-counselling' is not of value. But the contact between therapist and patient would not normally include a co-counselling element.

Self-responsibility

Self-responsibility means that the client has the right to make his own choices — to choose the road on which he wants to travel. The more he can be encouraged to make his own decisions, and the less he becomes dependent upon the counsellor, the better. The ability to be 'self-responsible' will vary with every client and is influenced by the nature of the problem and the emotional effect it exerts on him. Self-responsibility assumes a different aspect when the client is emotionally unstable or of an age at which the full consequences of decisions may not be fully appreciated. But even in these circumstances it may still be possible to guide the client, *within the limits of his understanding*, along the road of self-responsibility.

It must always be borne in mind, however, that there are few situations in life when for any one of us free choice is absolute. We are all constrained by forces which tend to push us in certain directions while different forces block our progress in others. This is reality. Part of counselling may be to help the client face up to the forces that he feels constrain him. He may be able to do something about some of the obstacles; others may be insurmountable. This is particularly relevant in rehabilitation where the patient's condition may be an obstacle that cannot be removed. Counselling may generate enough energy for the client to seek a new direction for his life in order to cope with his disability.

Transference and Countertransference

Transference is a term employed by psychoanalysts to denote, '. . . the transfer by the patient to the analyst of emotional tones, of either affection or hostility, based on unconscious identification'.[21] Although this definition refers to 'analysis', counsellors should also be aware that similar feelings may be directed by the client toward them. These feelings may be linked to relationships past or present, and the counsellor is put into the role of the significant person. If the counsellor reacts to these projected feelings, this is called 'countertransference'.

Counsellors, in contrast to psychoanalysts, do not deliberately foster transference. In psychoanalysis much use is made of transference and of working through it. But the counsellor should be aware that the client may be investing feelings in him that would be more appropriately directed toward another person. These feelings are more likely to develop in psychoanalysis than in counselling, partly because of the depth at which analysts work, but also because of the greater frequency of contact. Therapists in rehabilitation who have frequent, sometimes daily, contact with patients may experience transfer of feelings more than counsellors who see clients at weekly intervals. Intimacy of physical contact is another factor which may contribute to transference. Patients who are seriously disabled, at least in the early stages of rehabilitation, are usually quite dependent, physically. This dependency is very likely to re-create feelings associated with early childhood. But these feelings may be a mixture of love and hate — classical transference feelings. The child grows through dependency to independence and this growth is often beset with problems. Parental constraints and sanctions foster a gradual independence or a permanent state of bondage. When a person, because of illness or accident, becomes once more dependent, his feelings are likely to be in conflict. One part of him — the child — may enjoy the dependent role, while the other part — that which has grown up — may rebel. Rebellion often creates angry feelings. Psychoanalysts will interpret these feelings to the client: therapists may be well advised not to. To acknowledge them may be sufficient. By so doing, the therapist is opening the way for the client to discuss his feelings at that moment. This supports the point made on page 25 that counselling deals more with the present than with the past and more with the conscious than with the unconscious.

Trust

> No lesson seems to be so deeply inculcated by the experience of life as that you never should trust experts. If you believe the doctors, nothing is wholesome: if you believe the theologians, nothing is innocent: if you believe the soldiers, nothing is safe. They all require to have their strong wine diluted by a very large admixture of insipid common sense.
>
> Lord Salisbury in a letter to Lord Lytton 1877

Lord Salisbury did not include counsellors among the people not to trust. If we set ourselves up as experts we could very well be included, particularly if we think of ourselves as ones who know all the answers. Yet an expert is one who is skilled by experience. And part of that experience is knowing — and freely acknowledging — that we do not have any answers, let alone all of them. This (often unspoken) premise establishes the counsellor as an honest person in whom the client may place his trust; in whom he may have confidence. It must be very alarming and awe-inspiring to be in the presence of someone in whom all wisdom resides! In seeking someone in whom to place his trust, the client looks for confidence, credibility and understanding. That someone must not abuse the trust placed in him.

Therapists, by nature of their roles, have already had invested in them a great deal of trust. The patient who, after a crippling accident, is being encouraged to stand and walk, trusts the therapist. This physical trust should not be underestimated, for very often it can lead to deeper emotional trust. Indeed in certain experiential group exercises this physical trust aspect is developed before going on to explore and verbalise feelings. To fall backward, with eyes closed, into the arms of another person, displays a great deal of trust — in both people. The client who talks to a therapist about his fears and frustrations of his inability to walk, is placing his trust in her. But trust is a two-way process. The catcher must feel confident that he will catch the person falling into his arms and that he will be able to hold him. The therapist who is teaching a paralysed patient to swim must feel confident in her ability to cope. Therapists are all too aware of those patients who do not fully trust. They are tense and fearful; they do not relax or co-operate fully. Trust with those patients has to be established gradually. The trusting patient can make things so much easier for himself and for the therapist. The client, in counselling, also has to learn to trust. Some are more able to do this than are others. The patient who has had an injury 'guards' the injured part. The client who has been emotionally hurt guards his emotions to prevent further hurt. It may take time — a great deal of time — for him to experience the healing that trusting, within the counselling relationship, can bring to his hurt emotions.

Zeal

One definition of zeal is, 'Ardour in the pursuit of an end or in favour of a person or cause: active enthusiasm.' (*Shorter Oxford English Dictionary*.) Therapists, if they are to mobilise the patient's inner resources to overcome his handicap, must be enthusiastic. This enthusiasm is conveyed to the patient in the way treatment is carried out. Patients who have lost their enthusiasm can often be stimulated into fresh action and progress by the enthusiasm of other people. The therapist who includes counselling as an integral part of her repertoire of skills is surely possessed of zeal in her desire to treat the 'whole person'.

Zest

'Keen relish or enjoyment.' Counselling, in common with all work, should be enjoyed. The pleasure we derive from it may be just the spark that the client needs to help him rise above his disability.

Summary

This chapter has covered eighteen important aspects of counselling philosophy. One topic — 'openness' — was touched on but not discussed in depth. Counsellors should be open in two dimensions. A window is a useful analogy. A window allows people to look into a room or out from it. If curtains are drawn, the window might as well be a brick wall. If it is dressed with lace, the vision is partly obscured. A window not so obscured invites passers-by to look in and admire. Counsellors are like windows. Their vision of the client's world can be crystal clear, partially obscured or effectively curtained by emotional trappings. Windows so obscured make for difficult counselling. If the counsellor is unable to see the client clearly, neither can the client see the counsellor clearly. If both are working in the dark, they may both get lost. The open counsellor who has stripped off some, if not all, of those things that obscure, will encourage the client to be open. The more one becomes aware of self, the more clear one's window becomes and the more clearly one shall see and be seen by others.

This chapter has been more than a dissertation on counselling philosophy. Many of the topics have been written up with the intention of challenging the reader to continue the process of self-knowledge which is so essential if counselling is to be effective. Let Charles Dickens have almost the last word in this chapter.

> When you're a married man, Samivel, you'll understand a good many things as you don't understand now; but vether it's worth while goin through so much to learn so little, as the charity box boy said ven he got to the end of the alphabet, is a matter o' taste.
>
> (Mr Weller in Pickwick Papers.)

May the journey through 'A' to 'Z' have been worthwhile.

Notes

1. Rogers, C.L. (1961) *On Becoming a Person*, Houghton Mifflin Co., Boston.
2. Shertzer, B. and Stone, Shelley C. (1980) *Fundamentals of Counselling*, Houghton Mifflin Co., Boston.
3. Dean, H. and M. (1981) *Counselling in a Troubled Society*, Quartermaine House Ltd, London.
4. Hamilton, G. (1962) *Theory and Practice of Social Casework*, University Press, New York.
5. Davison, E.H. (1965) *Social Casework*, Baillière Tindall, London.
6. Gilmore, S.K. (1973) *The Counsellor in Training*, Prentice Hall Inc. Englewood Cliffs, N.J.
7. Stewart, W. (1977) *A Guide to Counselling*, Wessex Regional Health Authority.
8. Stewart, W. (1983) *Counselling in Nursing: a Problem-Solving Approach*, Harper and Row, London.
9. Hollis, F. (1966) *Casework: A Psychosocial Therapy*, Random House, New York.
10. The British Association for Counselling, Standards and Ethics Committee.
11. Patterson, C.H. (1974) *Relationship Counselling and Psychotherapy*, Harper and Row, New York.
12. Krumboltz, J.D. and Thoreson, C. (1976) *Counselling Methods*, Holt, Rinehart and Winston, New York.
13. Taken from the programme of the Second International Congress on Patient Counselling and Education, held at the Hague 1979 and quoted in 8 above.
14. BBC 'Principles of Counselling'. Radio programmes.
15. Stewart, W. (1979) *Health Service Counselling*, Pitman Medical, London.
16. Katz, R.L. (1963) *Empathy*, Free Press of Glencoe/Collier Macmillan, Ltd., London.
17. Reik, T. (1949) *Listening with the Third Ear*, Farrar, Strauss and Co., New York.
18. *Brewer's Dictionary of Phrase and Fable*, Avend Books, New York, 1978.

19. Marteau, L. *Ethical Standards in Counselling*, British Association for Counselling. Bedford Square Press of the National Council for Voluntary Organisations.

20. Drever, J. (1969) *A Dictionary of Psychology*, Penguin Books, Harmondsworth. Quoted in 8 above.

21. Miller, B.F. and Keane, C.B. (1978) *Encyclopedia and Dictionary of Medicine, Nursing and Allied Health*, W.B. Saunders, Philadelphia.

3 THE PRACTICE OF COUNSELLING*

A Model of Counselling

The previous chapter presented a number of important aspects of counselling philosophy. This chapter considers these concepts within the six stage Wessex Model of counselling, which I have developed myself, and named after my home region. The stages are:

Stage 1	Meet the Client
Stage 2	Identify the Problem
Stage 3	Explore the Problem
Stage 4	Action Plan
Stage 5	Implement the Action Plan
Stage 6	Evaluation

The approach throughout this book is a problem-solving one. The reader should not infer from this that it is the counsellor who *solves* the client's problems. Problem-solving in counselling cannot be equated to solving mathematical problems where there is a 'right' answer. Egan[1] points out that counsellors need to

> understand and appreciate the complexity of any given problem situation. Oversimplification of problems followed by superficial solutions help no one. On the other hand, they [counsellors] need to avoid being overwhelmed by the complexity of problem situations. Even in the face of chaos, they must be able to help the client do *something*.

The reader has already been introduced — on page 31 — to one problem-solving model, where the same point — bringing order out of chaos —,was raised. It is psychologically important that the client goes away from the first contact with the counsellor feeling that something, however little, has been accomplished, and that some light has been able to get through. An underlying hope of any counselling, but especially when a problem-solving approach is used, is that the client will be able

*A substantial part of this chapter has been taken from my previous book, *Counselling in Nursing: A Problem-solving Approach*, Harper and Row. London 1983.

to apply the model which has been used to other problems he may face in the future, and thus be more able to cope with life.

People who are new to counselling often feel as clients feel: 'Where do I start?' 'How do I start?' 'What do I say?' This is why this model of counselling is presented; it begins — as the King, in Alice In Wonderland, said — at the beginning and goes on till it comes to the end; then it stops. It is a 'progressive' model that begins with the client, and continues systematically until counselling is terminated.

Working to a model does not mean that it has to be adhered to rigidly. A model should provide some basic guidelines; but they should be guidelines and not constraints. Working to a counselling model, however loosely, can help to ensure that one does not start thinking of a solution as soon as the problem is presented: equally, that one does not encourage the client to start planning what to do before he has had adequate opportunity to explore all the ramifications of the problem. One of the difficulties of presenting a counselling model on paper is to convey that it is a dynamic and not a static process, neither does it always follow neatly from start to finish. Another difficulty is to convey that unspoken awareness of when it is time to move on to the next stage. There is no clearly identifiable point at which to move on. Rather, it is a blending, a merging of what is taking place, that provides a natural impetus for forward movement. This unspoken awareness — so essential in counselling — is more easily demonstrated in a teaching group or by listening to interviews.

Stage 1 Meet the Client

The first stage of the model starts with the client. Meeting the client is probably the most vital stage; for it is upon the foundation of this first contact that any hope of productive counselling is built. In these early contacts the counsellor and client set out to establish a relationship in which both feel comfortable and able to work together in an area which is causing concern to the client. What has been said so far makes it sound easy and matter-of-fact but, in reality, the first contact may be difficult. Some clients talk quite readily about themselves and whatever it is that is causing them concern. Others have great difficulty expressing themselves and every word seems to be drawn from the depths, with long silences punctuating brief comments. The client may be feeling anxious, apprehensive or nervous about the need for counselling and the counsellor who, by his attitude, demonstrates that he understands these feelings, will help the client understand them also; understanding will pave the way for a fruitful relationship. Having said this, counselling is generally a verbal exchange, and there are some people who find it difficult to accept that 'talking' can bring the degree of relief they are seeking. If counselling were just talking, perhaps their reservations would be justified. But counselling is more than talking. This will be dealt with in greater detail later on.

The Counselling Contract

When counsellor and client have established that they feel able to work together, it is usual to enter into some form of 'contract' or agreement about how they will proceed. This is particularly important when it seems that more than one session is required. Some readers may jib at the word 'contract'; but what it does imply is an undertaking, on both sides, of how the affair is to be concluded. The client will agree, in broad detail, the area to be tackled, although there may be certain details that he does not wish to touch on, at least not until the relationship is firmly established. So, the contract is a setting of boundaries and expectations. Some clients do not want to set boundaries; for them counselling needs to be free-ranging. Such trust places a tremendous onus on the counsellor who, unknowingly, may tread on uncharted land; the client, because of his emotional disturbance, may resent this intrusion. Some boundaries are usually helpful.

In addition to the boundaries to exploration, there are the boundaries of time. How long will each session last? How frequently will counsellor and client meet, and where? In a fee-paying service the fee will be discussed and agreed. There needs to be a tentative agreement reached on how many sessions should be aimed at and how they will be assessed. A part of the contract should be the mentor relationship that the counsellor has, and its purpose.

Stage 1 Skills

This section introduces four principal skills which operate throughout counselling.

1. Awareness of the uniqueness of the client.
2. Rapport.
3. Empathy.
4. Listening and questioning.

It could be argued that only listening and questioning are skills, and that the others are qualities. Be that as it may, they have been included here because they are crucial elements in the first stage. Rapport and empathy have been covered in Chapter 2. The premise of this book is that the majority of therapists — of whatever discipline — can learn the skills of counselling if they have a genuine desire to do so. But, like any other skills, much practice is required, and a willingness to undertake a great deal of scrutiny of one's performance as a counsellor. This constant examination and re-examinaton inevitably leads to a great self-awareness, and hand-in-hand with this comes more understanding of people as clients.

The Unique Client

It may seem unnecessary to state that every client is unique. Just how this uniqueness shows itself needs to be expanded. There are some obvious areas such as work, male/female, status and so on, and we all attach different emphases to all of these, but there are other areas which, at first glance, may not be so obvious.

Personality. This book is not the place to enter into a lengthy discourse on personality types and how they are reputed to behave; but suffice to say that because everyone has a different personality, it is fairly obvious that there are likely to be some clients whose personalities would not be compatible with the counsellor's own. There may be clients with whom he feels he could be friends, but others with whom he could not. But counselling is not, in the strict sense of the word, friendship. The counsellor has to be friendly, but the difference between friendship and counselling is in the reason for the contact, rather than in the quality of the relationship.

Character. An aspect of personality is character — that sum total of a person's qualities that influences the way he behaves towards others. A facet of character is how one person treats other people, influenced by his moral attitude and his ethical values. Of all aspects of character, it is possible that moral attitude is the one that has the greatest potential for conflict between two people. It would be very unlikely that two people would come together — or remain together — in friendship if their moral codes were vastly different. Yet, in counselling this situation may very well arise. That is why it is essential that the counsellor develops the ability to suspend his own judgements so that they do not confront the client's, thus creating conflict.

Motivation. A person's motivation towards significant areas of his life is something else that contributes to his uniqueness. There is a tendency for some people to assume because they have achieved a certain thing, that everyone else should likewise be able to. Unless the counsellor has taken account of what motivates him, he could mistakenly apply pressure on the client to move along a certain route, propelled by the counsellor's motivation rather than his own. This may work for a time, but unless the 'will to change' comes from within the client, change, if it does occur, is likely to be short-lived.

Experience. The last area to be covered in this consideration of the uniqueness of the client is the vital area of his life experience. It is extraordinary, but true, that two children of the same parents may emerge from their home giving the impression of having experienced two significantly different up-bringings. If this can apply to siblings, how much more may it apply to those who are not related? Two people can look out of the same window and see two dissimilar worlds. Two students can listen to the same lecture and hear quite different explanations of the topic. How we perceive the world around highlights our uniqueness. In the same way, what has occupied people's waking hours exerts different influences. The very nature of a person's daily occupation is a major factor in creating him as he is. Most people are slotted neatly into occupational pigeonholes, and are given — or don of their own free will — a set of expectations in keeping with a specific occupation. Having donned this cluster of expectations, most people find that this role takes over to a degree, and it is often difficult for people to break out of their roles. It is also difficult for other people to see the person behind the role. When considering the client, it is essential to look beneath his role, to discover what makes him unique.

Listening and Questioning

Some people mistakenly think that all a counsellor has to do is listen. Although listening is essential, it is not a passive but an active process involving all the sense and not only the ears. In any communication between people, four factors have to be considered.

1. *Use all senses.* Listening demands an attitude of readiness and openness, and an expectation to hear something. Many people listen but do not always hear. Counsellors have to learn to listen 'between the lines'; to hear the emotions linked to the words. Brammer[2] speaks of 'attending', and gives four principles:

1. Eye contact.
2. Relaxed posture.
3. Natural gestures.
4. Verbal statements that relate to what the client has said.

To this could be added 'position'. The distance from or proximity to each other is important. If the counsellor sits directly in front of the client this may be too uncomfortable, as may sitting too close. Generally speaking, a comfortable position is where the chairs are not too far apart and at a slight angle to each other. If the client is not comfortable with the distance, he will, unless the chair is fixed, adjust the distance. Should he do so, this should tell the counsellor something. That is why it is necessary to use all senses.

2. *Language.* A substantial part of communication is non-verbal. It is worth pointing out at this stage that speech arises from the conscious mind while non-verbal language is, to a large extent, from the unconscious. Thus, two levels are in operation. In counselling, both counsellor and client may find themselves responding to each other's non-verbal communication and not to the verbal. If what is being communicated non-verbally matches the verbal, the messages are said to be congruent. However, if they are incongruous, conflict will be produced in the receiver. The response he makes is then likely to be to the non-verbal and not to the verbal. If this conflict between the two elements of communication is not resolved, counselling will surely break down. Thus it is incumbent on all who engage in any form of counselling to be aware of how their inner worlds — those secret parts, consciously secret, or unconsciously hidden — influence relationships.

3. *Understand and be understood.* It may seem unnecessary to state how essential it is when communicating that each person understands what the other is saying. So often misunderstanding occurs because one or the other has not made himself understood. It is frequently necessary to wait for feedback, to make certain that there is understanding. The fact that one person does not fully understand another is often due to unclear thinking on the part of the speaker, rather than on some lack in the hearer.

4. *Meaning.* People who come for counselling often feel themselves to be in a jumble because their emotions are jumbled. The person who is incensed with anger may be incoherent. A person distressed with grief

may not be able to find any words at all. Strong emotions distort the thinking process. Part of the skill is to get the client to talk and then to encourage him to continue talking, not necessarily in a non-stop flow, but talk interspersed with listening and thinking. This is achieved by making comments, passing observations and asking questions.

5. *The skill and art of asking questions.* The counsellor asks questions to:

1. Seek clarification.
2. Encourage exploration.
3. Elicit information.
4. Establish facts.
5. Establish that understanding has taken place.
6. Gauge feelings.
7. Demonstrate his own understanding.

The counsellor does not ask questions with the intention of prying nor to cause embarrassment or confusion to the client. Questions should not intrude. They should not deliberately offend, neither should they be offensive. They should not be conjured out of the counsellor's fertile curiosity. It is generally agreed that open-ended questions — those which encourage the client to expand on a theme — are more useful than closed questions. Open questions encourage the client to express what he is thinking and feeling. Closed questions are useful where facts are required. But even when information is needed, too many direct, closed, questions can be off-putting. Framing open questions is not always easy; it is something that needs a great deal of practice. A very useful book on questioning skills is included in the references at the end of this chapter.[3]

Note Taking

In certain situations some notes are essential, if only to keep the key issues before one's eyes. Such notes need only be single words, enough to act as refreshers later in the session. Single words or short sentences can usually be written without taking one's eyes off the client for too long. Referring to the notes from time to time may give the client confidence that what has been noted is there to be used. Note taking may also be used effectively to slow up a very talkative client. The client should be made aware of the purpose of the notes and of their confidentiality.

It is by the counsellor's use of the skills outlined in this section of the chapter, and the way he communicates, that he is able to lead the client gently, but with assurance, into identifying the problem.

Stage 2 Identify the Problem

In this second stage of counselling, the client is helped to identify which specific problem, or part of the problem, can be tackled. During the first stage the counsellor may have helped the client to arrive at a fairly accurate assessment of the situation and he may feel that it would be useful and helpful for the client to tackle the problem along a certain line. But when the client is asked, 'What do *you* feel is the most pressing problem you would like to tackle first?', the answer may be quite different from the counsellor's idea. That is why it is always wise to let the client choose which area to concentrate attention on. This might be an appropriate place to refer back to the discussion on the contract (p. 44). There the client's choice acts as a boundary; now it is a definite though indistinct pathway forward.

Some clients may not be able to identify what their problem is. They may be in too vast an emotional jungle. What they need is for the counsellor to tread the way with them, cutting aside some of the tangled undergrowth to let in some light. Just listening to what the client says may be enough; and from this, certain possible avenues may emerge. Because the client is uncertain and possibly confused, any suggestion of what the problem is should be offered tentatively and not with any certainty. Phrases such as, 'It would seem as if . . .', 'Could it be that . . .?', 'This is what it looks like to me . . . is that how you feel?' may help him to clarify his thoughts and feelings. Put in this way, he has the opportunity to reject what he is hearing if it does not seem quite right. He may not find it quite so easy to reject openly a statement such as 'Your problem is that . . .'. 'Now I've heard you, this is what I think should be done.'

Ownership

'It's all her fault', said Mr Taciturn, as he faced the counsellor. 'She leads me a dog's life. I can't think why. I've done nothing to upset her.' Mr Taciturn has difficulty owning up to the problem; owning up to the possibility that perhaps he had some part to play in the difficult marriage. Many people, when under stress because their emotions are in turmoil, cannot see that they have contributed to the problem: they try to push it away, onto someone else. Egan[1] says, 'In sum, a problem situation is not clear until the client owns it in some way. If the client is hesitant to own it, then the helper can encourage him or her to do so.'

Stage 2 Skills

Stage 1 skills continue throughout counselling, but in later stages these skills acquire new emphases. Listening, for example, becomes more active and directed. It is not uncommon for the client to repeat something he has previously related. It is possible that at the first telling it did not register with him that he had told it. At the time, his emotions may have been running at too high a level for it to register that this point had been told. Since the first telling, new thoughts and feelings may have surfaced and now *they* need to be talked about. Another possibility is that he and the counsellor were not in complete rapport; empathy may have been transient: his message may not have been sensitively received. That is why, in the later stages, listening assumes a fresh importance.

Reflecting. Here the counsellor reflects back to the client (as does a mirror) the factual content of, on the one hand, what he is saying, and, on the other, the feelings *as he perceives them.* Any reflection of feeling must be tentative. 'You said that you would never be able to have children and this has knocked the bottom out of your world, is that it?' This is focusing on the facts but linking the feelings to them. Brammer[2] points out, 'When a helpee is expressing strong emotion, it is so obvious to both, that reflecting is unnecessary. The more subtle feelings, however, are often disguised behind words. The helper looks for those hidden feelings that enable the helpee to recognise them more clearly.' Not only may the counsellor reflect the facts and feelings by putting them into his own words, he may use the same words as the client used. This has the effect of letting him hear again; and hearing them may release feelings hitherto kept in check.

Mary was talking to Peter about his relationship with the head therapist.

Mary: You say he's an absolute pig to work for, is that right?
Peter: I didn't say that, did I? What a horrible thing to say about someone. I may have thought it.

This led to a fruitful discussion of how so often our lips say what our hearts mean.

Another aspect of reflecting is linking what the person is saying with what he is doing, or has done. 'You say you don't mind your wife having this friendship with another man, that it is only platonic, but every time you mention this man, your fists clench, as if you were angry. Is that worth looking at?' Brammer[2] points to some common errors in reflecting:

1. *Stereotyped responses:* '. . . repetitive style gives the impression of insincerity or an impoverished word supply.'
2. *Timing.* Not every statement has to be reflected. 'Usually it helps to nod acceptance or give a slight "uh huh" or "I see," to encourage continuation until a reflection seems appropriate.'
3. *Depth.* The reflection must be appropriate to the feeling being expressed and to the level of awareness of the client.
4. *Language.* Suit the words to the intellectual understanding of the client.

Simple words can generally be understood by everyone.

Paraphrasing. Paraphrasing, according to one dictionary definition, is 'a free rendering or an amplification of a statement.' It may condense or it may expand the words used. In general conversation many assumptions are made about what has been said. Counselling is not an 'ordinary' conversation. Paraphrasing helps to ensure understanding.

Words are vehicles to convey feelings. So not only is it necessary to understand the client's words, we must also try to understand why particular words, in preference to others, are used. If the client has been expressing his thoughts with difficulty, then is a good time to paraphrase. Letting him hear the meaning as understood by someone else may help him to clarify more precisely what he does mean. It also demonstrates that the counsellor is really attending. Paraphrasing, well done, encourages the client to continue.

Summarising. Summarising, like paraphrasing, when well done, is not an intrusion; but it should not be overdone. Summarising may be used at any time during a session and is useful to highlight recurring themes. A useful technique is to invite the client to summarise what he has been saying. Brammer[2] lists the following as important elements in summarising.

1. What is said (content).
2. How it is said (feelings).
3. Purpose, timing and effect of the statements (process).

Egan[1] says,

> A good summary is not a mechanical pulling together of a number of facts; it is a systematic presentation of *relevant* data. The helper

makes some decisions as to what is relevant but bases this decision on listening to and understanding the client.

Egan goes on to say that summaries are useful

1. For starting a new session. Not that the threads can be picked up exactly where they were left, but to give the client an opportunity to choose which direction to travel.
2. When a session is going nowhere.
3. When clients get stuck. 'A summary of the principal points they *have* made can help them to see the "bigger picture" more clearly and therefore help them move to dynamic self-understanding.'

A summary at the end of a session provides an opportunity for both counsellor and client to think about the next session.

Specificity. Getting the client to be specific may, at times, be quite difficult. But it is essential if he is to come to terms fully with whatever is causing him concern. The opposite of specific is 'general' and so often the client will escape into generalities and vagueness. A generality, common in everyday speech, is 'you'. The client who says, 'You never know when people approve of what you're doing', when encouraged to rephrase it to 'I never know when people approve of what I'm doing', will usually be able to perceive it in a different light. Personalising it in this way makes it pertinent and real. In one sense, this is similar to 'owning the problem'. Being specific opens the way for a realistic acknowledgement of feelings. Owning such feelings, and not merely reporting them, opens the door to explore them. While this may be uncomfortable for the client, it is vitally necessary.

Sometimes feelings are expressed before the counselling relationship has been established firmly enough for an exploration of those feelings. Then it might be wiser not to explore them; if they are central to the client's problem he will return to them. That is why specificity is introduced in the second stage. It does require the client to be prepared to examine himself closely and not to hide behind the facade of generalities. To do this requires confidence, not only in himself but also in the counsellor. The client may fiercely resist all attempts to encourage him to be specific, particularly about his feelings. Being able to talk about one's feelings is something not everyone finds easy to do; perhaps not all have learned how. If this is so, the client may need to be led gently into this learning experience. Most people know how anger or sorrow feels but some feelings require much finer tuning. This is where the counsellor may adopt a teaching role. It is important, of course, that the counsellor recognises within himself when he evades being specific by escaping into general statements. All the while he colludes with the client by allowing him to talk about feelings second-hand, as if they belonged to other people and not to him, constructive counselling will be limited. 'Is this how you feel?' or 'Is that something like your situation?' may be enough to bring the interview back into focus from the 'then and there' to the 'here and now'.

Maintaining Momentum. During the early stages of counselling, as client and counsellor are getting to know each other and as the client spends time telling his story, there may not be any pressing need for the counsellor to find ways to keep the interview on the move. Later on, however, when the tale has been told and the problem has been identified, or partially so, and as counselling enters the exploratory stage, it may happen that the process slows down or comes to a halt. Comments such as 'and then?'; 'what happened?'; 'what was the outcome?'; 'tell me about . . .'; 'what were your feelings at the time?' are all aimed at moving the interview forward — gently, not pushing it. But there is a natural time for a session to end. If momentum slows down, there may be the appropriate time to stop, by summarising what has taken place.

Silences. One way of maintaining momentum, although it may seem a paradox, is the constructive use of silence. So often, what could be a constructive silence is ruined by an over-anxious counsellor, unable to tolerate the silence, or possibly feeling that the client cannot tolerate it. Silences may arise from a blockage within the client; here the counsellor may be able to suggest something to the client, but he should be allowed time to think and to feel. Silences may also arise as a result of the interaction between the counsellor and the client. Perhaps he has been pushed too far, too quickly, thus causing him alarm. In this instance, silence is a retreat. If he is not listened to he may well retreat into silence. Something the counsellor says may set up emotional vibrations which he finds difficult to handle. There are comfortable silences and uncomfortable ones. In the former, a comment such as, 'That feels really comfortable. I wonder what was passing through your mind just then?' may well open doors that hitherto have been barred. With uncomfortable, negative, silences, it may be less easy to get things going again. It depends what created the silence. If the counsellor feels that he has done something to create the silence, and tests this out, that may be sufficient to move things on. Silences which are allowed to drag on may demoralise both counsellor and client. If the counsellor feels that the silence arises from within the client, a comment such as, 'This silence makes me feel . . . Are you finding it difficult to put something into words?' leaves the client free to choose how he will respond. He may not have felt the silence as uncomfortable but this could lead to a fruitful discussion on feelings. Every gap in conversation does not have to be filled with words. Some of the most constructive work is done during silences.

Stage 3 Explore the Problem

Stepping Stones not Stumbling Blocks

Exploration requires great sensitivity and skill. The aim is to help the client explore different aspects of whatever problem is confronting him. It is probably the most difficult stage. It is also the most delicate. It is so easy to cross the line between genuine exploration and blatant nosiness. In this stage it is possible, by trying too hard, to put stumbling blocks instead of stepping stones in the path of the client. In this stage, where unknown territory often has to be trodden, the counsellor has to be more aware of the client's need for empathic support during times when exploration may be difficult or traumatic. From the counsellor's point of view, it is here where he, himself, is most likely to feel in need of the support of a mentor, particularly where exploration is slow. This applies especially to on-going counselling, when discouragement may become very real to both counsellor and client.

During the previous stage of identifying the problem, the client may have reached a new understanding of what his problem really is. As together counsellor and client looked at some possible avenues, light may have begun to shine through some of the chinks which have been created. Counselling does not necessarily involve probing into the deep recesses of the dim and distant past. Past and present are bound together but counselling is more concerned with the present and the very recent past. Exploration of the emotions of the present frequently opens doors to the emotional contents of the past. The client, to come to terms with the past, may need to explore the past within the present counselling relationship.

Exploration — A Dual Activity

It should be emphasised that exploration is very much a dual activity, involving both client and counsellor. Sometimes the client may lead the way; at others it is the counsellor who will move in a certain direction, always realising that such leading is tentative. He must be ready to retreat the instant he becomes aware that he is no longer alongside the client. Leading in this way must be done very gently. It must be leading, not pushing.

Broadly speaking, the counsellor sets out to help the client explore significant areas in his life, as well as the significant people. It is also necessary to help him explore how these areas and people interact with each other. Alexander, married with children and parents still alive, worked in a factory. He also had a part-time job as a barman in a public house and he played string bass in a jazz group. He had a health problem in that he had been having tachycardia. One way of helping him to explore what seemed like a fairly formidable list would be:

Significant people	*Significant areas*
Wife	Work
Children	Part-time work
Parents	Group
Workmates (factory and pub)	Health
Group	

Exploration revealed that he had the part-time job and played in the band because his wife could not manage the household budget effectively. The children were noisy and unruly (he blamed his wife but she counter-argued that he is hardly ever at home). So he escaped by becoming involved in outside activities. He detests work and would prefer to be a full-time musician, but he feels trapped in domesticity. He regards tachycardia as a sure indication that he is going to die young.

The nurse working with him helped him to see possible links between these different factors which created a picture of someone whose present medical condition may have been influenced by his way of life. As they explored these various studies, she was conscious that Alexander was unwilling to enter into any exploration related to his parents. Several times she 'led' him towards this. The third time he said, 'You obviously want me to talk about my parents. I don't want to. Please leave it there.' Not all clients will be as forthright as he was, but at least the nurse knew that no useful purpose would be served by pursuing this. Counselling may not always produce neat answers.

When Alexander visited his GP he had been told, 'You are overdoing it. Something must go.' Alexander could not accept this sound practical advice, but as the nurse helped him explore the relationship between significant areas and people, insight came. 'I suppose I'm doing all these things to escape from a home where I don't feel a great deal of love. Yet, in reality, if I go on like this I'll end up possibly not able to work at all. Then I'll really feel I'm in prison.' As a result of talking it through, he decided to give up the jazz band, the activity he considered the most stressful.

Stage 3 Skills

Here and Now: Then and There. In stage 2, the counsellor may have used specificity to encourage the client to be explicit. In stage 3 he may want to use another skill — here and now — to look at the interaction between himself and the client. Some clients, like those who generalise and need help to be specific, may be helped to examine what is actually happening in counselling. Clients who have a tendency to talk about feelings *in the past*, rather than now, may be helped if the counsellor can point to something in the 'here and now' — something that is actually happening between them — to help to identify present feelings. As specificity contrasts with generality, so 'here and now' contrasts with 'then and there'. The principal difference is that in the one the client is encouraged to own his feelings and not to generalise; in the other, he is encouraged to own his feelings as they exist *at that moment*. At the same time, the counsellor may show the way by talking of his feelings in the interaction.

When Alexander was talking to his counsellor, she said, 'When you talk about your wife, you sound as if you're talking about a little child. Just now you used the same tone to me. I felt really very small.' This brief exchange helped Alexander to realise that in his relationships he often treated women in this way. In other words, the nurse used how she felt to help him see that other people could possibly feel the same way.

People who always talk of events and feelings in the past and never in the present, may be helped to do so by comments such as, 'I find it difficult, listening to you, to know how you really feel right now. Everything seems so remote.' This confronts the client to ask himself, 'how do I feel?' He may feel angry, surprised or hurt at this suggestion. But that reaction can be used effectively to demonstrate the difference between the here and now and then and there. It is worth stressing again that if the counsellor is able to use what is happening between them, a great deal will have been accomplished. Some people refer to this skill as 'immediacy'. Speaking of immediacy, Egan[1] says,

> Through this skill you engage in direct, mutual talk about what is happening between you and the client in the counselling relationship so clients can overcome blocks to more effective involvement and see

more clearly both the productive and unproductive ways they tend to relate to others.

Self-disclosure. Self-disclosure means that the counsellor decides to reveal something of himself to the client. Disclosures must be used with discretion. Inappropriate or mistimed disclosure may increase rather than decrease the client's anxiety. Accurately used, however, self-disclosure can be positive and helpful and may assist in reducing the aura of omnipotence that sometimes surrounds counsellors. One of the dangers of self-disclosure, is that it can remove the focus from the client, especially if the disclosure is lengthy. Another danger is that the counsellor can come over as in need of help as much as the client, particularly if what is disclosed is a 'problem' to the counsellor. Self-disclosure may thus be used for self-gratification; the counsellor wants to talk about his own life rather than listen to the client.

Egan[1] suggests three principles be applied to self-disclosure:

1. Selective and focused. 'Helper self-disclosure is appropriate if it keeps clients on target and does not distract them from investigating their own problem situations.'
2. Not a burden to the client. 'Helper self-disclosure is appropriate if it does not add another burden to an already overwhelmed client.'
3. Not too often. 'Helper self-disclosure is inappropriate if it is too frequent. This, too, distracts the client and shifts attention to the counsellor.'

Peter was talking to Roy about his father's recent death. Peter was having great difficulty expressing himself until Roy said, 'My father died four years after mother. When he died I felt I'd been orphaned. Is that something how you feel?'

Peter sat for several minutes in deep silence before saying, 'You've put into words exactly how I feel. May I talk about my childhood and how Dad and I got on together?'

This would seem to satisfy Egan's three principles.

Confrontation. Confrontation is not fisticuffs! There are times when it is wiser to ignore than to comment, but there are times when it could be valuable for the client to know how the counsellor feels about some part of the interaction. This is one aspect of confrontation that is similar to the 'here and now' interaction. Another is where the client may benefit from being confronted with the possible outcome of his behaviour or some contemplated course of action. In this sense, confrontation is helping him look at reality, or at least at reality through the eyes of the counsellor. If confrontation is not physical fisticuffs, neither is it verbal fisticuffs. Any confronting is best put in a tentative way, as a suggestion, rather than as a statement of fact and then only after careful deliberation. It should *never* be used as a retaliation. The aim of confrontation is certainly not to make the client feel small, nor to 'get at him'. If it is carried out with as much respect, interest and understanding as any other part of counselling, filtered through caring, it will usually be well received. It is better to focus on some aspect of behaviour than on some aspect of personality. Finally, confrontation is generally only used when the relationship is firmly established. If the client is not certain of the counsellor, he may perceive his comment (valid though it might be) as an unwarranted attack. The other side of this is that the counsellor must know the client well enough to make a judgement of how the confrontation will be received.

Penetration. Feelings may be identified at various levels. It is quite likely that in the early stages of counselling, the counsellor will be involved mainly with the client's superficial (not unimportant) feelings. But as counselling progresses, he may have to help the client get at feelings that lie beneath the surface. Normally, getting in touch with deeper feelings can only be achieved as the counsellor demonstrates an awareness of how the client is feeling — sad, anxious, fearful, angry, happy, excited, and so on.

The principal difference between exploration of surface feelings and penetration to deeper ones is that quite often feelings on the surface are expressed without too much hesitation; deeper ones often remain unstated though they may be implied. The client may be dimly aware that they are there but needs help to make them explicit.

The client who is experiencing difficulty in trying to decide what to do with her home, now that her husband is dead and her children have all married, may need help to accept the fact that her true problem is one of loneliness.

To another client one might say, 'You say that you didn't want to come into hospital because it made you feel helpless. You also said that you had been in hospital as a child. Is there any connection with the way you feel now and the way you felt then?'

Penetration is generally best approached with a phrase such as, 'I wonder if . . .', 'Do you think that . . .?' 'It seems possible that what you're really saying (or feeling) could be . . .' It is always useful to ask, 'How does that sound to you?' Feelings may be misinterpreted.

Extrapolation. This is where the counsellor encourages the client to look beyond the immediate. It may be a looking back or a looking forward. By the client putting himself in different situations in the future, he can be helped to judge how he may react and feel. Likewise, by relating the past to the present, he may be helped to see that what he did and what he was in the past influences what he is and does now. Very often it is a case of putting up counselling Aunt Sallys, just for the client to experience knocking them down.

However, at this point it is possible to move from true exploration to pure (though disguised) prying, which then becomes offensive to the client who, because of his circumstances, may be very much a captive audience. If the counsellor listens accurately to the client's feelings, he will pick up cues that he is treading on inappropriate ground. On the other hand, it could be appropriate ground, but the timing may be inappropriate.

Images. The final skill to be discussed in stage 3 is the use of images to help the client get in touch with the feelings of his inner world. What imaging does is to cut through the intellect and release feelings attached to inner pictures. Susan was talking about her first term on her Master's degree course. 'I haven't got enough time to study, to read, to absorb all the lectures. I feel in a panic.' The counsellor sat for a few minutes in silence then said, 'I have had a picture of an expensive and precious plate but it is all cracked; not broken, but in danger of fragmenting.'

This was exactly how Susan did feel. The next stage was to help her imagine how the plate could be made whole again. This is an example of how counsellors can use images that are created within them to help clients identify their feelings. But it is more than merely identifying feelings. A person's psyche, through the use of inner pictures, will often show the way toward healing, as it did with Susan. As she continued to look at the plate she saw a jar of honey being poured over it; the honey removed the cracks. Honey, to her, represented love. When she discussed this with the rest of her group they all admitted that they too were feeling as she felt. That group became a very caring one.

William was talking about a feeling of oppression in his head. The inner picture he got was of a dried up walnut. As he continued to watch it, it gradually became smaller, then disappeared completely, and with it went his oppression.

Sandra was expressing feelings of loneliness, yet she did not seem a lonely person. Her inner picture was of a clearing in the middle of a large dark wood. In the middle of the clearing was a little girl in a green dress, crying bitterly '. . . my mummy and daddy have gone and left me here'. As she watched, the trees turned into cot bars and she was standing in a hospital cot, shaking it and screaming, 'I want my mummy, I want my daddy.' This image had released a memory of her at about 3 years of age, admitted for a tonsil operation. The feelings of isolation, loneliness and rejection were very powerful and she was able to see a little of how such feelings may have contributed to her feelings of loneliness in adult life.

Like all the skills outlined in the first three stages, imaging must be used sensitively and intelligently and be appropriate to the occasion and the client. Images are generally attached to powerful feelings; and powerful feelings, when released, may cause the client to burst into tears. Words then seem totally superfluous. So often, healing comes when blocked channels are cleared. One last illustration must suffice. Sandra (mentioned above) had been talking for some time about her difficulties. Her counsellor who had not been sitting with closed eyes, but had been using the imaging technique said, 'I get the impression of a giant whirlpool and you are caught up in it.' Sandra was thoughtful, then said, 'That's exactly how I do feel, though I've never identified it just like that. Yes, I am afraid of being sucked down by my job (as a nurse) and losing my identity. And in order to prevent this happening, I have to keep frantically busy.' This led to a fruitful discussion of her fears about being engulfed by her work.

Interregnum

So far in this chapter we have considered three stages of the model: meeting the client; identifying the problem and exploring the problem. These three stages deal with the process of counselling. But, as was pointed out earlier, achievement of insight is not enough. The next three stages consider ways in which clients may be helped to put into action some of what has been talked about in the previous stages. Part of the skill of counselling is helping the client to marshal his inner resources to live life more as he wants it. Some problems can be resolved with counselling help, others cannot. Part of the task of counselling is helping some people cope with situations that cannot be cured. When the client is ready he will be encouraged to move toward forming an action plan and then to implement it.

Perhaps I have given the impression that counselling follows neatly from stage to stage. This is not so. This is the principal difference between, for instance, a mathematical model and a counselling model. Mostly there is a great deal of movement between one stage and the next, particularly in stages 2 and 3. When the time comes to consider an action plan it may prove necessary to return to stage 3, as some different aspects of the problem are raised. Rather than consider the model as a linear one, it may be more helpful to consider it as circular, with the option of returning to previous stages as and when necessary.

This six stage model may be used with equal effect for on-going counselling — over a number of sessions — or for single sessions. In 'one-off' counselling, the stages are contracted, and in-depth exploration of the cilent's inner world may be neither possible nor appropriate. Nevertheless, a great deal can be accomplished in one session, even if only one central problem is clearly identified and worked on. If the client leaves with some sort of action plan worked out, and if he feels more at peace with himself, then that is as much as anyone could expect.

Counselling is like travelling from London to Brighton. It can be done by express train, car, bicycle or foot. For each of these modes of travel, the pace will be different. Some counselling interviews can proceed at a rapid pace; others are much slower. It is the client who sets the pace. Any attempt to force him to change from a walking pace to a run, in all probability, will result in 'client fatigue'. One client may be quite able to dash along; the nature of his problem and his emotional state may permit him to do this quite happily. Another person may want to talk, so as to view the countryside as it passes. If, somewhere along the road, he decides to hasten his pace, so be it. The skilful counsellor will be able to adapt to this change and still remain alongside the client.

Stage 4 Plan the Action

When, and only when the client feels sufficiently free from the forces that have been restraining him, will he be able to contemplate action. The aim is to help the client discover, then harness, his inner resources which have been locked in. Increased self-awareness and insight are often the keys that will release these resources. The action plan is divided into two stages: thinking it through and carrying it out. Inadequate thinking through may spell disaster. The client may feel so much better and more able to cope, that his enthusiasm and new-found confidence could run away with him, unless the counsellor keeps the emotional brake on. That is why a full exploration of the plan is essential. It slows down the pace, but it should not be allowed to drag on too long.

Identify Alternatives

In the first stage of the action plan, the counsellor helps the client look at ways of coping with his particular difficulty, by talking these plans through with him in an open way. Because the counsellor does not pass judgement, or try to force unacceptable solutions on him, the client will be more inclined to look with confidence at various alternatives. At first glance this may look the same as extrapolation, but the main difference is that here the focus of the exercise is the action plan. It is true that in the action-plan stage, extrapolation may need to be used if the alternatives are to be fully explored. This emphasises how skills are blended into each other, just as are the various stages.

Identify Goals

Identifying goals which may be achieved soon, if not immediately, and longer-term ones is a positive approach for the client, who even at this stage may not see how his problem is to be tackled. This is often a useful pencil and paper exercise. Short term goals are generally enabling ones that help towards achieving longer term ones. To leave a goal as 'I want to get well again' would be too daunting, too vast and difficult to grasp hold of; in much the same way as it is very difficult to grasp the concept of 'working to save the world from starvation'; it would be far more logical to start with feeding one person.

Egan[1] lists the following characteristics of goal-setting:

1. *Accomplishments.* 'I will learn to walk again.' is a workable goal for a person who has had an amputation.
2. *Clear and specific.* 'I will save one hundred pounds.'
3. *Measurable or verifiable.* 'Clients must be able to tell whether they have achieved their goals or not.' How is attainment to be measured?
4. *Realistic.* 'I will be working again within a month' may not be a realistic goal for an amputee.
5. *Adequate.* Goals that are set too high are unrealistic. Goals that are set too low are not adequate. Setting goals that are adequate depends on a clear identification of the problem.
6 *Owned by the client.* It is essential to ensure that the goals really are the client's and not the counsellor's.

7. *Client's values.* Counselling will remain ethical only in so far as it respects the client's values. Sheila was in conflict over an unwanted pregnancy. She was unmarried and could not count on the support of her parents. At the same time, she could not bring herself to have an abortion. It would have thus been against her values for the counsellor to have pressed for a termination; though it wasn't inappropriate for her to explore this as a possible goal.
8. *Reasonable time frame.* The client who sets the goal of 'I will learn to walk again' needs to go on to consider, 'when?' He may need help to arrive at a realistic time scale for this goal to be reached.

Egan concludes this section of his book with these words, 'A goal, to be workable, must meet all these requirements. If one is missing, it may prove to be the fatal flaw in a client's movement toward action.'

On page 31 the reader was introduced to a problem-solving model. Now might be a useful time to refer back to it, to see how this section on goals and goal-setting relates to that model.

Identify New Skills

Counsellor and client, together, may need to discover new skills if the client is to achieve his goal. A skill that has been implicit so far in this book is, 'how to get on with people'. Many people come for counselling because they are experiencing some difficulty with relationships. Contact with the counsellor affords a unique opportunity for the client to examine the way he relates to people and, if necessary, discover ways to make it easier to get on with them. Some clients come because they want to develop the skill of counselling. Some, because they want to learn more about their inner worlds. Others become clients because some circumstance of fortune or misfortune has temporarily thrown them off balance. Counselling, for them, may be to develop skills of coping with stress. There are many and varied life crises which prompt people to seek counselling. In short, people may need to develop skills to deal with difficult situations — careers, redundancy, retirement, illness — or with awkward people. This is a very broad generalisation, but it may suffice.

Joan lost the chance of many good jobs because she was too timid on the phone, especially with brusque men. She was helped to become more assertive.

Andrew, who had been made redundant, was helped to compose an impressive, but accurate, *curriculum vitae*.

Hand in hand with developing new skills must go the strengthening of existing ones. Existing skills may be operating fairly well or they may be lying dormant. During the exploratory stage the counsellor should be making — mental if not written — notes of skills and strengths that could be harnessed to deal with the problem and to reach the goal.

Referral

There may be times when the counsellor recognises that he does not possess the skills to deal with a particular client. Recognising one's limitations is a very necessary part of one's professional experience. Inability or refusal to do so could prove harmful to the client and possibly traumatic to the counsellor who may find himself swamped and out of his depth. Knowing to whom a client could be referred means that the counsellor should be in touch with someone, or some agency, who can advise. Therapists in hospital, as well as those working in the community, are in contact with social workers, who normally would be in a position to advise on which agency or person would be appropriate.

Passing a client on may pose problems for the counsellor, as well as for the client. The client will have to re-establish a relationship with another counsellor; the counsellor may feel lacking in some way that he had not been able to help this particular client. These feelings are very real and should not be dismissed as trivial, and in a way they are similar to those experienced by counsellors whose clients suddenly stop coming, with no explanation. While it is difficult to measure success in counselling, counsellors would be less than human if they did not feel something when clients terminate abruptly before the agreed time.

One possible reason for a premature termination is that counselling may have been non-productive; the client may feel he is getting nothing out of it. Another reason is that the relationship for that particular client has not been satisfying enough. It could be that the benefits do not outweigh the cost, whatever that means to the client. It could mean that the counsellor has become dissatisfied or discouraged with the progress being made and is giving out messages that he would like to terminate the relationship. It could also mean that the counsellor is out of his depth and doesn't realise it. Transference and countertransference feelings may be yet another reason, if the counsellor is unable to handle them constructively.

Renegotiate the Contract

Having devised the action plan, pointing the way ahead, the client and the counsellor may feel that the client can now implement the plan without assistance. Some clients may want to try to manage on their own and this may be what they need. For others, the real test would be putting the plan into action, and for them, continuing help may be necessary.

In the original contract it may have been agreed that there would be a fixed number of sessions or that when a certain stage was reached, the relationship would end. Having reached the stage of formulating the action plan, the client may then wish to continue; then the contract needs to be renegotiated. For those clients for whom an action plan is not appropriate — those who are using the relationship to explore their inner worlds — renegotiating the contract will normally take place at the end of the agreed time limit. When the new contract has been agreed, it is time to move on; to implement the action plan.

Stage 5 Implement the Action Plan

At the close of the previous stage it was suggested that some clients may decide to implement the plan without assistance. If this is so, the door to future counselling should be left ajar. For in time of difficulty, the client may want a few minutes of the counsellor's listening ear to help him over a rough patch — a counselling booster. Some clients may still need help to bring the plan to fruition.

Information

Before some clients can really think about putting the plan into action they may need a great deal of information. It is not suggested that the counsellor becomes the resource agent for this information. What would be of positive help, however, where the client needs specific help, is for them together to locate an information source. The client is then in a position to find out the information for himself. By so doing, his self-responsibility is being encouraged. Alan was starting up a business, following recovery from a long period away from work with angina. Rachael, his counsellor, did not know all the legal and business avenues, but she was there to help Alan think about them in a logical way. To help a client who is nervous, different situations can be 'role played'; by so doing, he may be encouraged to approach people he would not normally approach. Thinking round a topic is certainly one of the aspects of the action plan.

Achieving the Goals

It is vital that the first goal should be attainable. That is why in the goal-planning stages the goals are arranged so that those that look as if they are not too difficult to attain are given priority. Longer term goals, those that require more sustained effort are best left until later. If achieving goals also concerns relationships, it is very likely that the client will need continuing support from the counsellor. Goals that are not readily reached bring frustration in their wake. Non-co-operation of other people can, as it was in Alan's case, resurrect resentment and bitterness; these may then need to be worked on before real progress can be made. Alan became very tense, due no doubt to his anxiety about establishing a business. In order to relieve this tension he was encouraged to take relaxation lessons from a remedial therapist. This was another skill he acquired. But the necessity for it only became apparent when the plan was being implemented. Some goals are less easily achieved. In Alan's case he was never able to give up smoking, which had been one of his goals.

Agencies and Sources

As with information, the counsellor may be able to point the client in the direction of certain agencies where specialist help could be obtained. Alan made contact with the British Heart Foundation, and although there was no group which met locally, they sent him some useful literature. This was particularly helpful, for in it he could read how other people lived and coped with the same condition. Other clients may need to be put in touch with other agencies, specific to their circumstances. One agency that usually is able to offer assistance is the Citizens' Advice Bureau. Some areas have established special units that are able to provide information about organisations that are available to assist specific clients. Another source of information is the local Social Services Department. The Department of Health and Social Security and the Community Health Council will both provide advice and information on a wide range of topics, and they would be able to point the client in an appropriate direction to receive help. Details of these agencies are to be found in Appendices A to E.

Rachael used the problem-solving model (on page 31) to work with Raymond, Alan's son, who was expressing doubt over remaining at school; he wanted to leave and start work 'to help the family income'. This helped him to see that things were not as desperate as he had imagined. Some time later he decided that he would leave school but only when he had taken and passed at least five 'O' levels.

Decision-making

Another useful model is force-field analysis.* This is a decision-making technique designed to help an individual understand the various internal and external forces which influence the way he makes decisions. For most of the time these forces are in relative balance; but when something disturbs the balance, decisions are more difficult to make. Having identified the forces, the next stage is to devise strategies to help the client reach his goal. For a more detailed description of the model, refer to Appendix F.

Support

The client may need a great deal of support while he is implementing the action plan. Support means understanding, kindness, caring, being there when needed. In a counselling sense, support means making oneself available to listen and possibly to help the client with a particular stage of the action plan. Support for a couple with marriage difficulties meant that William was there to listen to each of them as they poured out their feelings when it became evident that the marriage was no longer workable. Support also meant, 'Help us, William, to tell the children'. Support was helping the children talk about their feelings of being torn in their love for both parents.

But support is not a permanent leaning post. If it were, the client might well be discouraged from establishing his own strengths. If it is a post on which the client leans, just as a young sapling may need a support until it becomes fully established, it must be gradually, and gently but firmly withdrawn as soon as he is sufficiently psychologically mature to stand on his own. Irreparable harm may be done to the client who has become over-dependent on counselling support. If this happens, the motives and needs of the counsellor must be seriously questioned.

Stage 6 Evaluation

Evaluation often brings about a reappraisal of the problem and of the areas for exploration. Evaluation, if undertaken with care and thought, can be an excellent learning device. If the client is an active partner in

---

* The force-field analysis model presented here is adapted from the ideas contained in 'A Handbook of Structured Experiences for Human Relations Training', Vol. 11, University Associates Publishers and Consultants. 7596 Eads Avenue, La Jolla, CA 92037, USA.

the evaluation exercise, both he and the counsellor will be able to learn from each other. It may not always be easy to state precisely what has been achieved. In contrast with some clinical conditions, feelings cannot be excised when they cause problems, but very often being given permission and opportunity to talk about them will start the cleansing and healing process. But it may be some considerable time before the full benefits are realised.

On-going evaluation gives both counsellor and client an opportunity to explore their feelings about what is happening and also to appraise, constructively, what should be done next. A terminal evaluation gives the client a feeling of completeness and also provides him and the counsellor with an opportunity to look at some of those things which did not go according to plan, as well as those which did. An evaluation well carried out, not only looks backward, it also looks forward. It provides the client with something positive to carry with him into the future and the counsellor with the satisfaction of a job completed.

Final Evaluation

One of the first tasks is to carry out a review of what brought the client and counsellor together. It is possible, particularly when counselling has taken place over a period of time, that the original reason has faded into insignificance, as more recent and more momentous themes have been explored. In a way, it is like taking a journey: the traveller knows from where he has come, and knows roughly the route taken; but looking back, the starting point has become obscured, partly through distance, but also through time. Unlike taking a journey, however, it is often necessary for both client and counsellor to look back in order to firmly establish the final position.

Start at the Beginning

A useful place to start is the original contract. Clients may have difficulty remembering exactly how they felt and reacted when they first presented their problems. Just as events fade from the memory, so do some feelings, particularly when progress has been made toward resolving the problem. It is almost as if the prevailing mood (at the time of evaluation) has always existed. It may seem that asking the client to look back could cause a set-back; retracing one's steps may reveal obstacles that were previously hidden. That is true; and in a sense this criticism of evaluation is justified. But at the same time, it would not be the aim of evaluation to dwell overlong on any one issue. In a final evaluation, more emphasis should be placed on the way ahead than on what has taken place.

It is useful to look at the problems which have been identified, specific aspects of them and how the problems were tackled. This also means having to look at the goals that were identified and the strategies adopted to achieve them.

Positive Growth

One of the things the counsellor can do, throughout counselling, is to encourage the client by pointing to areas of positive growth and to incidents that highlight the gaining of insight. Gains which seem small to the counsellor may be as mountains to the client. When Rachael reached the stage of evaluation with Alan, he commented that in the early days of contact with her he had suffered from

> some pretty foul moods of black despair. One of the things that really helped, was that you never once offered platitudes. So many people use to say, "Oh, you'll be all right; everything will work out." You never said that. It was the way you asked questions, as if you expected me to find my own answers, that gave me hope. Many times I felt as if I was drowning; then I would remember the tasks we had set; that spurred me on.

As Alan was talking, Rachael realised that here was another area of growth. He had never been one for 'this psychological stuff', but now he was talking at a feeling level.

The Counselling Relationship

The counselling relationship is the most potent force in helping the client. It must not be overlooked in the evaluation process. Let Alan speak.

> We'll be sorry not to see you again, Rachael. Pop in when you're passing, any time, we'll be glad to see you. One of the things I've learned from you is to trust people. I was bitter — about life in general — when you came. Now I can honestly say that it has gone. I think that bitterness was making me believe that everyone was against me. You respected me and this helped me to respect myself and my capabilities. We don't know much about you, really, but we think you're lovely.

But the gains are not always — indeed, seldom — one-sided. Counsellors gain something too. Rachael did. She learned more about herself. She had to learn patience, particularly when dealing with 'obstructive people' who were not helpful to Alan. When Alan was passing through one of his dark moods he said, 'I don't feel as if there is much to live for'. This made Rachael quite angry. 'It made me feel that I was wasting my time.' Through this she realised that she wanted to control Alan. 'I had to learn what it was to go where you wanted to go and at your pace.'

Success?

Success is not easily measured. A person who comes for one session and leaves saying, 'I feel better for having talked it over, even though there is nothing you can actually do', may then be more able to cope with her life.

But who measures success? The client or the counsellor? If the client is helped to live his life more resourcefully; if he has developed strategies to cope with some insoluble problem, is this not success? If the client has been able to reduce the frequency of the quarrels with his wife, through insight into his personality, is this not success? If the counsellor has gained more awareness of how he reacts to a particularly trying client and is then able to use this experience to help others, is this not success? Clients who have succeeded in climbing a few hills are more likely to want to tackle mountains, and are more able to.

Failure?

If success is difficult to measure, so is failure. When children 'go off the rails' parents often blame themselves. 'We could have done more.' 'Where did we go wrong?' are questions that are often asked. But they are to no avail. When counselling does not succeed, counsellors may be tempted to ask similar questions. 'Was there something I could have done?' 'Some stop I could have pulled out?' 'Some technique I could have used to ensure success?' Success and progress or failure — whose responsibility is it? Whose credit or whose blame? The counsellor has no prescription to follow and ultimately it is the client who must shoulder the responsibility for his own decisions and actions. While Andrew was receiving counsel from Roy, he stole a car and crashed it. He was killed. Andrew had a choice. Nothing 'made' him steal that car; it was his choice. It is certainly true that he may have cried loud and long for help and perhaps Roy did not hear him. Andrew's death made Roy re-evaluate: that was positive and constructive. But for him to have taken on his shoulders the responsibility for Andrew's actions would have been taking an unfair burden and most certainly would seriously have affected his counselling.

Shared Responsibility

The counsellor can never remain absolutely neutral or unaffected by the outcome of counselling. It would be all too easy when counselling ends without seeing positive results to pass all the responsibility on to the client. If the counsellor feels, 'If only he had been more open, more communicative, less defensive', and so on, this should lead to a full evaluation of his own contribution. Similarly it may be easy, when counselling ends positively, for the counsellor to accept all the credit, forgetting that whatever his contribution has been, it was the client who was in focus throughout; and whatever was happening within him, much more was likely to be happening within the client. If the counsellor experienced growth from conflict within the counselling relationship, much more did the client experience conflict and subsequent growth. To him then must go the credit for whatever success has been achieved. Likewise, lack of success must remain with the client. The counsellor shares both.

Recording

On pp. 21 and 48 reference was made to 'note taking'. For one's own professional development, some time should be devoted to making a summary of what has taken place throughout counselling. The model on which this chapter is based may be a useful structure for such a summary. It is possible that what is included in the summary may never be read by anyone else. But the fact that he has taken time and effort to commit it to paper may, at some time, be a useful resource for him, when pondering on a particular point in counselling. Experience can never be wiped out, but when experience is reinforced by evaluation, many of the interactions, the words, the nuances that so quickly fade from the memory, are captured in a way that experience by itself cannot do. If the counsellor feels that the final evaluation is proving too difficult, that may be because evaluating his own part in the process is eluding him. It is possible, for example, that some aspect of the relationship between himself and the client is proving a stumbling block. If the stumbling block is not removed it will remain an obstacle in the way of effective counselling. Stumbling blocks can be turned into stepping stones by an honest and in-depth evaluation, assisted by honest recording.

Summary

The practice of counselling, within the Wessex Model, is in six stages:

1. Meet the client
2. Identify the problem

3. Explore the problem
4. Plan the action
5. Implement the action plan
6. Evaluation.

The approach is basically a problem-solving one, but the importance of insight and self-awareness — for both client and counsellor — have not been neglected. None of the six stages is more important than any of the others and it has been suggested that the model be thought of as a circular one with linking loops, rather than a linear one.

The skills used in stage one form the foundation of good counselling practice and operate throughout the other stages. As the client's emotional understanding and awareness deepen, other skills are added to the primary ones of stage one. The skills of later stages help the client explore his deeper feelings and the way he reacts to the problem that confronts him. The first three stages deal with the process of counselling; stages four to six deal with the action.

The action plan is arrived at only after full discussion between client and counsellor. For the plan to succeed it must receive the full commitment of the client. Formulating the action plan requires as much skill as any of the previous three stages. Clients who are still enmeshed in the problem are unlikely to be able to think logically about action and less likely to be able to put it effectively into practice. Action plans arrived at after inadequate exploration are prone to failure. An important part of the action plan is formulating goals. These are best arranged in order of those that are easily attainable, or at least possibly attainable reasonably quickly. Short term goals which are attained enable the client to work toward and attain longer term goals. Part of attaining goals may be the use the client makes of resources and agencies outside of the counselling relationship. One of the resources may be that the client has to be referred to another counsellor for more specialised help in order to achieve his goals.

Both counsellor and client are involved in evaluating counselling as it takes place and when it is drawing to a close. If evaluation is neglected, the client is left with a feeling of incompleteness and the counsellor is impoverished in his experience. Evaluation, though time consuming and sometimes traumatic, when thoroughly and honestly carried out, is a most useful exercise for increasing counsellor self-awareness, the most essential component in the counselling relationship.

Notes

1. Egan, G. (1982) *The Skilled Helper*, Brooks/Cole Publishing Co., Monterey, California.

2. Brammer, L. (1979) *The Helping Relationship*, Prentice-Hall Inc., Englewood Cliffs, NJ.

3. Long, L., Paradise, L.V. and Long, T.J. (1981) *Questioning Skills for the Helping Process*, Brooks/Cole Publishing Co., Monterey, California.

Appendix A

The Citizens' Advice Bureau Service

This account has been prepared by the author from the booklet 'The Citizens' Advice Bureau Service'.

The aims of the Citizens' Advice Bureau are:

1. To ensure that individuals do not suffer through ignorance of their rights and responsibilities or of the service available; or through an inability to express their needs effectively.
2. To exercise a responsible influence on the development of social policies and services, both locally and nationally.

The service, therefore, provides — free to all individuals — an impartial service of information, guidance and support, and makes responsible use of the experience so gained.

The bureau service sees itself as the well-informed general practitioner of the social services, combining the roles of prevention, diagnosis and referral to the specialist consultants. It provides a friendly, non-statutory service of advice and help. Any member of the public may walk into any Citizens' Advice Bureau and ask for help, information or advice. Help will be given to fill in a form, or explain a new piece of legislation and how it is likely to affect the inquirer's own circumstances. Staff will make telephone calls and draft letters. The bureau will stand between the inquirer and the organisation, government department, authority or individual with whom he is at odds. The points of view of each is put to the other and this, in the majority of cases, results in a solution acceptable to both sides. A growing number of bureaux are becoming involved in tribunal assistance and in representation at County Courts. Specialist advice sessions, when solicitors or accountants, for example, deal with inquirers' problems, are organised.

The Citizens' Advice Bureau Service is made up of about 900 full- and part-time bureaux throughout the United Kingdom. Each bureau is a local self-governing unit, organised in the community for the citizens of that community. The day-to-day administration of a bureau is the responsibility of the bureau organiser. The staff may be paid or voluntary, full or part time. Training — initial and on-going — is provided for all staff. Local authorities provide almost all the financial support in the form of grant aid. This does not influence the independent stance of the bureau serving the local community.

Appendix B

Hospital Information Unit

This account was prepared by Robert Gann, Librarian, 'Help for Health', Wessex Regional Library Unit, Southampton General Hospital.

Help for Health began in 1979 as a British Library project which investigated the need for information about the voluntary sector in health care. From this research it seemed that health-care staff were constantly seeking the addresses of self-help groups, details of the help provided by voluntary organisations or the educational literature produced by patient organisations, but had no readily available and accurate source of this information. The Help for Health Information Service was set up to answer these needs and is now funded by the Wessex Regional Health Authority. It is a unique service and forms the largest collection of self-help information in the United Kingdom.

Patients and disabled people in the community need information to enable them to understand their condition, to cope with it at home, and to make full use of the voluntary and statutory resources available to them. They may wish to use voluntary organisations for practical help with accommodation, transport, recreation, holidays, employment. With problems such as mastectomy, colostomy, spinal injury, bereavement, counselling by people who have gone through the same experience could be of great support to the patient. Help for Health is an information service which can alert partients, and health-care staff acting on their behalf, to voluntary organisations, self-help groups and publications to help them to understand and cope with health problems.

Help for Health is:

A *resource centre* with the addresses of over 2000 national and local patient organisations, many offering specialist counselling, and a major collection of patient-information materials, largely in book and leaflet form.

An *inquiry service* answering 300 inquiries a month from health-care staff, social workers, voluntary bodies, patients and members of the public. Inquiries are received by telephone, letter or in person. The service is staffed by a qualified librarian and a clerical officer.

A *publisher* producing information sheets, a newsletter and a series of guides to information on a variety of health problems.

Nurses, and in particular health visitors, regularly form the largest group of users of the Help for Health Information Service.

Appendix C

Social Services Within the Hospital

This account was prepared by Ian Allured, Assistant Principal Officer (Health), Hampshire Social Services Department.

The National Health Service Act of 1974 states that social work help should be available and accessible to patients and their families who themselves ask for help, or who are referred at any stage of their treatment.

To facilitate this service, hospital-based social workers are employed by the local authority social services department, thus providing the hospital patient and his family with direct access to the resources of the social services department. In addition, the patient will have a continuity of social worker as the support will continue from the health-based worker when the patient is discharged home where this is seen as necessary.

Social workers are based within the hospital so as to be active members of the multidisciplinary team, and to provide an overall assessment of the patient's total situation and to help plan for any needs the patient or his family may have, and to help ensure that the appropriate community resources are mobilised to ensure as successful a discharge home as possible.

The social services department thus offers the following broad range of resources:

1. A social-work service for personal and family counselling — especially where the patient and/or his family are having to adjust to considerable changes in their normal functioning and personal circumstances, or where the illness is exacerbating existing problems.
2. A wide range of domiciliary and residential services.
3. Knowledge of statutory and voluntary resources within the community.
4. Experience and resources relating to the following main client groups: children; the elderly; the physically handicapped; the mentally ill; the mentally handicapped.

Most hospital social-work departments have a completely open referral system whereby referrals are welcome from any source, but as a matter of courtesy it helps if the patient is made aware of the referral and is in agreement with it.

The actual day-to-day running of social-work offices within hospitals may vary from authority to authority but the above general picture should act as a guide to the range of services available. If in doubt the hospital social work office or the local social services area office will be able to provide more specific information.

Appendix D

Social Security Matters

This account was prepared by Mrs G.M. Kempster, Regional Information Officer, DHSS, London West Region, Basingstoke.

The nurse, from time to time, may encounter clients who are experiencing some difficulty over their state benefits. The notes pages of each allowance book answer many questions. More detailed advice can be obtained from the local Department of Health and Social Security (DHSS) office. The address of the issuing office should always be on the allowance book. Advice can always be obtained from the local DHSS office as well. If the nurse does not know their whereabouts, look them up in the local telephone directory under 'Health and Social Security, Department of'. They are open to the public 09.30 to 15.30 hours, Monday to Friday, but are available to answer telephone inquiries between 08.30 and 17.00 hours. It is not usually necessary to call in person at the office unless urgent advice or action is required.

The social security benefit system is complex — providing a range of benefits, some of which are dependent on National Insurance contributions; some are means-tested and some simply payable in particular situations, such as severe disability. Many people are not aware of their rights and may be missing out on help available. It would be impossible for the nurse to have full knowledge, but she may find it useful to carry with her (or have access to) two booklets, both of which are obtainable, free, from any DHSS office. These are 'Which Benefit?' and 'Help for Handicapped People'. They provide a brief guide to the benefits available in different situations such as disability, unemployment, etc., and will point out where to go for further guidance.

Appendix E

Community Health Councils and How to Use Them

This account is summarised by the author from a statement by: Mr Ken M. Woods, Secretary, Southampton and S.W. Hampshire Community Health Council.

Community health councils were established by Parliament in 1974 to give the public a voice in the affairs of the National Health Service (NHS). A community health council may be thought of as the local public watchdog on NHS matters. Its services are funded by central government and are free to the users. A community health council — composed of 24 lay people — has three main roles:

1. To play a significant part when dramatic changes in services are undertaken. An example would be closure of a hospital.
2. To inform the public about the plans, ambitions and problems of the district health authority. On occasion it provides details on aspects of regional proposals and decisions.
3. To offer information, guidance and advice to people who experience difficulty in dealing with some issue related to the NHS.

In addition to offering advice on available services, where and how to use them, what standards are reasonable, or unreasonable to expect from the NHS, community health councils advise on the correct procedure when a member of the public wishes to complain about some aspect of the NHS.

A person may make use of the information, guidance and advice offered by the community health council by contacting (by telephone, by letter or in person) the appropriate community health council office. The address may be found in the local telephone directory under the heading 'Community Health Council'.

The general aim is to ensure that every inquiry receives an answer from the most appropriate source, even though the inquiry or complaint concerns a department or organisation other than the NHS.

Access to community health councils, which exist to ensure that members of the public receive the best possible service from the NHS, is informal and confidential.

Appendix F

Force-field Analysis

The client asks himself these questions:

1. What is the goal I want to reach?
2. What precisely is it that I want to achieve?
3. Is the goal realistic?
4. If it is not realistic, why not?
5. Can I identify some definite behaviour which needs to be changed?
6. If the behaviour involves someone else, what strategy can I devise to achieve this?
7. What effect will my goal-change have and on whom or on what?
8. How can I measure the change when it takes place?
9. When I have achieved my goal I shall be . . .
10. When I have achieved my goal I shall do . . .
11. The degree of risk in making a change is . . .
12. The advantages of making a change are . . .
13. The disadvantage of making a change are . . .

Helping forces

14. Can I identify internal and external forces that would help me achieve my goal.

EXAMPLES OF INTERNAL FORCES: Type of personality — optimistic, cheerful, outgoing, studious, caring, intelligent, thoughtful, intuitive, imaginative.

Age.

Health.

EXAMPLES OF EXTERNAL FORCES: Family, friends, locality, job, finance, housing, career, mobility, commitments, hobbies.

15. Can I identify internal and external forces that would work against me achieving my goal?

Any of the internal and external forces listed above may, in certain circumstances, act as restraining forces.

16. Which would be the easiest helping force to strengthen and work on to assist me to reach my goal?
17. Which would be the easiest restraining force to start diminishing its influence?
18. What strategy or strategies can I invent to achieve the aims in 16 and 17?

Repeat 16 and 17 as often as necessary with different forces.

The underlying principle is that by strengthening the helping forces and diminishing the restraining forces, a decision will be easier to make, because energy, which has been trapped by the restraining forces, has been released.

19. Have I achieved my goal?
20. Has my original goal changed in any way? How? Why?

4 COUNSELLING IN REHABILITATION: SAMENESS AND DIFFERENCE

Introduction

This chapter will follow the same layout as the preceding one. There we looked at the basic concepts and principles of what could be called 'pure' counselling. Now it is time to discuss how counselling may be applied in rehabilitation. We shall also examine how similar and how different is counselling in rehabilitation compared with counselling in other areas of application. It could be argued that counselling is the same wherever it is used, and to a degree this is true. That is why the principles were introduced where they were, to form a base from which to consider their application in this specialised field. But there is a sense in which the particular area of work calls for — indeed demands — a modification of certain of the principles previously discussed.

An analogy may be drawn from medicine. A person who trains as a doctor learns skills and acquires a body of knowledge that is basic to his profession. When he starts to practise, he will discover that he has to modify his approach according to the particular community in which he practises. An African community, by virtue of its resources and provisions for health-care, will require him to use his skills in a different way from a more sophisticated and affluent Western community. His skills as a doctor are used in both settings but how they are used is influenced by the specific setting. Counsellors are influenced by the specialised settings in which they work. If this applies to people employed as counsellors, how much more does it apply to people who are not so employed but who use counselling as part of their repertoire of skills? Therapists in rehabilitation are one such group of people. Not for them the luxury of regular 'counselling' sessions arranged to a planned appointment system and a timetable that can be arranged so as to allow adequate time for analysis and recording. For them, counselling is likely to be fitted in between physical treatment, or possibly in the patient's home, constrained by the knowledge that too much time spent with one patient deprives others. Yet therapists have a unique opportunity to assist their clients. To them is entrusted the physical treatment of some condition upon which, so often, is focused deep emotional hurt. Counselling, used in conjunction with whatever other skills the therapist is using, prepares the way for emotional healing to take place. Emotional healing must, inevitably, influence physical healing.

Stage 1 Meet the Client

Who is the Client?

In counselling, counsellor and client come together usually because it is the client who seeks help to deal with a problem. The patient who is involved in a programme of rehabilitation also needs help but — and there the similarity ends — he will not have been referred specifically for counselling help. Yet, counselling may be crucial for full recovery. All therapists will be sensitive to the importance of their first contact with patients. Somehow, within a very short space of time, they must convey that the patients can trust them to design and carry out a plan of treatment that will eventually lead to the maximum recovery. There can be little doubt that therapists rely heavily on the quality of the relationships they establish with their patients. These relationships are influenced by the amount of contact they have with each other. The intimacy of this contact is another factor which influences relationships and is a major difference between counselling and rehabilitation. The amount and degree of physical contact between counsellor and client will vary according to the particular technique being used; some counsellors use physical contact as a way of helping clients get in touch with feelings. But whatever technique is used, counsellors have no remit for physical treatment in the way that therapists have in rehabilitation.

The Contract

Therapists may not think of making contracts with their patients, yet there *is* an unspoken agreement. The patient will be expected to attend the physiotherapy department, for example, every day for a stated period during which time he will carry out exercises prescribed by the therapist. For her part, the physiotherapist will prescribe and supervise the patient's treatment and will assist him, as and when appropriate, toward the goal of independence. So the idea of contract does exist, though it may not be made as explicit as it generally is in counselling. But how does counselling fit into therapy? Does the patient assume that in addition to the physical treatment he will also be encouraged to talk about the emotional problems linked to his physical condition?

> And I think that some of us, at any rate, need someone who is known to be ready to act as a counsellor or a sort of social consultant — not a social worker, that's too professional, and not a parent — that's quite a different relationship. But it must be someone who doesn't diminish your dignity.[1]

Many people feel that their dignity has been diminished by their disabilities. Their dignity may be further chipped away by the way people relate to them. Professionals may also be guilty. They may create the impression that they alone can solve the patient's problems. Where the patient is regarded as an active partner in the rehabilitation process, his dignity will be enhanced, not diminished. Who better than the therapist — of whatever discipline — to act as the counsellor? What better time to spend a few minutes in active listening, with a few choice questions, than when the patient is expressing his frustration at the slowness of his recovery? Would a more ideal opportunity present itself to talk with an anxious relative, who has accompanied the patient, while the patient is safely in the hands of another therapist in the hydrotherapy pool? or to listen to the elderly husband of a patient who is having speech therapy following a stroke? The opportunities are there: very often we need to grasp them. 'But,' some may say, 'I don't have that sort of time.' Time is a very real problem which besets all who would try to make counselling a reality and not an unrealistic ideal. But a great deal can be done in a very short time; and if counselling is combined with treatment, time is not wasted. One difficulty is that of being overheard; but again, it is surprising how intimate a conversation two people may have without being overheard. In the early stages of therapy if the therapist says something like, 'If you feel at any time you want to have a good moan, get something off your chest, I'll try to be a good listener and help you talk' this will let the patient see that listening is also a part of therapy; counselling then becomes a part of the contract.

Stage 1 Skills

In Chapter 2, empathy and rapport were considered at length and in Chapter 3 their use was implied in several stages of the model. It hardly need be repeated just how fundamental these are in the counselling relationship and in rehabilitation. This chapter will concentrate on the *uniqueness of the client* in rehabilitation; the uniqueness of being a patient. Just as no two people are alike, no two people will react the same way to crippling disease or injury. Most of us could recall many instances of people who have succumbed to what other people would regard as trivial events, while others have triumphed over major tragedies. Very often those who rise above tragedy seem the most unlikely so to do. It is difficult to say why this should be: that is what makes for uniqueness. This is not the place nor have we the time to enter into a lengthy discussion about the psychology of illness or disability, but it is worth stating my belief that every illness, accident of birth or traumatic event, exerts an entirely different effect on different people *and everyone responds differently*.

There could be a tendency for us to think 'closed thoughts' about people and their disabilities. By this I mean, we slot them into 'disability pigeonholes' and expect those with similar conditions to feel the same and to react in the same way. But this is not so; for although the same condition may be common to a number, there any similarity ends. What radically changes every 'case' into a 'person' is the body in which the event takes place and the different feelings experienced. The woman who is recovering from a hysterectomy will require different emotional support than will the parents with a spina bifida child. Though the counselling skills may be the same, the way they are used, and the different emphases given to them, means that each and every person must be recognised and related to as the unique individual he is.

Listening and Questioning

The importance of listening has already been alluded to in this chapter but there is just one point which should be elaborated — listening to the emotions expressed in the words. Some patients referred for rehabilitation — those recovering from strokes, head injuries and other neurological conditions, to name but a few — experience difficulty with words. Therapists — of every branch — know the frustration transmitted by such a patient as he struggles, first, to grasp hold of the word then to express it. Listening in these circumstances assumes new meaning. There is intense desire to produce words, and accompanying frustration when either the words will not come or they are jumbled making understanding difficult. Buried within the disability are other emotions which exert a powerful and often distorting effect on the search for words. People who have no speech impairment often experience difficulty when trying to express how they feel but generally they can be encouraged to do so. They can be encouraged to tell of their fears and worries that possibly the condition will worsen, or that something else more dreadful may happen. They can be helped to talk of their anxiety over their loved ones and how they will manage should sudden death strike. They can be helped to talk of the joys of recovery. The speech impaired person may have similar feelings but he is locked in by the words that he can express only with difficulty.

If the patient is not encouraged to express his fears and worries, as well as his anger and bitterness — or whatever other feelings are present — recovery and adjustment will be affected. Healing comes not only from without — as a result of external treatment — but from within, as hurt feelings accept healing. When physical treatment takes place alongside emotional healing, rehabilitation is complete.

Stage 2 Identify the Problem

To help a client identify the problem is a crucial stage in counselling. When patients are involved in a programme of rehabilitation, part of the problem has already been identified. But, as was stated previously, treating the actual physical condition may not be a problem: how the patient is adjusting, may be. So, in this stage the therapist must allow time for the patient to express and talk through his feelings. If the therapist does not give him 'permission' to talk and express his feelings, who will? He may need to be led into this by a few words of encouragement such as, 'I wonder how you are coping with . . . '. He may choose to talk about the physical side of coping; but how he talks about this will provide useful clues to his emotional coping. The main thing is to get him talking: about himself and his condition, not about trivialities, unless these can lead into something more productive. Time overspent on trivialities is time wasted. The patient will generally have no difficulty in finding people to talk about the weather: therapists must demonstrate that they are willing to talk about the deeper things that influence therapy; happy topics should not be excluded.

Another useful door to lead the patient toward — in the hope that he will open it and talk about his feelings — is to enquire, 'How did your wife (or nearest relative or whosoever) cope when you had your accident?' An equally useful comment would be to enquire about some practical issue, 'How are you managing for money?' Being able to talk around some of the activities of daily living, and what he can and cannot do, will provide the therapist with some useful leads as to how the patient views the whole subject of his rehabilitation.

Ownership

This is no less important in rehabilitation than in any other counselling, though once again the emphasis is different. In counselling, the client may need to be brought to a realisation of the part he plays in a relationship that does not work: the patient may need help to realise the vital part his attitude towards therapy plays in the rehabilitation relationship. The patient may also need help to accept and own the fact that some of his feelings towards himself are negative and that as such they will hinder his progress. But before he can own his feelings he must identify them. After identifying them, and owning them, he may need help to see how precisely they affect his attitude toward his disability, his treatment, and everyone concerned with him. Once having owned that, yes, he does feel angry and hostile and as a result he does have displays of bad temper that upset his whole family, he will begin to see his feelings in a different light. A person who owns a Rolls Royce car does not feel guilty and ashamed of it, neither does he hide it away. Feelings need not be wrapped up in guilt and hidden away either. Feelings are an essential part of every one of us. Many of us need help in handling our feelings so that they work *for* us and not *against* us.

Stage 3 Explore the Problem

On page 54 this sentence appears, 'Exploration requires great sensitivity and skill.' Therapists are acutely aware just how sensitively physical exploration of tender areas must be carried out. Patients who are tense can be relaxed by gentle fingers and hands. Patients with massive injuries and disabilities have emotional scars that the most sophisticated technology can neither detect nor heal. Gentle exploration of them may. Feelings cannot be excised; but kindly understanding may act like the honey that healed Susan's cracked plate (p. 59). Exploration may expose; but only to allow true healing to take place.

Exploration of feelings is often psychologically painful and because it is, we tend to shy away from it. Exploration of feelings linked to physical pain and trauma is doubly painful. Counsellors often help clients explore psychological pain but because therapists work directly with physical pain, they are in a far better position to help the patient deal with his inner pain.

Stage 3 Skills

Here and Now: Then and There. Counsellors are often able to use the counselling relationship in a constructive way by pointing to something that is happening in the 'here and now'. Therapists may also capitalise on the rehabilitation relationship to help their patients understand a bit more what is happening within themselves. Therapists often become the focus of the patient's negative feelings toward therapy and whatever life event has made therapy necessary. In a sense this is 'displacement' (refer to mental mechanisms p. 25).

A very natural response is to retaliate, verbally if not physically. If, when on the receiving end of displaced, negative feelings, one says something like, 'You're obviously feeling a lot of emotional pain and this makes you want to hit out at someone, and I just happen to be in the way', this will tell the patient that his feelings have been recognised but that they are not being taken personally. A remark such as, 'My goodness! you are grouchy today; you feel like a prickly pear and I can't get near you' may encourage the patient to talk about his feelings *as they are at that very moment*.

Self Disclosure. Not all negative feelings arise either within the client or the patient. Janet left home having had a disturbing row with her husband. The first patient she visited (she was a community OT), after several minutes said to her, 'Janet, you're very quiet today. Are you annoyed with me?' This caused Janet to take stock. 'I'm sorry, Mrs Andrews. Simon and I had a row before we left for work and it's played on my mind. Thank you for bringing me out of myself. My feelings could easily have got in the way of your treatment.'

It is worth repeating the warning; having made a disclosure, return the focus to the patient, even though the patient may wish to continue acting as the 'counsellor'. If Janet had not been able to rise above her feelings, and had they continued to get in the way with other patients, she might have needed to seek counselling help for herself.

Images. The use of images is a powerful means of helping the client to get in touch with the feelings of his inner world. This technique may be used with effect in therapy, particularly in dealing with pain and trauma. Psychological pain may be located anywhere in the body but often it lodges in the vital organs. And just as actual pain causes stress and distress, so psychological pain causes emotional stress and distress. The imaging technique can help identify the course of the pain and then its location. Having done this, the client can be helped to lessen the effect of the pain by allowing his psyche to bring healing in its own unique way. There is nothing magical nor mysterious about this technique, for what it does is to tap into the subconscious, bypassing the intellect, thereby releasing energy which acts directly on the area of the body under stress.

Assagioli,[2] speaking of the power of concentration, propounds a psychological law thus,

> Images of mental pictures and ideas tend to produce the physical conditions and the external acts that correspond to them.

When the patient produces an inner picture of the pain and is then encouraged to imagine how it may be transformed, he is putting to work powerful, healing forces. Let Roy relate his experience of this inner healing.

> Over a period of four months I had consultation, with five GPs, for trigeminal neuralgia. For the first time in my life I required a daily intake of drugs in a more or less vain attempt to control the agonising pain. The drugs may have been responsible for a stimulation of my mental facilities at that period. Also my reading was leading me into an area of search with meditation. Both of these would no doubt give me a slightly more attuned state of inner thoughtfulness. However, the actual memories of my therapeutic experience are these.
>
> Being in a familiar place, and feeling no apprehension towards the therapist, gave no delay in becoming semi-relaxed. Full relaxation was not possible by the state of my mind, the pain, depression, anger, insecurity, frustration and the overall feeling of not being a person of worth.
>
> All the kind words that come from persons who try to help, those you instinctively know are genuine, are only helpful in a very minor way. Kindness is only half-received by one who is full of self-pity. My first feelings were of not being convinced that anything could relieve my pain and that it may help the therapist more than me. (As a counsellor I know that some sessions have more benefit for me rather than for the client.) Being negative in attitude didn't delay my mental imagery. On closing my eyes, almost at once I was able to see bright colours but unable to control the change of shapes and not able to see clear outlines of anything which had sense or reason. Coloured bands and shapes moved so fast that in some cases before being able to describe the colours two or three others had been and gone. I'm sure that the predominant colours were dark grey, red and silver/gold. In the centre of what felt to be my forehead a very bright beam of light came towards me. It started in a very thin spot of white light which, when coming closer, opened out and became hot light. It gave a great feeling of fear, that if the light was allowed to enter my forehead it might burn me, or that it was some of my own energy which was being returned to me. I didn't wish to receive the energy.
>
> Although I was concentrating on mental pictures and trying to make

these shapes go into forms, I was fully conscious of my surroundings and what was said to me, also the heat coming from the therapist's hands on my head. I was only slightly aware of time. (I'm sure that many people being helped feel guilt at using too much of the helper's time. These guilt feelings must retard the process of getting well, in many.)

My most vivid recollection was of being told to swallow my pain. Dark black clouds went down my throat very fast, without taste but with a sensation of swallowing a type of bile.

After recovery from any type of unpleasant experience the safety mechanisms of the mind quickly blot out the very bad, painful memories, which leaves, in most cases, an unclear or incomplete outline of events. But before the session was ended I was aware that the pain in my face had lessened and by the end it had disappeared completely. With it went many of my negative feelings and I was left feeling very calm.

I understand that many people find imagery, or mental pictures, easy to evoke. In my case actual pictures don't come instantly and even with suggestion from the therapist it is only images of a seemingly free nature which appear. For example, if I were told to imagine a summer garden, maybe I could evoke the colours of summer but an actual scene would elude me. That makes me believe that every person should be allowed his own free expression without rushing things along.

Roy's account, written many months after the event, relates more the impressions and feelings of the patient than of the technique which is possibly the least didactic of all approaches to counselling and therapy. People who want to become proficient in the use of imagery would find it helpful to study the use of symbols. Several books are included under the general heading 'imagery'.[3] Also included is the address of an organisation that specialises in the teaching of an approach which concentrates on the use of imagery.

Stage 4 Plan the Action

Therapists, by nature of their jobs, are involved in encouraging the patient to some form of action. From the moment the person becomes a patient for whom planned rehabilitation is likely, some form of action is envisaged. But, action designed *for* the patient is not always accepted *by* him.

The benefits of treatment are not always appreciated because the whole concept of rehabilitation is foreign to the patient's experience. Understanding of what is involved in treatment must be more than an intellectual assent. For a rehabilitation programme to work, there has to be an emotional acceptance of it by the patient. Rejection — total or partial, by way of inattention to carrying out the programme — may thus result from not enough attention being given to ensuring the patient's commitment to the action plan. Some patients will 'obey' and comply; others will rebel, simply because they have not been consulted and because they do not understand the goals set for them. When strong feelings get in the way, goal-achievement is threatened. That is why exploration of the patient's feelings toward his disability is essential throughout rehabilitation.

Identify New Skills

Many patients have disabilities that mean the learning of new skills, either to earn a living or in order to improve the quality of life. Therapists are generally adaptable and innovative and adept at improvising: these are all characteristics of an enquiring mind, so essential in rehabilitation. So this stage of identifying new skills (or awakening disused ones) is one which most therapists would tackle without too much difficulty. But caution needs to be exercised. There is a great deal more to acquiring a skill than intellectual ability or manual dexterity. Motivation plays a vital part and motivation has an emotional component. Motivation — incentive or drive — determines behaviour. Yet motivation is difficult to measure. We can observe *how* a person is motivated (by what he does) but not *why* or *what* motivates him. A child who practises many hours a day on the piano is motivated to become a top-rate pianist. His behaviour is obvious: what drives him is not so obvious. In the same way, what motivates one person to overcome severe disability by hours of hard work, while another person, with similar or less disability, succumbs, never to rise, is difficult to determine. One may assume that the rewards received by the latter are not enough to drive him on. But having said this, it would be as equally difficult to determine the satisfying rewards for the former as it would be to gauge the dissatisfying rewards for the latter. The unknown factor is probably emotional. The person who is not defeated by tragedy has somehow harnessed his emotions to work for him, while the other person's emotions work against him. A counselling approach to the setting of goals and helping the person explore, understand and express his feelings may make a world of difference between victory and defeat. We must recognise that although goals may be physically attainable, they may yet be unrealistic because they are emotionally trammelled.

Thus, goals and the skills or means necessary to reach them, are interrelated and both are powerfully influenced by feelings. Feelings that are ignored will surely impede the best conceived action plan.

To plan the action, for the therapist, *is* different from counselling, in the same way that identifying the problem is. The patient's disability is the presenting problem, that is true, so in one sense the 'problem' has been pre-identified. But as we have already discussed, the patient may need a great deal of help to identify factors which, unless they are dealt with, could become problems. If one follows the counselling model as it is presented, the action plan can only come after the other three stages. In reality, thinking around the action plan is usually where rehabilitation starts, following hard on the heels of the assessment. This is necessary, for physical treatment often has to be commenced long before the patient is aware of what is happening. But this does not apply in all cases. Many people are fully aware and need to be involved in working out their own action plans.

Stage 5 Implement the Action Plan

In rehabilitation, thinking around the action plan and implementing it may be difficult to separate. Normally the therapist will be as involved in the second as in the first, whereas in counselling the client may decide to 'go it alone'. Nevertheless, there are certain categories of patients who do carry out their own rehabilitation and who require little or no help from therapists. Those patients who have little contact with therapists should be assured of support — physical, material and emotional — as and when required. It could also be suggested that except for a small minority — those who are unconscious and other totally dependent patients — every patient is expected to carry out some part of the treatment for himself or, when living at home, with the aid of relatives. If these patients neglect their 'homework', leaving everything to the therapist, progress is slowed down. Total involvement is vital.

Information

Patients who are receiving minimal help from therapists may, nevertheless, require a great deal of information if they are to be effectively rehabilitated. Many patients report being totally unprepared for the after-effects of, for example, planned surgery. While it may be perfectly true that someone did explain what would happen, and how the operation may affect them, the anxiety of the forthcoming operation probably had the effect of preventing them from hearing what was said. But to reiterate what has been said several times in this book, telling someone is not sufficient; we have to ensure that what we said has been understood. Part of this understanding is to help the person explore what he has been told, and we can achieve this by allowing him to talk and to ask questions and in turn to ask questions of him. The purpose would certainly not be to drown the patient in a flood of what he might feel or experience following a particular intervention, but on the other hand, it is not sufficient to tell a patient who is to have major abdominal surgery, 'You'll feel a bit uncomfortable for a few days until the stitches come out.' Asking the patient how he thinks he will feel will usually provide a useful road into his understanding.

Relatives are often in need of information and straightforward advice on how to manage someone who is being rehabilitated. They are frequently the ones who have to cope with the patient's fears, anxieties, frustrations, moods and awkward behaviour, when rehabilitation is carried out from home. That is why they need someone to whom they can talk. The therapist would be the ideal person, but recognising the difficulties of limited time, coupled with limited staff, other people may have to provide the information and advice needed. Some of the appendices to this book could be used to direct relatives to appropriate information and advice sources.

Stage 6 Evaluation

It was suggested on page 67 that on-going evaluation is an essential component of counselling. This view is supported by Brechin and Liddiard,

> evaluation . . . should not be something that is entered upon at the end of an intervention to see whether some particular method of treatment or therapy has or has not worked. Rather, it should be an integral part of the total process of intervention.[4]

Time for evaluation, built into every session (it need only be a few minutes) will encourage the patient to feel that he is a very definite part of the process and that what he thinks and says is important and that he is an active partner and not a passive recipient.

Where counselling has taken place over a number of sessions, and most certainly at the end of a rehabilitation programme, a final evaluation is desirable. Many of the points dealt with in pages 67–71 apply with equal relevance to this chapter. Very little more need be said. Counselling rarely results in miracles. More commonly the client feels that he is now able to live on better terms with life. Therapists in rehabilitation often work near miracles and may feel justifiably proud of their achievements. But, as was pointed out on page 70, therapist and patient, just as counsellor and client, share in both success and failure. The one should not lead us into complacency; the other must not drive us to despair.

Summary

This chapter followed the outline of the Wessex Model of Counselling which was presented in the preceding chapter. This model, although designed for on-going counselling, may be used with equal freedom in a single session. Many of the topics covered in chapter 3 have been dealt with here — *as they apply in rehabilitation*. This was thought to be essential; it was considered not sufficient to present a model without attempting to apply it. In this way, several areas of similarity and dissimilarity were discussed.

There are more similarities than differences between 'professional' counselling and counselling in rehabilitation. The principal similarity is that the concepts and principles of counselling are equally appropriate in rehabilitation. The principal difference lies in the reason for the relationship. Clients normally seek counselling help of their own free will; rehabilitation is forced upon people by virtue of some event which in its wake would bring severe and permanent disability unless ameliorated by effective rehabilitation. Rehabilitation and counselling go hand-in-hand. The one attends more to physical treatment. (Not exclusively, for there are many patients, particularly in the fields of mental illness and mental handicap for whom physical treatment plays a secondary role. But even in these areas, a great emphasis is often placed on physical activity, while other aspects are relegated to second place.) The other works with the patient's feelings. They interact with each other.

It could be argued that both counselling and rehabilitation are relationships, for both counsellors and therapists rely on the quality of the relationships they establish with clients and patients. If this is so, then everything that has been said so far in this book about counselling applies, with minor modification, to rehabilitation. Professor David Metcalfe, of Manchester, said, when addressing an audience of therapists at the King's Fund Centre in 1982, 'Since we work directly with the disabled, we are right to want to be able to use a counselling approach.'[5] And, as has been emphasised throughout these four chapters, counselling offers a way of reducing '. . . fears and frustrations . . . and also helps promote feelings of self worth, acceptability and satisfaction with life . . .'.[6]

Notes

1. Brechin, A., Liddiard, P. and Swain, J. (1981) *Handicap in a Social World*, Open University Press, Milton Keynes.

2. Assagioli, R. (1980) *The Act of Will*, Wildwood House, London.

3. *Images*

(a) Assagioli, R. (1980) *Psychosynthesis*, Turnstone Books, Wellingborough.

(b) Cirlot, J.E. (1978) *A Dictionary of Symbols*, Routledge and Kegan Paul, London and Boston.

(c) Bayley, H. (1974) *The Lost Language of Symbolism*, Ernest Benn Ltd, London.

(d) Jung, Carl, G. (1979) *Man and His Symbols*, Aldus Books, London.

(e) Wickes, Frances J. (1977) *The Inner World of Choice: A Jungian Approach to Psychotherapy*, Coventure Ltd., London.

(f) The Institute of Psychosynthesis. Highwood Park, Nan Clarks Lane, Mill Hill, London NW7.
This Institute produces a range of inexpensive books covering a whole range of topics which could be loosely grouped together under the heading 'Transpersonal Psychology'.

4. Brechin, A. and Liddiard, P. (1981) *Look at it This Way: New Perspectives in Rehabilitation*, Open University Press, Milton Keynes.

5. & 6. Both these quotes are taken from an article by Sally Burningham which appeared in *Remedial Therapist* 29 October 1982 Vol 5 issue 5. The first quote was from the opening speech by David Metcalfe, professor of general practice at Manchester.

The second quote is from a paper given by Brigid Breckman, a stoma care sister at St Peter's Hospital, London.

5 SELF-AWARENESS

The Concept of Self-awareness

The concept of self-awareness centres on the word 'self'. One definition of self is, 'Usually in the sense of the personality or ego, regarded as an agent, conscious of his own continuing identity.'[1] Thus it could be deduced that the self is (to quote from the same source, under the heading 'personality') 'the integrated and dynamic organization of the physical, mental, moral and social qualities of the individual, as that manifests itself to other people' and (under 'ego') 'An individual's experience of himself, or his conception of himself.' While both of these sub-definitions pertain, they do not fully explain the essence of self.

Cicero said, 'The spirit is the True self — Mens cuiusque is est quisque' (De Republica VI; 26). If he is correct then the self transcends both personality and ego. Yet there is a definite place for recognising that both do have a place in self. Self may be thought of from a developmental standpoint. The new-born baby — we assume — has no idea of self but he quickly learns to recognise his own body as something separate and distinct from his mother's. As his world enlarges, his 'self' concept changes. How he interacts with other people, and the pleasure or displeasure he derives from these interactions influence his self-image. By the time he is adult, he knows fairly well his physical self, his relationship to other people and his place in society. Paradoxically, however, he is, generally speaking, less aware of his true inner self than he was as a child. Children have a great facility for getting in touch with their own inner worlds and with other people's. Socialisation — including education, which concentrates on 'learning' rather than on 'being' — tends to lessen the individual's awareness of his true self. This is because he becomes caught up in society's various expectations.

Self and Others

Part of socialisation is how we live with others. The world revolves around the tiny baby, but as he grows older he must learn to revolve in harmony within the orbits of other people's worlds. This learning process is frequently painful; for many of his own desires — and with them sensitive feelings — are subjected to the desires of other people. So often these suppressed desires and feelings carry with them tiny parts of his true self thus ensuring a reasonable fit with other people.

Self and Roles

Part of fitting into society are the roles we are allotted or which we adopt. Examples of these are the school-child, adolescent, mother/father, husband/wife, neighbour, and the innumerable occupational roles. The degree to which we identify with these roles means that so often we become nothing more than a conglomerate of expectations. Other people expect us to behave strictly according to the role book and if we don't, they very often do not know how to respond. People who over-identify with roles, often find it difficult to break out of them: yet it is essential that we do. The man who, in his youth, was athletic and strong, may experience great crises when, because of age, he is no longer able to participate in feats of strength and endurance. The girl with a lovely figure, who wins every beauty competition, may pass through a crisis when she is faced with the truth that her youthful beauty has deserted her and has not yet been replaced by the different beauty of age. These are examples of how we may invest too much emotional energy in roles at the expense of developing our true selves. Roles are important, of course, for through them we have a well-defined place in society. But just as an actor, on stage, plays a part then discards it to become himself, so must we. We must be the director of the players; they must not — as so often they do — control us. Assagioli[4a] refers to roles as 'sub-personalities'. William James refers to them as 'various selves'. We shall return to the idea of sub-personalities later in the chapter.

The Personal Self

What has been discussed thus far could be put under the heading 'personal' or 'conscious' self; that self to which we and others have access without too much difficulty. It is a self made up of body, emotions and mind. This self is governed more by acquired knowledge than by self-awareness.

To most people their bodies are important and, as has been pointed out already, are an important part of their roles. But is the body the true self? Most people would say, 'no'. They would instinctively feel that they are more than just 'body'. The body passes through various stages of growth; it may become diseased and deformed; it is often tired and eventually it will wear out and die. Is the self held prisoner by an ageing and decaying body? Or is self something above and beyond the body?

What of emotions? Is self ruled by vehement, commanding or overpowering emotions such as hate, love, greed, grief, anger, revenge? Strong emotions and feelings, at most, are fleeting. Can we then say that self is as fleeting and unpredictable as these emotions? Emotions may lift us to great heights and inspired by noble feelings of love we may achieve great deeds. But dark despair can cast us into the depths. Is this the self, unstable and vacillatating? Or is self a part of us above and beyond our emotions?

Mind offers no more assurance than body or emotions. What a wonderful faculty is the mind. As Macaulay said, 'The highest intellects, like the tops of mountains, are the first to catch and reflect the dawn.' High intellects are capable of achieving greatness but once again the question is asked, 'Where in mind is the true self?'

Our wonderful bodies, best emotions and highest intellects are not worthy temples of our true selves. Scrope Davies, writing circa 1831, reminds us that 'Babylon in all its desolation is a sight not so awful as that of the human mind in ruins.'

The Central Self

If there is one self, made up of body, emotions and mind — the personal or conscious self — then by implication there must be another self that is internal and transpersonal. Various writers have expressed similar views. For Jung, self is the totality of the psyche. Adler describes the 'creative self'. Assagioli talks of the 'transpersonal self'. To paraphrase their ideas about this 'inner' or 'other' self, the following definition is suggested.

> *The personal self is that which separates us from other people.*
> *The inner self is that which joins us to other people.*

Cicero defines the self as spirit — that divine essence of life which is present in every person. This begs the question, 'what is spiritual?' Spiritual must not be limited by thinking of it only as 'religious', however noble and wonderful this may be. Spiritual expression may find an outlet in religious worship, but for another person it may be in the pursuit of beauty, art or music. There are many and varied forms of expressing the inner self. We have already considered the idea that both thought and emotion may be of such a nature that they are able to lift us up into realms beyond the earthly. While Cicero's idea of the spirit may be correct, the other idea of the two selves is still valid.

Jung[2] says

> The self is a union of opposites . . .. The opposition between light and good on the one hand and darkness and evil on the other is left in a state of open conflict . . .. The self, however, is absolutely paradoxical in that it presents thesis and antithesis and at the same time synthesis.

This quote gives the impression of conflict resulting in completeness. In other words, the self is constantly striving to balance the two opposing forces of our natures.

Eastcott[3] says,

> We have spoken of outer and inner worlds; we have also outer and inner selves with which we inhabit these two places. Mystery veils the inner self, just as it guards the inner world and the inter-dependence of these two selves or 'halves' of our being is one of the agelong problems of mankind.

Both Jung and Eastcott point us along the road towards a two-self person. One with which we are in touch, the other of which we are aware, yet which is veiled in mystery. Both, as Eastcott stresses, are interdependent. Is there a way that the mystery behind the veil may be revealed? Or if not revealed in its entirety, may we become more aware?

To seek an answer to these related questions we need first of all to ask another. What is the function of this inner self or the 'central self' as it will now be called?

The Influence of the Central Self

To help us think about the function of the central self, an analogy may be drawn from astronomy. The centre of our solar system is the sun which has three main qualities: energy, warmth, light. Around the sun, and totally dependent on it, and influenced by it, a number of major and minor planets revolve. When considering the central self, the analogy is continued thus:

1. The sun is the central self.
2. The revolving planets are different parts of our personal self — our sub-personalities.
3. Each sub-personality is made up of three parts: body, emotions, mind.

Just as the earth (to take one of the planets) rotates on its own axis and at the same time revolves around the sun, so each sub-personality 'planet' constantly rotates around on *its* own axis, and revolves around the central self. This brings every one of the three parts of each sub-personality within the focus of the central self, there to be influenced by the three main qualities of energy, warmth and light.

Continuing the analogy, it is suggested that while the three main qualities of the central self are inter-related, and influence all three parts of every sub-personality, each quality has a special affinity with one of the three parts: energy with the body, warmth with the emotions, light with the mind.

Energy — Body. In the natural world the sun's energy is stored by plants. The central self radiates energy to the 'body' part of each sub-personality.

Warmth — Emotions. The warmth of the sun encourages trees to leaf, flowers to open and living creatures to rejoice. The warmth from the central self acts upon our emotions in the same way.

Light — Mind. Light chases away darkness. The penetrating light of the central self illumines the dark recesses of the mind.

This beautiful picture, regrettably, is marred by the indisputable fact that very often the sub-personalities resist strongly the influence exerted by the central self. That is what Jung referred to as the good and evil. If only we could, unreservedly, surrender to the influence of our central selves . . .! At the same time, however, just as each of us is made up of many sub-personalities, so each sub-personality is acted upon in a different way by the central self. Sub-personality 'A' may be more 'body' than emotion or mind and when the person gives the central self permission — a deliberate act of will — certain facts about 'body' will gradually be revealed. These then require to be brought within the influence of the central self and to be acted upon by it. For sub-personality 'B' emotions may be in conflict; for 'C', mind may be the problem area. But nothing is ever static. Change produced in one area often necessitates change in another. So whatever has been accomplished, there is always more to achieve. There is no such state as total conflict replaced instantly by total harmony: there is always a dawn. Gradually, however (and it may take a lifetime), the conflicting areas can be brought into harmony with the central self as we continue the quest for self-awareness.

Assagioli[4b] relates self-awareness to the three parts of the personal self and is emphatic that for awareness of self to be productive, the person must 'dis-identify' with body, emotions and mind. This means affirming,

> I have a body but I am not my body.
> I have emotions but I am not my emotions.
> I have a mind but I am not my mind.

This dis-identification is not something which is done only once; it is a continual re-affirming. But it does have the effect of opening the channels of communication between the central self and the sub-personalities.

The central self can also be thought of as a powerful communications satellite, receiving, decoding and transmitting signals to and from all the sub-personalities. For just as the planets in the solar system influence one another, so each of the three parts of each sub-personality are related: they have to be, for together they make up the personal self. So each needs to know what is happening within the others. Some may not like what is happening in another, particularly when change produces a threat, and will send strong signals expressing their resistance. The result is conflict and confusion. Conflict resolution if left to the personal self is likely to result only in partial resolution. This is because the warring factions have no mediator. When the central self functions as mediator, every sub-personality is allowed a proper hearing. They are then influenced by the central self and mediation results in resolution. When this process is repeated many times over, self-awareness is greatly enhanced.

Body Awareness

To this stage in the chapter we have discussed self and awareness of self in a general way. Now it is necessary to spend time discussing some of the practical issues. If Assagioli is correct — that in order to become more aware of self we need to understand the interplay between body, emotions and mind — then it would do no harm to continue our discussion by concentrating once more on these three aspects of the personal self.

Our bodies are precious for they are the means whereby we live; but however precious they are, they are only instruments. Yet many people relate to their bodies as if they were their true self. We must achieve a balance between lavish attention and total disregard. But always it must be remembered that our central selves are not our bodies. It is necessary, in the pursuit of self-awareness, to become more aware of how we relate to our bodies for they are the main focus for sensation and experience.

Sensation

The main areas of sensation are in the five senses plus the kinaesthetic, a sense which is less well observed by most people. In the quest for self-awareness we need to know how and in what particular circumstances any one of our six senses influences us. It is worth re-emphasising that when I speak of the body, emotions or mind that they are not totally separate and independent. Indeed, quite the reverse: they are totally interdependent.

Visual Sensation. When considering visual sensation, for example, related to self-awareness, we may find it a useful exercise to discover which colours attract us and which repel us. Having discovered this, we could go on to explore the significance of both groups. This is where the imaging technique, outlined in the preceding chapter, is useful. Visualise a preferred colour and observe it carefully. It may take a particular shape which may then lead you on an interesting and fruitful inner journey. Coupled with this, if you carefully *observe* and *feel*, the mood evoked by both the colour and the journey will, together, add another dimension to what is happening. Visual sensation is not just colour. It may be the quality of light — bright/dull, or it may be concerned with specific objects, designs or shapes. It is not suggested that there is anything pathological in people who concentrate on visual sensation — or any of the other points we shall consider — but *for some people* awareness of self may be seriously hampered if they cannot free themselves from some aspect of body, emotions or mind which controls them.

Taste, Smell and Hearing. Taste, smell and hearing, as with sight, may all be used imaginatively to increase awareness by concentrating on what brings pleasure or aversion. The sensation of hearing may be used as a powerful means of awareness. All manner of sounds may evoke memories, moods and feelings. The same process may be used with sounds as with colours. There is one aspect of sound which is worth mentioning, that of music. Music is a well-known therapeutic agent and may be used in a positive way as a self-awareness agent. Music may take us on an imaginary journey where many significant people and situations are encountered. Some may be in actual memory form, others in symbolic form. Events from our past may be clothed upon with feelings evoked by the music. Doors which before may have only been glimpsed may suddenly swing open, unlocked by a musical key. While this free-floating experience is often productive, at other times we may need to concentrate on the five elements of musical structure: rhythm, tone, melody, harmony, timbre, then ask, 'What emotions, what images are evoked?'. Where in the body does the music vibrate? It is a well-known fact that certain tones cause vibrations in certain parts of the body and it is conceivable that the choice of music we prefer to listen to is influenced by the pleasurable sensations created in our bodies.

Assagioli[4b] points to the fact that music can be a cause of emotional disturbance. Music programmes which are so arranged that the listener alternates between height and depth, without time to adjust, can cause confusion. Concerts that are over-long can create emotional indigestion. Raucous and unremitting musical sound can produce severe disorientation. So, while music may be therapeutic, it may also be deleterious. But it is one medium that can be used positively in the search for self-awareness as we struggle to understand not only our likes and dislikes, but why and how particular music affects us emotionally.

Touch. Touch can soothe and also inflame great passion. Touch can relax tired and tense muscles; it may also cause a person to shrink away in fear. We can enjoy being touched, embraced, hugged, cuddled or we can detest these touchings. Rowan,[5] speaking of humanistic therapies and the part touching plays says, 'As babies we all had strong needs to be touched and cuddled. If these were not met, we may go through life looking for the touch we missed.' In another part of the same book, *The Reality Game*, he says,

> Many humanistic practitioners touch the bodies of their clients, whether out of ordinary human sympathy, encouragement to regress, provocative massage designed to bring out feelings, re-enactment of birth, etc . . .. In opening up the whole inner world which has been blocked off, we use a lot of gratification (whole body massage, cuddling and comforting, giving of bottles or breasts, immersion in warm water, group rocking and lullabies, affirmation of good qualities and general loveableness, and so on) because we find it to be highly therapeutic and very effective in producing real change, if used in the right way.

This quotation has been included in full because of its particular relevance in rehabilitation where the opportunity for body contact is ever present. What this extract does show is just how far counselling has moved away from the psychoanalytical model, where touching by the therapist, or touching of the therapist by the client, is taboo. In humanistic therapy, touching is 'OK'. People who want to use touch in their counselling must have acquired a high state of self-awareness in all three aspects of body, emotions and mind, lest their own limitations hinder the client in his quest for self-awareness.

Kinaesthetic. Kinaesthetic sensation is the last of the senses to be discussed and it has particular relevance for all therapists in rehabilitation. Most people rarely give any consideration as to how muscles work in order to produce movement. All manner of complex movement is engaged in to which, until some event comes to intervene, little active attention is given. Yet, when disaster strikes and the person of necessity becomes involved in rehabilitation, he will have to become aware, possibly for the first time, of the inner sensations that control weight, position and movement. The awareness of muscular sensation, for example, is of particular importance when teaching people how to relax. Some have great difficulty in developing the awareness of muscular tension. Not only is this awareness necessary in being able to relax, it plays a vital part in teaching patients to re-use muscles that have become damaged, either by accident or by surgery.

Similarly, many patients who are being rehabilitated need to be re-educated in how various parts of their bodies are positioned in relation to other parts and how they function in relation to one another. This re-education would include being aware of body weight and its distribution. Thus we see that this particular awareness of self has a special relevance in rehabilitation.

Emotional Awareness

When considering emotions as a part of the personal self, or of the particular sub-personality under scrutiny, it is necessary, first to identify which emotions or feelings are generally prevalent and, secondly to discover just how and under what circumstances those emotions influence us. It may not always be easy to think of particular emotions, other than some of the more obvious ones, such as love, hate, jealousy, mirth and so on. To facilitate the study of emotions the 'Emotional Awareness Wheel'

Here are a number of suggestions as to how the 'Wheel' could be used.

1. At its basic level, as a straightforward awareness of words
2. By considering each emotion in turn from love through to ecstasy and thinking about the circumstances, situations, events and times in which they have been experienced.
3. By considering the words in their pairs and the emotional impact they make.

Figure 5.1: The Emotional Awareness Wheel

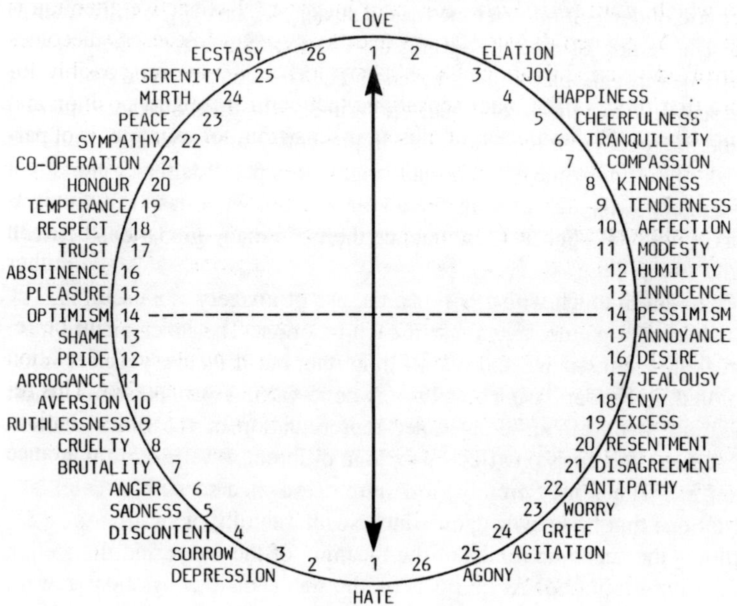

(Figure 5.1) is presented. 26 pairs of emotions and feelings are arranged in progressive order around a circle. The feelings are divided into two groups — 'light' and 'dark'. They could also be thought of as 'positive' — those feelings that make us feel 'good' — and 'negative' — those feelings that make us feel 'bad'. If the terms 'good' and 'bad' are not acceptable, positive feelings could be thought of as those that make us feel comfortable while negative feelings are those that make us feel uncomfortable. But feelings influence behaviour, so positive feelings generally help us to get on with other people, while negative feelings have the opposite effect.

The 26 pairs of words have been numbered for ease of reference and they have been so arranged that starting from number 1 — love — there is a gradual lessening of emotional tone through to 'innocence' which marks the end of the first quarter. The second quarter is a gradual increase of dark emotional tones to the strongest, 'hate'. The third quarter is a lessening of tone to 'optimism'. The fourth quarter is heightening of tone through 'pleasure' to 'ecstasy'. The first quarter could be thought of as 'Autumn'; the second quarter, 'Winter'; the third quarter, 'Spring'; and the fourth quarter, 'Summer'. In presenting any model one runs the risk of getting some of it not quite right. It is possible that some of the pairs of words are not semantic antonyms. But what has been aimed at are emotional opposites. In practice there are many gradations between any two poles.

To get in touch with emotions, the use of imagery is a useful aid, by imagining a picture to represent each emotion. The inner picture may, at first, seem strange and not a fitting one, but if its every aspect is explored, its deeper meaning will surely be revealed. Every person is almost certain to have a different inner representation of the same emotion because each emotion affects people in different ways. An example may suffice. The word 'serenity', to Andrew, evokes a scene of a calm lake (not one that he knew), upon which swim a family of swans. As he explores the scene he thinks of the meaning of the water and the feeling of being supported. As he floats on the water, his feelings float upward to the clouds that dance across the sky. He becomes one of the clouds only to realise that it represents a specific worry that has been on his mind for some time. He thinks that if he learns to relax more he will be able to rise above his difficulty. Coming back to the lake, he thinks of the water, its depth, its colour and the life contained in it. He realises that the water reflects his various moods. He also considers the bounds of the lake and how the water is contained; he relates this to the boundaries of his own life and realises that certain of them he finds irksome.

He explores the depth of the lake and there finds mud, a reminder of something that has been and is now different. Within the mud there teems a wild life that provides food for the creatures that inhabit the lake. And growing in the mud are plants that would probably not be able to grow anywhere else. He discovers quite a bit of garbage which has been discarded by picnickers (his sub-personalities?), but each bit of rubbish tells him something about himself. Rising out of the lake is a tree which he climbs and he looks down on the lake, to see a different view, light and shade and breadth that had escaped him. He realises that the lake is himself and that his personality is not unattractive, that it is highly productive, but that it does have a depth that, if explored, will reveal certain facets of himself that may not always please him. On the other hand, growing out of the depths there is something wholesome. But as he continues looking, the surface of the lake is disturbed, agitated by something. There he stops. His imagination had started to take him across the dimension toward agitation. Perhaps another day Andrew will want to explore that word also.

By using the Awareness Wheel it may be revealed that there is a high tendency for the person to seek experiences that bring peak feelings — ecstasy and elation are two examples. Danger often brings a sense of elation but in the wake of peak experiences frequently comes the opposite feeling. Some of us seek a peak emotion in order to stave off its mate. As we try to evoke events and situations when these feelings have been previously experienced, we may realise that they are more frequent than we first thought. Then we need to identify how we feel when that particular feeling has passed, and what we do to adjust our emotional state.

While some people actively seek peak experiences and feelings, others seem to live on negative feelings. Helping such a person to identify situations and events which evoke negative feelings, may also mean encouraging him to identify people who spark off these feelings. The person may need help to be able to move from the acutely negative aspect along the dimension toward the positive. The move may only be a few gradations but the change may make all the difference to his emotional balance. Deep feelings, explored within the safety of the counselling relationship have therapeutic potential of tremendous import. Very often we are hindered from moving toward positive feelings because one or another of our subpersonalities binds us. Counselling may be the key to open the lock.

Mind Awareness

Two aspects only of mind will be considered: thinking and imagination. Jung[2] classifies thinking as one of the functions of consciousness; the others are feeling, sensation and intuition. The first aspect of thinking to be considered is *what* we think. Some of our thoughts are quite spectacular, even bizarre. Thoughts have the habit of flitting in and out of our consciousness at amazing speed. They can linger or they can become so lodged in our minds that they pester. Thoughts can be under our control or they can be like a will-o'-the-wisp, leading us a merry dance into dangerous areas. They can be silent like the grave or as noisy as a busload of chattering children on the way to school. Thoughts are such changeable things and yet they can be so persistent as to exert a powerful influence on our behaviour. They can lift us to lofty heights or to depths of despair and degradation. The thoughts that mainly occupy a man's mind, declare in bold letters the sort of man he is. So, in our quest for self-awareness we need to be thoroughly familiar with our thought life and how our behaviour is influenced by it.

Thoughts are closely related to feelings; that is why it is difficult to consider one facet of the personal self without also considering the other two. A useful exercise is to relate thoughts to the Emotional Wheel. When considering sympathy, for example, in what direction do our thoughts take us? And what direction when its opposite, 'antipathy', is considered? It is very likely, when this exercise is carried out, that it will be almost impossible to distinguish thought from feeling. Situations and events remembered will bring feelings with them, but thought may then take us away beyond what we have actually experienced. Thought may be both historic and futuristic. Futuristic thought borders on imagination which will be considered later. As with emotions, thoughts may be classified as positive or negative, but once again, an emotional content has been introduced. What we think — of ourselves, of other people, of situations and circumstances — influences emotions which in turn influence our behaviour.

We may make the excuse, 'I can't help thoughts coming into my mind.' This is true, but only to a degree. We can take active steps to prevent them lodging in our minds. Dark, negative thoughts may be dispelled by light, positive ones. Racing thoughts may be slowed down by relaxation and meditation — an exercise of will — which emphasises once more the inter-relationship between body, emotions and mind. Many people harbour hurtful memories of events or people and around these memories their thoughts often revolve. Memories may be of distant or recent origin.

Evoked memories often bring with them the pain of the moment, but of equal importance, the associated feelings are brought to the surface. Two feelings which commonly surface are resentment and bitterness. Most of us indulge in negative thinking from time to time but people who dwell on things negative, for long, also experience feelings that are on the dark side of the emotional wheel. Just as racing thoughts may be slowed down by relaxation and meditation, so by the use of imagination it is possible for a person to move from extreme negative feelings toward the opposite pole.

Imagination

A great deal has already been said about imagination: imagery is imagination. To use imagination creatively we must be prepared to let our imaginations exercise control over our minds, albeit temporarily. Assagioli[4b] says, 'The imagination, in the precise sense of the function of evoking and creating images, is one of the most important and spontaneously active functions of the human psyche, both in its conscious and in its unconscious aspects or levels.' Many people find the use of spontaneous imagination easier than conscious or directed imagination. Yet, it may be necessary to use both. The person who dwells on a negative memory may be helped to move toward the positive pole by a deliberate and conscious process of 'imaginary desensitisation'. The actual situation is evoked in his imagination and he describes it in as much detail as he can recall. This would include his feelings at the time, and afterwards. He is then encouraged to 're-play' the scene, this time making his reactions more positive; his feelings will become less intense. Where the event involved another person (or people) he should be encouraged to adopt a more friendly attitude. After a series of 're-plays', each time adopting a more positive stance, he is almost certain to experience a change of feeling which will indicate a move some distance away from his original feeling. The next stage is to get him to evoke positive situations in his imagination and at the same time to try to experience the feelings which they generate. The final stage is for him to meditate on one of the positive feelings and let his spontaneous imagination take him into realms of thought and feeling as far distant from the negative pole as the farthest star is from the earth.

There are three other areas that are worthy of exploration: intuition, meditation and dreams. It is not my intention to deal with these in this book, not that they are inappropriate but they come more within the realm of pure psychotherapy than within counselling in rehabilitation. To describe them, and their associated techniques, is really outside my scope here. Readers who may be interested in learning more about these subjects are directed to the references where, under the heading 'Meditation, Intuition and Dreams',[6] several books are recommended. John Rowan[5] gives a very useful introduction to some of these techniques used by humanistic therapists.

Self-awareness in Rehabilitation

The discussion so far in this book has centred around the basic idea that for any form of therapy to be effective, it is vital to gain the patient's confidence and commitment. Both of these are influenced by how the patient perceives his role and by his attitude toward his disability. By inference, the more insight the patient is able to develop, the more complete will be his rehabilitation. But the development of self-awareness in rehabilitation is not an end in itself, in contrast to other forms of counselling or psychotherapy. In rehabilitation the focus is on helping the patient adjust to his disability (because he wants to and not because the therapist desires it). In order to achieve this adjustment, some patients may need a great deal of help to become more aware of the relationship between their disabilities and their emotions.

If the awareness of self is important for the patient, it is vital for the therapist. It would be ludicrous for a person who is not suitably qualified or experienced to carry out complicated physical treatment with patients. People in all branches of rehabilitation are skilled professionals and as such may rightly claim the respect and confidence of their patients. Counsellors, too, are trained and experienced professionals. A great deal of their training — both initial and on-going — is related to self-awareness. For how can they guide their clients in their quest if they, themselves, are not actively seeking self-awareness? It would be a case of the 'blind leading the blind' and just as dangerous. Thus the therapist who engages in counselling — and the development of self-awareness as an essential part of it — should, herself, be treading this same pathway toward awareness of self.

Summary

This has been a wide-ranging chapter, covering many topics dealing with self-awareness. Self-awareness is not a state that is ever achieved in the absolute. The most anyone may say is that he is treading this pathway;

but it is a journey of a lifetime. The prospects are infinite. Today's self-awareness is tomorrow's shadow, as we move one more step towards perfect truth and absolute awareness of self. No two people reach precisely the same spot of awareness. Just as two people, on looking out of a window, may describe two dissimilar views, so in self-awareness. What is obvious to one person may, as yet, be obscure to another. One person's pressing need may be considered trivial by someone else. Thus self-awareness is not a concrete fact that can be learned, like 2 + 2 = 4; but it is as high as the stars and as deep as an ocean: it is as boundless as the world.

This sounds poetic but I make no apologies. Self-awareness, because it cannot be measured and standardised, does have a certain poetic mystery about it. Although it cannot be quantified it certainly can be qualified: it can be detected in the way we conduct ourselves and in the way we relate to other people. The idea of self, as presented here, may not accord with other people's views. Self as two — personal and central — may be too foreign a concept for some people to accept. But those who cannot, may accept as valid the idea that the self is made up of body, emotions and mind. So, even if the whole cannot be accepted, part may be seen as relevant. There can be little doubt but that in addition to the trinity of body, emotions and mind, many of us do place great stress on the roles we play in life, or what have been referred to as sub-personalities. Some of these sub-personalities have long since outworn their usefulness, yet they linger on and exert a powerful, though unconscious, influence on our behaviour. Awareness of their influence lessens their control over us.

People, who by circumstance, are forced into the role of 'patient' are then expected to behave in a certain way. Part of the so-called 'difficult' behaviour many patients then exhibit, may be nothing more than a fight against the imposed role. They do not wish to adopt this sub-personality. Some patients adopt it too successfully and over-identify with it so that it begins to dominate them — something sub-personalities will do. Release, through awareness, may come as the trinity of body, emotions and mind of this particular sub-personality of 'patient' is explored.

The techniques outlined in this chapter (as well as those mentioned in the references) are suitable for helping patients to understand and come to terms with what is happening within them, arising from their disability and its aftermath. While talking things through is undoubtedly therapeutic, the therapist can show the patient how he may use the power of imagery to get in touch with feelings that often lie deeper than words. For therapists in rehabilitation (for whom time is often at a premium) any technique which the patient can use on his own, supported as necessary by the therapist, is beneficial. It is not using therapist time, except in talking through and offering guidance as to the next step. It demonstrates to the patient that he *is* an active partner in his own rehabilitation. It offers the patient a valuable technique for dealing with his feelings now and in the future. All of these must contribute to the patient's well-being and a satisfactory rehabilitation.

Notes

1. Drever, J. (1966) *A Dictionary of Psychology*, Penguin Books, Harmondsworth.
2. Jung, Carl G. (1968) *Psychology and Alchemy*, Bollingen Foundation Inc., NY.
3. Eastcott, J. (1978) *The Silent Path*, Rider & Co., London.
4. (a) Assagioli, R. (1980) *The Act of Will*, Psychosyntheses Research Foundation, London.
   (b) Assagioli, R. (1980) *Psychosynthesis*, Turnstone Books, Wellingborough.
5. Rowan, J. (1983) *The Reality Game*, Routledge & Kegan Paul, London and Boston.
6. *Meditation, Intuition and Dreams*
   (a) Perls, F.S. (1976) *The Gestalt Approach and Eyewitness to Therapy*, Bantam Books, New York.
   (b) Grof, S. (1979) *Realms of the Human Unconscious*, Souvenir Press, London.
   (c) Ferucci, P. (1982) *What We May Be: the Visions and Techniques of Psychosynthesis*, Turnstone Press, Wellingborough.
   (d) Garfield, P.L. (1976) *Creative Dreaming*, Futura Publications, London.

6 BODY-IMAGE

The Concept

The discussion in this chapter will pick up many of the threads of the preceding chapter on self-awareness. There is an inevitable overlap between 'self' and 'body-image' and although some of the themes may reappear, they will be treated in a different way.

Fisher and Cleveland[1] point to two different aspects of the 'self-concept':

1. The whole range of complicated attitudes and fantasies an individual has about his identity, his life role, and his appearance.
2. The attitudes which an individual expresses about himself verbally.

The self concept as described in this book would accord very closely to the first of Fisher and Cleveland's points.

Schilder[2] defines body-image as, '. . . the picture of our own body which we form in our mind; that is to say, the way in which the body appears to ourselves.' In other words, it is our mind's eye picture of ourselves. Schilder's work on body-image dates from the early 1920s but Critchley[3] (writing in 1950) traces the roots of the study of body-image back to Bonnier's work, around 1893, on 'coenaesthesia'. Coenaesthesia was referred to as, 'the sum total of sensations arising from without and within the body'. Somewhere (though its precise location cannot be stated with any degree of certainty but it is thought to be in the parietal lobe[3]) a part of the brain is responsible for being able to bring to our conscious awareness the total representation of our body. It is as if this awareness were then projected on to an inner screen[2] as a picture and we were looking at it through the eyes of an audience. Upon this screen will be displayed our physical shape and sensations — both external and internal — all of which are influenced by our attitudes, feelings, memories and experiences towards our bodies. Most people, when asked to close their eyes and move a finger, will have no difficulty in visualising this movement. Linked with this is the ability, with eyes closed, to point to, or touch, various parts of one's own body. Certain neurological and psychological conditions interfere with our body image; accurate touching then becomes difficult and often impossible.

Fisher and Cleveland[1] '. . . definitely consider the body-image to be a condensed formulation or summary in body terms of a great many experiences the individual has had in the course of defining his identity in the world'. Within this body-image we not only register our own thoughts and opinions about our body but the impressions we receive from other people of how they perceive us. As a result of other people's opinions we may carry around a body-image of an 'ugly duckling' (or if not a total 'ugly' some ugly part) or a 'handsome prince' or 'princess'. Whether we have a positive or a negative regard for our bodies (or parts thereof) has a distinct bearing on our total self-esteem.

Howells[4] relates negative evaluations of one's body to feelings of low esteem, insecurity, as well as anxiety over pain, disease and body injury. Wassner[5] reminds us that the individual's awareness of body-image is strongly influenced by the socio-cultural environment in which he lives. A point which she does not take up is that people reared in one culture may experience devastating 'body-image shock' when they move into a culture where different emphases are ascribed to various body areas. This has important implications in therapy where a therapist of one sex carries out treatment on a member of the opposite sex. If in the native culture this is taboo, all manner of body-image problems may be raised. Wassner goes on to say, 'Body-image is the root of identity, self-esteem and self-worth, the bases from which a man functions.' The ability to function within a particular society is, in part, influenced by its cultural values. For example, in a society where strength and fitness are idealised, failing strength may produce unwelcome and unacceptable changes in the individual's perception of himself because he no longer fits the ideal. These changes may be so resented that they produce emotional disturbances. That is when counselling may help.

The Nature of Body-image

Many factors contribute to the formation of the body-image. Critchley[3] identifies three cardinal groups of factors: visual, tactile and proprioceptive. Yet, as he says, none of them is essential. 'One can exclude the operation of all three and yet a body-image can remain.'[3] If Bonnier's idea is correct — that the body-image is the sum total of experiences arising from without and within the body — then to Critchley's three cardinal groups of factors must be added a fourth — internal sensations. For the purpose of this chapter, discussion will centre on the external and internal influences which together make up body-image.

The following analogy is offered as one way of making clear the body-image concept. Imagine that a baby is born with a built-in body-image 'printed circuit'. All the pathways are there intact, but not yet activated. Gradually, as he develops, various pathways are activated by external and internal impulses. By the time he is adult the circuit has been completely activated and he has a more-or-less clear body-image. External impulses arise from the senses; internal impulses arise from the internal organs plus the activity of the mind. All of these external and internal impulses are charged with emotions and they frequently cause distortions in the body-image.

When people have been the victims of crippling disease or accident, or exposed to mutilating surgery, or psychiatric illness, resulting in a change in either the body or the psyche, the body-image is forced to undergo a similar change if it is to be congruent with the 'new body'. This adjustment is often painful and emotionally disturbing. It is as if part of the printed circuit has 'blown'; for it to work properly again a by-pass needs to be built in. The person may be able to do all this by himself but he may need counselling help. The 'printed circuit' may prove to be a useful image to give him to work on: to try to discover the defective part and then to effect a 'repair'.

External Sensations

One of the delights of a parent is to watch a growing baby as he holds up an arm or a foot for his inspection. Very soon he will start to explore various parts of his anatomy. Inspection and exploration — visual and tactile sensations, as well as kinaesthetic and proprioceptive sensations arising from movement — are all part of the early stages of the developing body-image. At that age the baby will not understand that what he is looking at is his hand or foot, but gradually he will realise that they are his and part of his body. Hoffer[6] suggests that the foundations of one's body-image get under way by the age of six months. This assumption, however, would be difficult to measure, something which Hoffer admits. Nevertheless, the suggestion does have a certain amount of logic to it when one considers the dramatic amount of activity during the first six months of a baby's life. The early sensations of active movement are supplemented by movements of his limbs by other people. Visual, tactile and kinaesthetic/proprioceptive sensations are again brought into play. These early movements are built upon when he starts to crawl and then to walk.

> Movement stimulates the kinaesthetic sense which, along with touch, is crucial in the development of the body-image. Body-image influences perception of the environment by acting as a basic frame of reference for spatial judgements and it influences acquisition of motor skills through affecting the individual's ability to differentiate, control and co-ordinate body parts.[7]

Although this writer was speaking of dance therapy, what he says is pertinent in the development of body-image. Head[8] — a pioneer in the field of body-image — laid great stress on proprioceptive stimuli. His 'postural' model of body-image was developed almost to the exclusion of other sensations.

When considering visual stimuli, for example, it must not be overlooked that not all parts of our bodies are visible. Some are visible only with difficulty, by contorting ourselves or by the use of a complicated series of mirrors. Mirrors, of course, produce their own distortions of left/right reversal. Nevertheless, what we see of our bodies does play an important part in building up the body-image. Critchley,[3] however, points out that for blind people the lack of visual component of body-image is compensated for by tactile and postural hypersensitivity. So they do have a body-image.

Internal Sensations

External sensations are voluntary, sensory and motor. Internal sensations are involuntary, sensory and psychic. In the early stages of a child's development, many sensations are associated with the taking in of food and excreting waste. Associated sensations are of a tactile nature, some bring pleasure others bring discomfort. Just as with external sensations, it is difficult to be sure what is happening in the formation of body-image; so one has to postulate what the young child may experience within his body. From an adult point of view we could assume that just as we are aware of certain bodily activities of digestion, so is the baby. We feel hunger, and babies certainly do. And they very soon tell any listener when wind is causing them pain. But it is possible that the tiny baby possesses certain faculties which contribute to body-image awareness that are gradually lost as he grows older. Is it possible, for example, for the baby to be aware not only of the sensations associated with feeding, but also of the subsequent peristalsis as the food passes on its way? Under certain conditions — in a sound-proofed room, for example — we may 'hear' certain movements within our body, particularly heart sounds and blood flow. It is conceivable (although once again virtually impossible to test) that babies are aware of these sounds because they have not yet been crowded out by external auditory sensations. These internal sounds and sensations may very well form unconscious boundaries of body-image.

Boundaries of Body-image

If we did not have a clear awareness of our body-image there would be nothing to separate us from other people or from our environment. They, and it, could swallow us up, and we could become diffused as does a sea mist before a wind. Acutely disturbed psychiatric patients sometimes express feeling like this.

The most obvious boundaries are height, size (slim/fat) and general appearance — how we appear to ourselves and how we think we appear to others. Part of this is the regard we have for our bodies. One young lady, when asked about her body-image said, 'OK, from my neck down'. Some obese people feel a strong sense of disgust and loathing when they think of their bodies. Other people think of themselves as much slimmer than they really are; their body-image has obviously not adjusted to reality. Many people go to great lengths to change their body appearance and to make themselves more beautiful. 'Accentuation of the body-image is also brought about by such practices as the painting of toe-nails, the wearing of anklets, tatooing, sun-tanning . . ..'[3] Others undergo cosmetic surgery. All of these must, in some way, influence the body-image.

Clothing is another example of how the boundaries of one's body may be changed. Schilder[2] says, 'Clothes become a part of the body-image. The head-dress, for instance, enlarges the body and spreads it out.' The changing fashion of clothes must play havoc with a sensitive body-image! Change of attitudes is closely associated with change of clothing. Fisher[9] asks an interesting question. '. . . is clothing used by the individual to reinforce or deny certain body-image attitudes?' Clothes, then, may be a very definite boundary to body-image. Fisher also poses an interesting corollary. What happens when a person removes his clothing? Does a person who wears clothes as a boundary reinforcer feel exposed and vulnerable when he removes them? This question has implications for rehabilitation. A patient who does feel exposed and vulnerable when undressed, is likely to resist and resent this violence against his body-image. Resistance and resentment are almost certain to get in the way of effective treatment. Recognition of his feelings is one step towards helping him to feel less exposed and vulnerable.

In addition to clothing, other articles may extend and alter our body-image. The various fashions — including hair styles (of both men and women) and the often bizarre accoutrement of dress — all speak of a desire to extend (or diminish) the body appearance. Walking sticks, umbrellas, cigarettes (especially in holders), spectacles, the various 'tools of the trade' (the doctor's stethoscope) and so on, are all examples. A useful exercise is to think of a person you know well then see if the picture created includes any of the items mentioned, or any other item. A car is often one way in which we extend our body-image; for then the boundaries of the car become the boundaries of the driver. People whose body boundaries are extended by the body of a car must then make tremendous spatial judgements if they are to drive with due care and attention. It is possible that errors of judgement happen not when the attention wanders but when the body-image is at variance with the boundaries of the vehicle.

Passing fragments of thought must suffice to bring this section to a close. Do children become part of the body-image of their parents? If so, what effect does it have when their children are parted from them by great distance? And what effect if the children die? Do husband and wife incorporate each other within their own body-image? And what happens when one of the partners dies, or if they divorce? Do people who divorce not incorporate each other into their body-image? Are the houses in which we live part of our extended body-image? Do people who are confined in prison and in secure wards of hospitals experience a shrinking body-image? If so, what are the implications for rehabilitation for those who have been confined for a long time? Do they see themselves as Gulliver did in the land of Brobdingnag where everything and everyone was gigantic and, therefore, frightening? There are no definitive answers to these questions, but possibly in our various spheres of rehabilitation some answers may emerge to add new insights to this fascinating topic.

Changes in Body-image

Changes in body-image may be considered under three main headings: physical, neurological and psychiatric.

Physical Changes

From babyhood to old age our body-image has to make various adjustments to what is happening in our bodies. At one end of the age-scale we are developing quite rapidly in height, weight and strength; at the other end we again experience quite marked changes. In between these two age differences there is adolescence. Its accompanying sexual maturity brings dramatic changes; some of them are welcomed, others are so disturbing as to appear doubtful blessings. Adulthood brings with it different changes as new occupational and family responsibilities are taken aboard. Motherhood brings visible body changes to which women (and their partners) have to adapt. Critchley[3] says, 'In the former condition [pregnancy as distinct from pseudocyesis], little if any change takes place in the body-image despite the uterine dimension, while in the latter condition the swollen abdomen is probably clamant and ever present.' Work done by Benedek[10] and quoted in[9] would suggest that pregnant women incorporate the fetus into their own body-image unless there are strong feelings against the pregnancy, in which case emotional disturbance or even psychosis is likely. Women who cannot conceive are likely to experience great body-image conflict. In any pregnancy where the fetus was incorporated into the mother's body-image, the woman has to make a dramatic adjustment if an abortion takes place. She has to adjust to the missing part of her. If the pregnancy was an unwanted one, or if the fetus was not incorporated into the body-image, the woman still has an adjustment to make; but in the first case, I would suggest, the adjustment is greater, and may take longer.

Perhaps at no other time in her life is the woman subjected to such dramatic body-image changes as during the menopause. It is at this stage of her life when it seems that she is neither young nor is she yet old. Are the women who 'grow old gracefully' those who have successfully incorporated these changes into their body-image?

Men also experience body changes to which the body-image must adjust. Sexual difficulties, especially, create problems for many men; for most men's perception of masculinity centres around virility and potency. Thus, men who are infertile not only suffer emotionally, their whole concept of body is affected. Impotence and other sexual problems that interfere with a satisfactory sex life have a strong influence on the body-image.

Although men do not have a menopause, in their middle years of life body changes do occur. The man who once prided himself on his strength and endurance, now has to adjust to — if not exactly being a weakling — a body that does get tired much more quickly. Old age brings with it other changes — some welcome (like increased leisure and an increase in wisdom), others are not so welcome. A man who has been the 'breadwinner' now has to adjust to being a 'pensioner' and all that means in reduced activity.

All the changes which have been mentioned — for both sexes — may seem to require nothing more nor less than an emotional adjustment. But each change has very clear implications for body-image. No change can take place to, or within our bodies, without making some emotional impact. And, as was pointed out earlier, body-image is influenced by emotions of all kinds.

Neurological Changes

Distortions of body-image consequent upon neurological disturbances were the earliest body-image phenomena studied. A great debt is owed to those pioneering neurologists. Patients with certain neurological conditions may be unable to distinguish the left side of the body from the right; they may not acknowledge that parts of their bodies are paralysed. Some distortions are so unusual and bizarre as to '. . . indicate quite sharply that the individual is no longer thinking about his body the way he thought of it previous to his illness'.[1] These bizarre distortions may go as far as the individual believing that his body has disappeared or an inability to recognise his own fingers, to name them or to point out an individual digit when so directed.[1] In a study by Teitelbaum, quoted in[1], patients who had been hypnotised and were then directed to forget everything about their body, when they 'awoke' were not only unable to name parts of their body, they had problems doing certain tasks — naming objects, drawing geometric figures, naming articles of clothing, judging length, thickness and parallel lines. 'The most important result of the [Teitelbaum] study is that it lends support to the proposition that a relatively intact body-image is an anchor point or foundation necessary for the performance of certain judgments and skills.'[1]

The most well-documented body-image studies are to do with phantom limb phenomena — the illusory feeling that the missing part of the body is still there. Although these phenomena are usually associated with limb amputations, the experience can occur when any part of the body is removed. Pain is frequently experienced. Fisher and Cleveland[1] assure us that,

> with time the phantom limb usually shrinks and finally pretty much disappears. The phantom limb is usually felt initially to be outside the stump and then it gradually decreases its size and retracts and may in later phases, before it completely vanishes, be experienced as inside the stump.

Fisher and Cleveland quote research carried out by Dr William B. Haber in which he studied twenty-four male soldiers with unilateral above-elbow amputations. One of the tests he got them to do was to draw a picture of the phantom, relative to the stump. Half of the subjects drew pictures where the phantom extended beyond, or was even detached from, the stump. A Rorschach test revealed that those subjects who had extended/detached phantoms also scored low on boundary definition. That is, they had poor body-image. This study raises an interesting point. People who have a poor conception of body-image, and who experience a phantom, may be helped to define clearer boundaries, and so retract the phantom, by the use of the active imagery technique. Schilder[2] and Howells[4] suggest hypnosis as a way of helping patients who experience prolonged and distressing phantoms. The imaging technique, although having certain characteristics in common with hypnosis, is not identical; and it is a technique that the patient can be taught to carry out for himself.

Although most of the phantom studies have been on limbs, Schilder does say that phantom breast and phallus have been observed. Critchley[3] also says, according to the findings of Dr L.G. Kilch, '. . . phantom feelings are rare after a breast or an ear, but common after enucleation of an eye, excision of the rectum, or laryngectomy.' Speaking of the phantom rectum, Howells[4] says that this is quite common after rectal excision and that the phenomenon '. . . seems unrelated to age or sex, rectal pain, pathology of the disease, type of operation or healing rate of the perineal wound'. Children also experience phantoms. Howells[4] states (referring to the work of Hoffman[11]) that the phenomenon does not develop before the age of six years '. . . and this is thought to be related to the absence of a stable body image prior to this time'. While this may be true as a generalisation, a paediatric nurse teacher related how a boy of three years of age experienced great problems with a phantom, following a below-knee amputation. At that age, however, it would be difficult to determine precisely if the resultant pain was the main problem rather than a true phantom.

Pain is a common feature of the phantom phenomenon, and its severity varies from patient to patient. Some experience constant pain for several weeks; for others, the pain is experienced in peaks. Howells[4], speaking of 'psychological reactions to loss of a limb' says,

> persistent pain sometimes reflects the difficulty which certain rigid or compulsively self-reliant persons have in coming to terms with the facts of their loss [and] underlines, yet once again, the importance of providing adequate guidance and emotional support to the amputee.

Pain can be increased by having aggressive or violent thoughts or simply by watching violence on the television screen, or by concentrating on bodily damage.[4] Howells also reports that 89 per cent of people are still likely to experience the phantom after a year, but that the wearing of a prosthesis helps to retract the phantom limb back into the stump, thus indicating that the body-image has incorporated the prosthesis.

A study of 31 male and female subjects with various types of amputations, between the ages of 6 and 22 years of age, was carried out by La Fleur and Novotny.[12] Using a 'draw a person' test they concluded that, '. . . 17 of the 18 subjects (94%) who drew figures with four complete extremities were wearing a prosthesis'. This indicates a successful incorporation of the prosthesis into the body-image. They go on, '. . . [the] increased tendency to draw four complete extremities was evident the longer the amputee had worn a prosthesis'. In addition, congenital amputees, more frequently than the others, drew four extremities and labelled the prosthesis extremity 'real'. This study supports the view that the person who has had an amputation needs time to adjust his body-image to the change in this body.

A point that was touched on in several of the studies mentioned, but never developed, was that successful integration of the body-change into the body-image appears to be directly related to the re-establishing of self-esteem and self-worth. In other words, the lost part has ceased to stick out like a sore thumb.

Psychiatric Changes

In a review of body-image studies, McCrea *et al.*[13] have identified four categories of distortions manifested by schizophrenic patients as reported by Fisher and Cleveland.[1] The four categories are:

1. Masculinity/femininity. The distortions may be that the patient considers himself to be half male and half female. Or he may believe that he possesses the body of a female; or a female, the body of a man.
2. Body disintegration. The patient may experience loss of various parts of his body; e.g. the intestines.
3. Feelings of depersonalisation. Experience of unreality of part of the body or of his total body; as if he were an alien.
4. Loss of body boundaries. The patient feels that things happening to other people are happening to him. Injury to others is injury to his body.

Fisher and Cleveland, in their opening remarks to the chapter dealing with body-image in neuroses and psychoses, refer to a comment by Fenichel[14] to the effect that distortions in body-image frequently herald schizophrenic regression. They continue,

> This preoccupation with body function and the frequent reporting of perceived gross changes in body structure serve as adequate testimony to the radical shifts taking place in the body-image as these illnesses develop. Both the intensity and near universality of these kinds of body-image phenomena in mental illness raise the question as to the nature of the relationship between body-image and degree of emotional discord.

One female schizophrenic patient, on looking in a mirror, said to a nurse, 'Where am I? I can't see myself.' The same patient said, 'Is it me talking or is it you?' These distortions must have been very frightening for the patient.

One central theme runs through many of the accounts of bizarre body-image fantasies — violation of the body boundaries. 'The boundaries are either obliterated or become so plastic and vague as to be worthless either as a defence against all perceived threats or as a reference point to be used in distinguishing self from the other world.'[1] And Schilder[2] remarks that the schizophrenic patient often feels that his body is 'spread over the world'. Fisher[9] says, '. . . a psychotic person may maintain clearly delineated body boundaries as long as he continues to feel that he is a significant person with a meaningful role in the world.' The last part of this quote is significant for anyone engaged in counselling. If the person being counselled is able to feel a 'significant person' within the relationship, this may help to maintain his feelings of self-esteem and self-worth and so prevent loss of body boundary.

A person may 'convert' emotional conflict into one of a variety of physical symptoms, none of which has any organic basis. Among the symptoms are blindness, deafness, and paralysis of a limb.

The psychoanalytic view of distorted body-image, particularly in such hysterical conversion states is that '. . . a body part rendered non-functional by a conversion symptom is typically one to which unconscious sexual significance has been assigned and the incapacitation of the part represents an attempt to block the expression of sexual wishes.'[9] It would appear from a study of the literature that in almost all neurotic and psychotic states, distortions of body-image may occur. Fisher continues, '. . . schizophrenics and neurotics were characterised by significantly more sensations of body smallness than a matched normal control group . . .’. This observation is linked to the preceding paragraph. Where a person feels small, by comparison with something or someone, he also feels insignificant and of little worth. Anything that can be done to restore his feelings of positive self-esteem are also likely to help him grow in emotional stature.

Normal Changes

We thus see from this briefest of surveys of body changes — physical, neurological and psychiatric — that the body-image may undergo quite dramatic alteration. But it must not be thought that all distortions of body-image are pathological. So in order to correct this impression — if it has been created — this section will close with a discussion of ‘normal’ distortions.

When deep relaxation is induced, the person often states that he feels very heavy; that his body, or parts of it, became very large, or very small. He may become aware of sensations within his body. He may hear strange sounds and see strange ‘lights’ and patterns. He may experience feelings almost of hallucination. He may have the sensation of floating in space and that he has become detached from his body. All of these are normal distortions. They may occur to any of us as we hover in the hypnagogic state between being awake and dropping into sleep. When in sleep, strange distortions may be experienced and many of these experiences are alarming and emotionally disturbing. The border between what is normal and what is pathological is a very narrow one, and these feelings experienced in dreams, or near dreams, are what many mentally ill people — particularly psychotic patients — experience, only more so. The intensity and the frequency and the degree to which these experiences then start to influence a person’s life is one of the characteristic differences between normal and pathological. But it is important to remind ourselves that the needs of what is considered pathological lie within the normal. Body changes — external and internal — are all likely to produce distortions in body-image. Some people need a great deal of emotional support in order to accommodate body changes within their body-image. Those who cannot may well wander over the border into the no-man’s land of the pathological.

Summary

The concept of body-image, though not new, does not always receive attention in the literature of the various professions represented in rehabilitation. If one considers the areas covered in this chapter — which in no way exhausts the subject — perhaps more attention does need to be paid to the study of body-image, particularly as it relates to rehabilitation. Therapists, of all professions, work intimately with patients who are likely to experience changes and distortions in their bodies and, therefore, of their body-image. The therapist who understands the interplay between body and body-image, and how an integrated body-image influences recovery, will provide another avenue for fruitful exploration between herself and the patient. In the preceding chapter attention was drawn to the unique privilege that most therapists enjoy of physical contact with their patients. Patients who are experiencing emotional problems, related to their disability, may be helped to a better adjustment by the therapist working simultaneously with the body and with the body-image, using imagery techniques. People who experience distortions of body-image could be said to be 'out of touch' with their bodies. Physical contact — of the sort mentioned by Rowan in the preceding chapter — may be what the patient needs to help him get back in touch with his estranged body.

From the studies mentioned in this chapter, it would appear that there is no part of the body that is insignificant in the formation of the body-image. A corollary of this is that there is no part of the body which may not suffer from distortion, brought about by disease or trauma of some kind. Fisher and Cleveland[1] and Fisher[9] have both developed various detailed questionnaires to test body-image awareness. They also use the Rorschach ink-blot test. It is not suggested that therapists should involve themselves in administering these complex psychological tests; that is not the purpose of mentioning them. What these questionnaires and the results of the studies show, is that some people have a high awareness of their body as being distinct from all other people's and from the environment. Others have a low awareness, and because of this it appears that they are open to all manner of influences. On the dimension between these two extremes, of very high and very low, there are innumerable gradations. One of the principal observations, is that people with a high body-image awareness (or as Fisher and Cleveland call it 'barrier score') are more likely to incorporate satisfactorily body changes into their body-image than are those with a low awareness. An obvious implication for therapists is that recovery from disease or accident (if effective rehabilitation does depend to some extent on integration into the body-image of the disabled part) will be influenced by whether a person has a high or low body-image awareness. Coupled with either a high or a low body-image awareness are the attitudes the person has towards his body. People who are reasonably satisfied with their bodies are likely to have a high regard for them. While they may feel very keenly any assault on their bodies, and may experience distortions, they are more likely to make a better adjustment — in terms of time and incorporation into the body-image — than the person who has a poor body regard. These two correlates — body awareness and regard — could be two important factors in how well a person responds to rehabilitation.

An interesting observation (which supports the findings of La Fleur and Novotny cited on p. 120) is made by Polivy.[15] She suggests that following mastectomy, a decline in body-image only occurs several months after the operation. Whereas in women who had biopsies, which did not lead to operation, there was an immediate adjustment in body-image. She attributed this to denial on the part of those who had suffered the loss of a breast.

Denial is '. . . a primitive psychological mechanism, by means of which the unconscious mind struggles to push down out of awareness any thought which might cause pain to the organism.'[4] In order for the patient to adapt to the new state, he must work through and with the fear of what has happened as well as what may happen.

How the person regards himself, as well as how he compares himself to certain significant others, is discussed by Feldman.[16] He extends the study of body-image to include the individual's 'ideal' body-image (Figure 6.1). Feldman uses a repertory grid technique of 15 constructs related to 10 body parts of: self, mother, father, partner (either actual or 'elected') and ideal self: thus giving 150 elements. The method is one which has considerable merit for counselling in rehabilitation. The following modified scales are offered as a means of helping the patient and his therapist arrive at a clearer understanding of how the patient regards his body. Although the scales do not relate specifically to people with disability, the enterprising therapist will have little difficulty in converting the scales to include parts of the body affected by disability (Figures 6.2 and 6.3).

Another point that emerged from Feldman's study was how close or how distant the person views his body in relation to mother, father, partner and ideal self. The following scale makes use of this idea.

The following suggestions are given on how to use the scales.

1. The person completes the scales in the order, 'ideal self', 'personal self', and 'body distance' without referring one scale to the others.

2. The person compares 'personal self' with 'ideal self' and discusses any comparisons about which he feels dissatisfied.
3. Discuss the 'body distance' scale, particularly those areas of the body with scores 1 and 5. The results of this scale should be compared to the results of the other two scales.

An example may suffice. Andrew's scores on the dimension 'weak–strong' of the 'Personal Scale' were:

Figure 6.1: Body-image Awareness Scale — Ideal Self Scored on a Scale 1–5

IDEAL SELF

1	Face	Mouth	Hands	Skin	Belly	Sexual organs	Buttocks	Breasts	Teeth	Person	5
Kind	|	|	|	|	|	|	|	|	|	|	Cruel
Pleasant	—	—	—	—	—	—	—	—	—	—	Unpleasant
Ugly	—	—	—	—	—	—	—	—	—	—	Beautiful
Masculine	—	—	—	—	—	—	—	—	—	—	Feminine
Weak	—	—	—	—	—	—	—	—	—	—	Strong
Upsetting	—	—	—	—	—	—	—	—	—	—	Makes others feel nice
Large	—	—	—	—	—	—	—	—	—	—	Small
Worthless	—	—	—	—	—	—	—	—	—	—	Valuable
Shows feelings	—	—	—	—	—	—	—	—	—	—	Conceals feelings
Active	—	—	—	—	—	—	—	—	—	—	Passive
Cold	—	—	—	—	—	—	—	—	—	—	Warm
Gentle	—	—	—	—	—	—	—	—	—	—	Tough
Sexual	—	—	—	—	—	—	—	—	—	—	Unarousing
Clean	—	—	—	—	—	—	—	—	—	—	Dirty
Damaged	—	—	—	—	—	—	—	—	—	—	Whole

Source: Adapted by the author from the study of M.M. Feldman (1975).

Face	Mouth	Hands	Skin	Belly	Sexual organs	Buttocks	Breasts	Teeth	Person
1	4	5	2	3	1	3	3	2	3

When the scores were compared with his 'ideal self', the main discrepancies were in 'face' and 'sexual organs'. He scored 'face' low because he was very short-sighted and needed to wear 'heavy glasses with thick, ugly lens'. He did have problems with his sex life in that he did not feel assertive enough in his love-making.

His 'body distance' scores were:

Figure 6.2: Body-image Awareness Scale — Personal Self Scored on a Scale 1–5

PERSONAL SELF

1	Face	Mouth	Hands	Skin	Belly	Sexual organs	Buttocks	Breasts	Teeth	Person	5
Kind	—	—	—	—	—	—	—	—	—	—	Cruel
Pleasant	—	—	—	—	—	—	—	—	—	—	Unpleasant
Ugly	—	—	—	—	—	—	—	—	—	—	Beautiful
Masculine	—	—	—	—	—	—	—	—	—	—	Feminine
Weak	—	—	—	—	—	—	—	—	—	—	Strong
Upsetting	—	—	—	—	—	—	—	—	—	—	Makes others feel nice
Large	—	—	—	—	—	—	—	—	—	—	Small
Worthless	—	—	—	—	—	—	—	—	—	—	Valuable
Shows feelings	—	—	—	—	—	—	—	—	—	—	Conceals feelings
Active	—	—	—	—	—	—	—	—	—	—	Passive
Cold	—	—	—	—	—	—	—	—	—	—	Warm
Gentle	—	—	—	—	—	—	—	—	—	—	Tough
Sexual	—	—	—	—	—	—	—	—	—	—	Unarousing
Clean	—	—	—	—	—	—	—	—	—	—	Dirty
Damaged	—	—	—	—	—	—	—	—	—	—	Whole

Source: Adapted by the author from the study of M.M. Feldman (1975).

	Mother	Father	Partner	Ideal self
Face	1	5	3	5
Sexual organs	5	2	5	4

This showed a strong identification with his mother's 'face' and with his father's 'sexual organs': in neither part did he approach his 'ideal self'. In discussion, it emerged that he rated himself to be like his father whom he always regarded as not very masculine and very weak; he did say that his father had strong hands. He rated his own hands '5'.

Using the imaging technique Andrew put himself (or was guided) into various situations where he could compare his 'personal self' with his 'ideal self'. This, with discussion, helped him to move some way toward a more acceptable body-image.

Therapists in rehabilitation, as do their patients, have to realise that the patient's former 'ideal self' may no longer be fully attainable. He may have to readjust his ideal, particularly if some of the body areas on the scale have been affected by disability. This chapter is concluded with a résumé of the principal characteristics of body-image.

Figure 6.3: Body Distance Scale

Near = 1
Far = 5

	DISTANCE FROM			
	Mother	Father	Partner	Ideal Self
Face	_ _ _ _	_ _ _ _	_ _ _ _	_ _ _ _
Mouth	_ _ _ _	_ _ _ _	_ _ _ _	_ _ _ _
Hands	_ _ _ _	_ _ _ _	_ _ _ _	_ _ _ _
Skin	_ _ _ _	_ _ _ _	_ _ _ _	_ _ _ _
Belly	_ _ _ _	_ _ _ _	_ _ _ _	_ _ _ _
Sexual organs	_ _ _ _	_ _ _ _	_ _ _ _	_ _ _ _
Buttocks	_ _ _ _	_ _ _ _	_ _ _ _	_ _ _ _
Breasts	_ _ _ _	_ _ _ _	_ _ _ _	_ _ _ _
Teeth	_ _ _ _	_ _ _ _	_ _ _ _	_ _ _ _
Person	_ _ _ _	_ _ _ _	_ _ _ _	_ _ _ _

Characteristics of Body-image

1. Regard. Does the person have a positive or a negative regard for his body? It is necessary to ask the question about specific parts of the body. Is he satisfied or dissatisfied? What would be his ideal? What body experiences make for pleasure or displeasure?

2. Size. The way a person judges the size of his body, or a part thereof, is influenced by emotions and attitudes toward himself and his body and his relationship to other people. Men tend to overestimate and women to underestimate body size.

3. Awareness. Some people have a high awareness while others have a minimal awareness. '. . . individuals do focus a good deal of attention upon certain body sectors and minimal amounts upon others; and these patterns make sense psychologically.'[9]

4. Boundary. How does the individual experience the demarcation between his body and the outside world (which includes other people)?

5. Spatial. How accurately is the individual able to judge body position? '. . . it has become apparent that the spatial dimension is probably part of a broader category related to one's ability to separate what is significant from its context.'[9]

6. Anxiety. Some people are very afraid of body damage while others seem unconcerned about such a possibility. Fisher[9] indicates that there is little firm evidence that general fear is necessarily related to fear of body damage.

7. Masculinity/Femininity. Fisher[9] states, 'With rare exceptions, the male wants to tell you he feels masculine and the female that she feels feminine. Social desirability effects are pervasive and have rendered most masculinity/femininity scales ineffective.' Fisher poses the question, is masculinity/femininity concerned only with the difference in feelings about the genitals? Do men and women have different body awareness and is their attention directed toward different parts of the body? Fisher cites a few differences. Girls seem to be more concerned than are boys about distortions of the legs. Women seem more dissatisfied than men about the lower parts of their bodies. Males who experience failure are more likely to relate this to sensations of diminished height: 'It made me feel small'. In story compositions, males — after the age of 13 — focus less on the body than do girls.

There are many aspects of the body-image concept that have not been touched on at all in this chapter; others have been introduced but the themes have not been developed. Some themes will be re-introduced in subsequent chapters where they relate to specific physical, surgical or emotional conditions.

Notes

1. Fisher, S. and Cleveland, S.E. (1958) *Body-image and Personality*, Van Nostrand Co. Inc., New York.
2. Schilder, P. (1950) *The Image and Appearance of the Human Body*, International Universities Press Inc./John Wiley & Sons Inc., New York.
3. Critchley, M. (1950) 'The body-image in neurology', *Lancet, 1*: pp. 335–41.
4. Howells, J.G. (ed.) (1978) *Modern Perspectives in the Psychiatric Aspects of Surgery*, Macmillan Press, London.
5. Wassner, A. (1982) 'The impact of mutilating or trauma on body-image', *International Nursing Review,* 29: 3, pp. 86–90.
6. Hoffer, W. (1952) 'The mutual influence in the development of ego and id: earliest stages', *The Psychoanalytic Study of the Child*, vol 3–4, International Universities Press, New York.
7. Corsine, R. (ed.) (1981) *Handbook of Innovative Psychotherapies*, John Wiley & Sons Inc., New York.
8. Head, H. (1920) *Studies in Neurology*, vol. 2, Oxford University Press, Oxford and New York.
9. Fisher, S. (1970) *Body Experience in Fantasy and Behaviour*, Meredith Corporation, New York.
10. Benedek, T. (1960) 'The organization of the reproductive drive', *International Journal of Psychoanalysis, 41*: pp. 1–15.
11. Hoffman, J. (1955) 'Facial phantom phenomenon', *Journal of Nervous and Mental Disease, 122*: p. 143.
12. La Fleur, J.F. and Novotny, M.P. (1981) 'Studies of human figure drawings by amputee children and verbalization of their general adjustment', *Nursing Research Studies*, Chapter 33. Krampitz, S.D. and Pavlovich, N. (eds.) The C.V. Mosby Co., St Louis.
13. McCrea, C.W., Summerfield, A.B. and Rosen, B. (1982) 'Body-image: a selective review of existing measurement techniques', *British Journal of Medical Psychology, 55*: pp. 225–33.
14. Fenichel, D. (1945) *The Psychoanalytic Theory of Neurosis*, W. Norton & Co., New York.
15. Polivy, J. (1977) 'Psychological effects of mastectomy on a woman's feminine self-concept', *Journal of Nervous and Mental Disease, 164(2)*, pp. 77–87.

16. Feldman, M.M. (1975) 'The body-image and object relations: exploration of a method utilizing repertory grid techniques', *British Journal of Medical Psychology, 48*, pp. 317–32.

7 DISEASE AND PAIN

The Psychological Effects of Disease

Guilt and Disease

It is worth mentioning here that some people experience marked feelings of guilt that their body is ravaged by disease, or that they have to undergo surgery or that they are the victims of trauma of some kind. These feelings seem to originate in religious attitudes; but by no means are such feelings experienced only by avowed religious people. Such feelings possibly have their roots in the idea that man is created in the 'image and likeness of God' and any assault on the body is masked blasphemy. Some people, who themselves are not the victims, feel outraged that God's creation should be rendered less than perfect, possibly by wilful neglect. If this attitude prevails and if these people are closely involved with the sufferer, such an attitude can have a marked negative effect on treatment and rehabilitation.

The Skin

Disease may attack any part of the body, including the skin. Our skin — the most extensive organ — whether exposed or concealed — is our contact with the outer world. Blemishes on it, particularly if they assume emotional importance, affect the whole body. It would be very understandable for people who have skin disorders to regard their bodies — and therefore their personalities — as repugnant, the 'leper complex'. One part of the skin is the hair: loss of it requires a substantial emotional readjustment. Men generally go bald gradually. But when disease — either of the skin or of some other part of the body — strikes, and hair loss is sudden, results can be quite devastating. For women, loss of hair is likely to be more emotionally disturbing than for men. Toupees and wigs can do a great deal to make the man or woman appear more presentable, but underneath the hair covering, there may still be a great deal of emotional disturbance. Other exposed areas of the body, head, face (including the eyes, ears, and nose) and hands, are all body areas sensitive to disease and deformity and may become foci of emotional disturbance.

Other Parts of the Body

When other parts of the body — chest, abdomen, sexual organs and limbs

— are considered, we realise that disease in any one of these is likely to produce its own problems.

The Chest. Diseases of the chest may affect both heart and lungs which are interdependent. The lungs take in breath without which life would not be sustained. The lungs are among the organs that cleanse and refresh the blood and in so doing get rid of waste products. Linked as the heart is to this process, and having associations with emotions (the heart being sometimes referred to, poetically, as 'the seat of affections') it is easily understood how any disease affecting the respiratory and circulatory systems may produce emotional disturbances. Such emotional disturbance may localise in any part of the body almost as if some part of the disease had been carried to the spot by the blood.

The Alimentary Tract. The alimentary tract has a special place in the body schema, for it has an opening at both ends. In psychoanalytic terms any orifice has sexual connotations. Be this as it may, the abdomen, with its associated organs, is always vulnerable to disease. The alimentary tract is concerned with taking in, processing, and getting rid of waste. Any disease that interferes with this process may create anxiety, concerned either with a lack of nourishment or with a build up of toxins. Both of these anxieties may be physiologically unfounded, but to the patient, this sort of logic does not always prevail!

The Urinary Tract. The urinary tract, especially the parts that are involved in the function of urination, has an obvious link with the sex organs. Any disease (or trauma) that intervenes in the urinary tract is likely, therefore, to produce sexual difficulties with which, if therapy is to be fully effective, the patient may need counselling help.

Disease by itself produces emotional dysfunction as well as changes in the body. Disease that results in surgery has a double impact: something that is not always taken note of when the most appropriate rehabilitation programme for the patient is considered. In the preceding chapter, the importance of body-image and how various conditions may cause distortions was discussed. All the studies quoted were of subjects who had suffered some sort of trauma of body or mind. There does not appear to have been any work done on body-image related to disease, except where it results in disability. It is possible that when the body is invaded by disease of a crippling nature, that the resultant internal body changes do affect the body-image. If this is the case, and surgery results, the patient then has a double adjustment to make. I do not attempt to provide answers to these questions; perhaps they may point the way toward future study.

Crippling Disease

There are many crippling diseases with which rehabilitation therapists are involved. Many of these diseases would have been suitable to focus attention on in this chapter. In making a decision, on which disease to concentrate, the following criteria were laid down. The disease must: be widespread enough to be a problem for society, attack most age groups, be disabling in its effects, produce pain and have implications for rehabilitation. The disease chosen was rheumatoid arthritis, and this will now be discussed in greater detail.

Rheumatoid Arthritis. Rheumatoid arthritis (RA) is a relatively common disorder. It affects a wide range of people of all ages and of all social classes. Treatment for RA is palliative rather than curative and its crippling effects have serious social consequences by way of unemployment, often with resultant poverty. Locker[1] says, '. . . it has been estimated that 10 per cent of persons have some form of arthritis and approximately one third of these will have rheumatoid arthritis.' The progressive nature of the disease pushes the patient along the dimension from impairment — characterised by functional limitations — through disability, where activity is severely restricted, to handicap.[2]

Ehrlich[3] comments that

> Disease never occurs in a vacuum. It develops in a person who becomes a patient by virtue of seeking medical assistance. The narrow approach of offering medical, surgical and physical measures can grant symptomatic relief and is often all that is necessary for the treatment of acute illness. In chronic disease, of which arthritis is an archetypal representative, the best designed measures may fail if the full gamut of factors working upon the patient is not taken into account . . . A long-range plan of management requires multi-disciplinary attention, not the least of which must be provided by experts in the psycho-social sphere.

While it may not be possible to provide professional counsellors as 'psycho-social experts', the provision of counselling expertise as part of the repertoire of therapist skills would be possible if a more determined effort were made to ensure that such skills were acquired. People with chronic disease, 'of which arthritis is an archetypal representative', have to carry the double burden of the symptoms of the disease and the social consequences of a crippling and disabling illness.

Disabled people may well question their value as people and feel that they have no more contribution to make to society. This self-doubt is likely to occur in those people who, by virtue of their condition, are no longer able to earn a living. It also applies where the person is dependent on others to maintain even the basics of everyday living. Locker[1] quotes a case of a man who, severely limited by a wheelchair, was afraid to go out for more than 30 minutes in case he needed to go to the toilet. The toilets in his area were difficult to get in and out of and as he said, his wife could hardly take him in. This dependence on someone to help him with such a basic function caused him to devalue himself. It also severely limited his social contacts.

The person with arthritis has already had to accommodate to a changed body-image: a change that arises from both internal sensations (that cannot be seen) and external and visible changes. Counselling as a therapist tool, carried out in conjunction with other forms of therapy, may very well help to slow down the devaluing process by maintaining the person's self-worth.

The Clinical Picture. 'Rheumatoid arthritis is a chronic systemic disease with inflammatory changes occurring throughout the body's connective tissues.'[4] Although the disease affects both men and women, women are more prone to develop symptoms severe enough to require medical attention. The disease is characterised by swollen, painful and inflamed joints. Some patients experience active episodes with lengthy remissions. The more usual picture is of increasing frequency of attacks with subsequent joint damage and deformity. In addition to the joint changes, there is atrophy of muscles, bones and skin near the joint. Because RA is a systemic disease, other connective tissues — in the heart, lungs, blood vessels and pleura — may become affected. Owing to the effect on the blood-forming organs of the body, anaemia may be present.

The management of patients with RA aims at: rest, relief of pain, minimising emotional stress, preventing or correcting deformities, maintaining or restoring function, independence and mobility.[4] Patient education (of which counselling is an essential component) is necessary if the patient and his family are to be active partners in the rehabilitation programme.

Discussion of medication and physical treatment are outside the scope of this book; there are other authors more qualified to deal with the clinical aspects.

There are two linked topics that will be discussed: pain in this chapter and stress in the following chapter.

What is Pain?

No one definition of pain would appear to be adequate. One definition is '. . . a feeling of distress, suffering or agony, caused by stimulation of specialised nerve endings'.[4] According to McCaffery, 'Pain is whatever the experiencing person says it is and exists whenever he says it does.'[5] Bond[6] reminds us that pain is not present in the unconscious state, even although the unconscious patient will register physiological responses to stimuli. Generally, painful experiences are those we would avoid if we were able. (There are people, however, who actively seek painful stimuli and appear to derive pleasure from the pain. This book makes no attempt to deal with this experience.) It is an extraordinary fact that people vary greatly in the degree of pain they experience when subject to similar experiences. When treating people who experience pain, it is necessary to take account of what they say and try to get them to be as specific as possible. Pain arising from an external source — such as trauma — is easier to locate and describe than is pain arising from a hidden source. And some pain is almost impossible to describe.

Responses to Pain

In addition to what the patient says about his pain, the observant therapist will learn a great deal by watching the patient's behaviour. McCaffery[5] lists 8 categories of behavioural responses to pain:

1. Physiological
2. Verbal statements
3. Vocalisations
4. Facial expressions
5. Body movements
6. Physical contact
7. General responses to the environment
8. Patterns of handling pain

1. Physiological Responses. The physiological responses to sudden and intense pain are characterised by the 'fight or flight' reaction — anger, fear and anxiety. When the pain passes, the fight or flight reaction goes into reverse, as it were, in that the pulse rate slows and the blood pressure is reduced. When pain is repetitive, or of long duration, the sympathetic nervous system adapts to the continual stimulus. When pain becomes persistent and chronic, 'stress reaction' occurs, in which the delicate blood chemistry balance is disturbed.

2. Verbal Statements. When people are under stress, what they say is very likely to be influenced by the anxiety they are experiencing. Just as one has to listen carefully to what a child says, and pick out the salient points, so one often has to with adults who are talking about subjects which are coloured by anxiety. McCaffery[5] (quoting various sources) says that research has shown that physiological measurements taken when a person is in pain equate with what the patient says about his pain. She goes on to say that in order to get at the full significance of what the patient is saying about his pain, six factors need to be noted:

(i) *Presence.* Not all patients readily admit to having pain
(ii) *Severity.* They may use a word of lesser degree — none, little, a lot.
(iii) *Tolerance.* When the patient asks for relief, he has probably reached his level of tolerance.
(iv) *Quality.* (Taken from McCaffery.)

jabbing	shooting	pressure	spasm
gnawing	stinging	hurt	contraction
stabbing	pinching	knife-like	hot (burning)
cramping	stretching	sharp	discomfort
throbbing	constricting	bright	sore
pulling	cutting	dull	vice-like

(v) *Location and Duration.* The exact part, extent of the area — deep or superficial. Children may need a great deal of help to localise the pain and for how long it persists. If possible, link the onset and the duration of pain to some event, such as meal time.
(vi) *Rhythmicity.* How often does the pain occur and how severe.

It is also necessary to establish just how significant the pain is to the patient. He may relate the severity of his pain to his own idea of prognosis. He may interpret persistent pain as indicating that his condition is not progressing satisfactorily, or that he will always suffer pain, or that the treatment (or operation) has not been a success. The tone of voice and the speed of speech are indications of underlying feelings. Listening between the lines to the underlying feelings is a constant process in any patient/therapist relationship.

3. Vocalisations. Vocalisations are sounds that are not language. Included are groaning, gasping, screaming and whispering. Vocalisations have a particular relevance when dealing with children who have not acquired the skill of language.

4. Facial. Facial expressions frequently mirror feelings. Eyes, teeth and lips are all indicators of inner states of pain.

5. Body Movements. The following body movements frequently accompany pain:

(i) *Immobility* of a limb or the whole body in order to minimise pain.
(ii) *Purposeless or inaccurate movements* may result from excess energy, from trembling, from fear, or from the patient's inability to help himself or to relieve the pain.
(iii) *Protective movements* may be consciously controlled (running away, jerking the part away) or involuntary (or automatic reflex). Both voluntary and involuntary movements are a type of flight reaction.
(iv) *Rhythmic movement or rubbing* may indicate the area affected by pain.

6. Physical Contact. Physical contact may be self-contact or contact from others. The patient may use his own touch to bring relief from pain; he may, however, want the contact from someone else. Contact offered may be passively accepted, by for example, allowing his hand to be held, or actively accepted by gripping the hand of the other person.

7. Isolation. Pain which is prolonged tends to draw attention to itself. The patient may become so withdrawn as to exclude other people from his world. 'Aside from the feelings of the pain experience, he may focus only on his body and those things done to him which might affect his pain'.[5]

8. Handling Pain. The way a person handles his pain is influenced by cultural expectations; it is generally more acceptable for a child to express feelings about his pain than for an adult to do so, at least in some societies. The person's own life experience also influences the way he handles his pain — how he has learned to cope with pain in the past. McCaffery also lists anger, powerlessness, fear and guilt as ways in which some people handle their pain.

Adjustment to Pain

Anxiety, depression and insomnia frequently accompany pain.[7] This is borne out by Rachman[8] who says, 'Chronic and acute pain phenomena may require different approaches. Chronic pain control has been linked to depression and helplessness, while acute pain has been strongly linked to the presence of anxiety.' Illis *et al.*[7] maintain that '. . . patients in chronic pain exhibit much the same symptom stages as described by Kubler-Ross[9] in fatal disease.'

Kubler-Ross suggests that the person facing death has to progress through a sequence of normal, healthy emotional stages, starting from the onset of illness to death itself. Sylvia Poss[10] points out that '. . . the person who is dying will have far greater work to do if he has to accomplish it against a background of physical pain and personal humiliation.' When people who are beset by chronic pain can no longer find a meaning in life; when they can no longer rise above the pain; perhaps then they are in the same position as is the person when faced with death.

The Stages

The model developed by Kubler-Ross has five stages. It must not be assumed that these stages are mutually exclusive, nor that once having progressed into one stage that there is no return to an earlier one. The stages are:

1. Denial and Isolation. The person who is faced with the prospect of death withdraws emotionally. This isolation is important if he is to marshal his resources to start to cope with what is happening to him. In this isolation it is difficult for other people to make emotional contact. The sufferer feels that no one really understands.

Illis *et al.* maintain that that a person with a condition that holds no prospect of permanent relief from chronic and unremitting pain is in this first stage. It is a stage that is characterised by anxiety. 'The patients are usually unwilling to accept the abnormality, do not wish to hear treatment plans which do not include a cure and return to premorbid stage, and often go from physician to physician accepting therapies which give promise of a cure.'[7]

2. Anger. The anger — of patients facing death as well as those facing a life of pain — may be directed inward, toward himself, or outward to other people or just toward life in general. But anger is unhelpful if it imprisons the person behind bars of bitterness. Anger is destructive if it is prolonged to the point where it antagonises those who would try to help but who feel constantly repelled by it.

3. Bargaining. The dying patient begins to accept the fact that he is dying, but he does so by trying to lay down conditions: 'I will, if . . .' 'Give me a little longer then I'll . . .' In a symbolic sense, chronic pain, understandably, may be associated with death and dying, particularly if the pain leads to curtailment of activities and interferes with relationships. If one takes this view, bargaining, as part of the process toward acceptance, begins to make sense.

4. Depression. 'This stage [of adjustment to pain] is characterised by profound depression [which] may last for years. These patients have given up and have resorted to complete inactivity, hypochondriacal fixation upon the pain, the hopeless, helpless feeling of depression and the misuse of drugs.'[7] This is a fairly depressing picture of a chronic pain sufferer and there must be many people who are not like this. But those authors found many who did fit this picture.

Sylvia Poss relates depression to the sense of loss that accompanies the realisation that the illness (and its outcome) can no longer be denied. Speaking again of the dying (but with poignant relevance to chronic pain sufferers) Poss draws attention to two different depressions: *reactive* — in which the person is talkative; where he needs reassurance; where he needs to express his feelings in words. *Preparatory* — in which the person is silent; where there is a need for the expression of sorrow; where there is a need for company and love, not for words.

Chronic pain sufferers may need a great deal of counselling assistance to help them through these stages of depression. If, as Poss suggests, there is a need for the patient in the reactive stage to express his feelings, and if he is not helped to do this, he may become locked in to his reactive stage in which '. . . feelings of guilt, shame or aggression are turned inward'.[10]

Support for the view — that patients suffering from chronic pain are likely to be depressed — comes from a study of 100 patients treated for chronic pain, located mainly in the back or extremities.[11] 'Of the 100, 25 were definitely depressed, 39 were probably depressed, 36 were not depressed.'

The authors attribute improvement of depression to one or more of: acceptance of the pain, mastery of the pain, improved understanding of chronic pain with more realistic planning, involvement of the family in the treatment programme, increased physical activity, withdrawal from the effects of analgesics and sedatives, happiness about leaving the rigour and stress of the pain centre, or a change in the biochemical process resulting from a combination of the above physical and psychological factors.

In another study[12] of 120 chronically ill patients (mean age 54 years) and 33 controls (aged 18–47), anxiety, depressions, directly and indirectly expressed anger, and more helplessness were present.

These studies bring to our attention just how important it is to recognise that patients who suffer from chronic pain may also suffer psychological disturbance, sometimes of quite a serious nature. It follows that if the alleviation of pain is to be as successful as is possible, due account must be taken of the emotional factors which accompany the pain.

5. Acceptance. Acceptance is the final stage of the adjustment to dying with dignity and without despair. 'Acceptance is not happiness, but a preparedness to die.'[10]

Acceptance, as applied to chronic pain sufferers, means that they '. . . have come to grips with their abnormality, accepted their limitations, and are able to be treated in a reasonable fashion'.[7] Illis goes on to say that patients become suitable candidates for 'interventional procedures' only after they have been brought to the stage of 'rational acceptance'. To conclude this section on acceptance, the reader is referred back to page 18 of this book where the principle of acceptance is discussed.

Management of Pain

Relief from pain is medically desirable. Prolonged pain produces harmful physiological effects in the body. These effects may seriously impede recovery from illness. If the physiological changes are not halted, they may prove to have fatal consequences.[5] Attention has been drawn[13] to how pain may cause a patient to withdraw emotionally from his surroundings. So, relief from pain is psychologically important for the emotional well-being of the patient.

The rehabilitation of any patient must take place within his total environment. Rimón[14] asserts that

> A patient with RA can only be understood within the total life dynamics of which he/she lives; therefore, the physiological, psychological and sociological approaches should be incorporated in a comprehensive treatment approach. Such an approach may retard the advancement of the disability, decrease adjustment problems and psychic despair and provide the individual with hope and confidence for the future, including possibilities for an improved state of health.

If pain is all-invasive, the management of pain, as Rimón suggests, needs to be all-encompassing. Rimón's approach corresponds very closely to that suggested in this book. Therapists of all disciplines are realising that physical treatment by itself is not enough to treat the patient. If his psychological and sociological needs are not considered, physical treatment will proceed on shaky foundations.

Believe the Patient

'All patients with pain need to have their symptoms treated seriously. To reject it as "imaginary" is both a semantic error and an affront to the patient.'[15] This comment is salutary. It is fatally easy for one person to dismiss another's pain as trivial or non-existent — 'all in the mind'! Certainly pain can be 'psychogenic' — having an emotional or psychological origin — as distinct from pain which originates from an organic condition. Two personal anecdotes illustrate different aspects of this.

In 1946, when many servicemen were still recovering from the stress of war, I was nursing a Royal Navy officer who was suffering from an acute anxiety state. He developed severe abdominal pains and presented every indication of an acute appendicitis. The pain he was experiencing was obviously severe. He was operated on but there was no internal evidence of inflammation. His 'appendicitis', and the pain associated with it, was of a psychogenic nature; his anxiety had located itself in his abdomen. But, to him the pain was real; he felt it and responded to it *as if it had originated from organic change*. The reality of pain should never be dismissed. In contrast to the naval officer was Gillian, a girl of 14 years, suffering from leukaemia. She had been off treatment for well over a year when she began to complain of pain in her abdomen. The doctors, unable to find any accountable reason for the pain, referred her to a psychiatrist who treated her for psychogenic pain. Two months later Gillian was re-admitted in severe relapse with a massive flare-up. She eventually died.

These two cases illustrate the danger of 'labelling' pain as being one type or another. In the first instance, the pain *was* of psychogenic origin, and the abdomen became the focus of the patient's feelings of anxiety. In Gillian's case, the pain *had* physical origins but because no physical cause could be detected, the pain was mis-labelled as psychogenic. This, as Merskey commented, 'is an affront to the patient.'[15]

The Principles of Pain Relief

McCaffery[5] lists thirteen activities that may be used for the relief of pain. Of these, only four will be dealt with here. They are:

1. The therapeutic relationship
2. Other sensory input
3. Rest and relaxation
4. The use of imagery

1. The Therapeutic Relationship. The relationship that exists between therapist and patient is a unique one. For in it the patient will invest a great deal as he works on his rehabilitation programme. It is unfortunate that often, in order to prevent disability, or to minimise it, the patient may need to be encouraged to carry out activities that cause discomfort or actual pain. This may put a strain on the relationship. (In a way this is similar to what happens in psychotherapy where the patient experiences emotional discomfort and sometimes actual pain as the therapist helps him to deal with some difficult inner problem.) But in rehabilitation, if the therapist acknowledges that she recognises the patient's pain, and is not insensitive to it, the bond of trust will not be too seriously threatened. A frank acknowledgement of the pain may be just enough to relieve the anxiety (which so often makes the pain worse) and thereby reduce the pain. McCaffery[5] makes the point that eye contact with the patient in pain is one way of conveying concern. For some therapeutic activities constant eye contact may prove difficult, but even intermittent eye contact is more helpful than none at all. The therapist who works hard to establish and maintain a positive relationship with her patients is working at a deeper emotional level than someone who, though technically an expert, treats only the physical aspects of the 'case' and not the complete person. In the former relationship anxiety will be dealt with before it reaches crippling intensity. In the latter, anxiety is likely to build up undetected and act as a barrier to therapy.

Another aspect of the relationship is helping the patient explore the pain, not only as to precisely *when* it occurs, and *how* he could describe it, as well as its duration (in fact all the points mentioned on p. 136) but *what the pain means to him emotionally*. The patient may be unhappy, for example, that the pain makes him irritable, depressed, or prone to say things he would rather not have said. The whole question of pain in RA raises the point of the so-called 'arthritic personality'. 'The list of personality attributes ascribed to patients with arthritis is long.'[16] Then follows a long list of attributes that most people would classify as 'difficult'. But as Shontz[16] says, other studies show that while people with arthritis do differ in behaviour from people who do not suffer from chronic illness, when compared with other groups of chronic sufferers, there were few appreciable differences. Rusk[17] says, 'Pain produces emotional changes even in well-adjusted individuals.' It is important, therefore, not only to recognise that the patient is experiencing pain, but it is essential to give time to help him explore what he feels the pain is doing in him and to him.

An aspect of the relationship with the patient is the physical presence of the therapist. Pain is felt only by the sufferer. This isolates him from other people because pain draws the person's whole attention to itself to the exclusion of other stimuli. This point has already been made in a slightly different context (p. 137). It was also pointed out earlier that anxiety often accompanies pain: the presence of some trusted person may help to lessen the anxiety and with it the pain. The therapist, too, has to cope with the patient's pain. It is not a comfortable feeling to know that what one is doing (for the patient's benefit) is causing him pain. How the therapist reacts to this feeling may well influence how she helps the patient deal with pain. The therapist who cuts herself off emotionally from the pain is raising an emotional barrier between herself and the patient. She may do this by refusing to talk about the pain (avoidance), by talking about other topics (diversion) when the patient clearly indicates that he wants to talk about his pain, or by just listening passively (rejection). Both therapist and patient may feel that therapy has failed — or is failing — if pain persists or worsens. Fear of failure generates anxiety. The whole question of failure must not be swept under the carpet. If it is, it will act as a negative influence in the 'therapeutic relationship'.

2. *Other Sensory Input.*

Distraction. McCaffery[5] says that there is a positive correlation between pain relief and distraction. Distraction, by concentrating the attention on other stimuli, has the effect of reducing anxiety because the focus is elsewhere than on the pain.

> The patient cannot talk about the pain if he is talking about something else, and he cannot rub an injured area with the same hand he uses to move a chess piece . . . the more actively the patient participates in distraction the more effective the distraction is likely to be.[5]

Active involvement then, seems to be the key in distraction. The patient should talk through what is happening rather than be just a passive observer. Activities that involve all of vision, touch, hearing and movement are more effective than activities that use only one sense. Distraction is more effective if the activity is varied: one activity, if used over a long period, tends to lose its power to distract.

Cutaneous stimulation. The touch of another person's hand often brings relief from pain, as may the application of heat or cold. Immersing a painful limb in warm water, or the whole body in a hydrotherapy pool is a well-practised method of relieving pain. Massage is also effective. None of these measures need be carried out for prolonged periods. Indeed, '. . . moderate intensity of cutaneous stimulation is often more effective than high intensity'.[5]

3. Rest and Relaxation. Pain produces fatigue: tense skeletal muscles also produce fatigue. Patients who suffer from chronic pain — and this applies forcibly to arthritic patients — are inevitably tense in those areas of the body where they feel pain. Anything that can be done to reduce tension also reduces fatigue and pain.

Adequate sleep is an obvious way to provide rest and relaxation but as Bond[6] points out, '. . . in chronic painful disorders lack of sleep may be a major contributor to the patient's suffering'. Most patients who suffer chronic pain are prescribed analgesics but few therapists — other than nurses, when the patients are in hospital — are with the patients when they are trying to sleep, even with the aid of sleep-inducing and pain-relieving medication. So, it seems that the patient should be taught techniques that he can use when by himself.

Relaxation, which reduces physical and mental tension, also promotes sleep. Patients who are taught to relax, frequently report that, although the intensity of the pain did not diminish, they could bear it more easily and did not need the same amount of medication.[5] The pain did not seem to bother them quite so much. Deep relaxation, taught and practised when pain is absent, produces a somnambulant near-trance-like state. Some of the Yoga relaxation techniques are easily learned and taught and are very effective in producing deep relaxation.[18] Some of the books recommended in chapter 5 also deal with relaxation methods. A therapist may need to spend two or three sessions teaching a patient how to relax properly, but several patients may be taught at the same time. And it is time well spent! Susan, a tense middle aged teacher, suffered from asthma. She had been on medication for years but at no time had she ever been taught how to relax. After one of my own workshops we spent a half hour going through one method of relaxation. She grasped the principles of progressive relaxation and was determined to practise the technique regularly. Although this illustration does not deal with chronic pain, the principle is the same.

4. The Use of Imagery. McCaffery uses the term 'Waking Imagined

Analgesia' and says of it, 'The patient's use of his imagination to decrease his perception of the intensity of pain is an ancient phenomenon.'[5] The use of imagery is more than just another form of distraction. The patient recreates pleasant events and tries to re-experience every feeling attached to them. 'With an active imagination, the body begins to respond as it did when the event occurred.'[5]

Le Shan[19] suggests that people with chronic pain inhabit the world of nightmare, where terrible things, over which they have no control and to which there is no end, happen to them. If this is so, it is possible that therapeutic techniques that can enter the bizarre world in which nightmares are enacted may hold another key to pain relief. Imaging is one of these techniques. Pain interferes with sleep and, following Garfield's thought, sleep may be disturbed by nightmares. Most dreams and nightmares, especially persistent ones, contain within them the seeds of emotional release. Thus, dream interpretation is another technique which may be used to advantage. This subject is not within the scope of the present book. Many of the books referred to in chapter 5 provide excellent references and guidance for anyone wishing to pursue further the use of dreams as a therapeutic tool. Support for the view that the use of imagery is effective in pain relief comes from several studies quoted in a paper by Achterberg-Lawlis.[20] But the patient must be willing to use his imagination. Neither this technique (nor any other) can be forced upon an unwilling patient. Those patients who do use this method, combining it with deep relaxation, may find that they have acquired a double-edged powerful way of reducing the pain of rheumatoid arthritis.

Summary

Disease, whether acute or chronic, is an invasion of some part of the body. No one part of the body can be affected without the remaining parts also being affected. The longer disease remains located in the body, the more influence the diseased part exerts. In chronic conditions there is the distinct possibility of the diseased part being 'cut off' as unclean and unworthy. Disease which is accompanied by unremitting pain is a constant reminder to the patient of what has happened, or is happening, to his body. For many people, the pain is a reminder of happier days before they became afflicted. The occurrence of disease and its associated pain is, therefore, to many, a black day on a calendar; a crossroads to which they have been pushed by some unseen force over which they had no control. And the painful road they now tread leads on only to a bleak land of pain which threatens to engulf them in its blackness.

The pain and the disabling effects of RA interfere with many of the patient's basic activities of daily living and there are many such people who feel increasingly isolated by their disability. Many of them suffer psychological disturbances such as depression, anxiety and a deterioration in their relationships with other people, something that emphasises their isolation and withdrawal into themselves.

Sufferers from RA need a great deal of physical, psychological and sociological support if they are not to become enslaved by what many of them feel is the tyranny of disease and pain. Many physical treatments give relief from pain, but others — because they aim at preventing disability, or at least delaying it — increase the pain the patient already has. This puts a strain on the relationship between therapist and patient. Therapy must attempt to deal with all aspects of the patient and not just the physical. In order for the patient to be at peace with himself, he may need counselling help to encourage him to express his feelings about his disease and disability. In the terms of Kubler-Ross, he may need to be helped to grieve and mourn in the same way as a dying person needs to do this, if he is to die with dignity and without despair. Indeed, it has been suggested that only when the patient has reached the stage of 'acceptance' is he suitable for pain amelioration treatment. While some patients may reach this stage unaided, many more are likely to require counselling support in order to work through their negative feelings. Acceptance is not resignation. Acceptance is a calm and positive acknowledgement of a fact. Resignation is a passive and negative giving in to a fact. The one contains hope; the other, only despair.

Therapists working with RA sufferers can offer a great deal by way of pain relief, other than the administration of pain-relieving medicines. All the studies quoted in this chapter point to techniques and methods that therapists may use to relieve pain. Many of the techniques mentioned can be taught to the patient so that he can use them when by himself. When patients feel that the therapist is taking an interest in them as people, they in turn will relate to the therapists as people. Within this relationship the patient can be helped to explore his feelings toward his illness. Exploration of feelings, carried out within a trusting relationship, has the effect of reducing anxiety and the depression that so often accompanies pain-producing disease. The RA patient who suffers chronic pain often feels depressed. Depression carries with it emotional pain and isolation. The patient thus suffers a double burden — pain and isolation. His pain makes him withdraw into himself and his isolation is enhanced by his depression. Where the patient is encouraged to explore these feelings, pain (exacerbated by anxiety) will be relieved. Alleviation of pain has a positive infuence in depression. Counselling can break the vicious circle of anxiety, depression and pain.

Within the therapeutic relationship, and in addition to helping the patient explore the meaning of his pain, the therapist may use the technique of distraction — a combination of sensory inputs — and cutaneous stimulation. The other techniques of relaxation and the use of imagery are certainly ones that the patient may use by himself and they appear to offer insight into the patient's inner world while at the same time they aid in the reduction of anxiety and pain. Neither relaxation nor the use of imagery is complicated, nor are they difficult to teach. They could quite easily be taught in a group. Some other pain-relieving techniques (and relevant references) include hypnosis[5,13,19,21], behaviour modification[5,11–13,22], biofeedback[11–13,20,22] and acupuncture[23–25]. These four techniques are all ones that most therapists could learn to use and thereby help to reduce pain of any kind, but particularly pain that arises from a chronic condition such as rheumatoid arthritis.

Notes

1. Locker, D. (1983) *Disability and Disadvantages: The Consequences of Chronic Illness*, Tavistock Publications Ltd., London/Methuen, New York.

2. Wood, P. (1975) *Classification of Impairments and Handicap*, World Health Organisation, Geneva.

3. Ehrlich, G. (1972) Evaluation and research in arthritis, Proceeding Preview, Twelfth World Congress of Rehabilitation.

4. Miller, B.F. and Keane, C.B. (1978) *Encyclopaedia and Dictionary of Medicine, Nursing and Allied Health*, W.B. Saunders Co., Philadelphia.

5. McCaffery, M. (1972) *Nursing Management of the Patient with Pain*, Lippincott Company, Boston.

6. Bond, M.R. (1978) 'Psychological and psychiatric aspects of pain'. In *Modern Perspectives in the Psychiatric Aspects of Surgery*, Howells, J.G. (ed.), The Macmillan Press Ltd., London.

7. Illis, L.S., Sedgwick, E.M. and Glanville, H.J. (eds) (1982) *Rehabilitation of the Neurological Patient*, Blackwell Scientific Publications, Oxford.

8. Rachman, S. (ed) (1980) *Contributions to Medical Psychology*, Pergamon Press, Oxford.

9. Kubler-Ross, E. (1970) *On Death and Dying*, Tavistock Press, London.

10. Poss, S. (1981) *Towards Death with Dignity*, George Allen & Unwin, London.

11. Kramlinger, K.G., Swanson, D.W. and Maruta, T. (1982) 'Are patients with chronic pain depressed?', *American Journal of Psychiatry, 140*: 6, pp. 747–49.

12. Westbrook, M.T. and Viney, L.L. (1982) 'Psychological reactions to the onset of chronic illness', *Social Science and Medicine, 16 (8)*, pp. 899–905.

13. Broome, A. (1984) 'Psychological approaches to chronic pain', *Nursing Times* (8 February), pp. 36–9.

14. Rimón, R.H. (1981) 'Psychosomatic aspects of rheumatic arthritis', *Psychiatria*

Fennica (1981) Suppl 97–101. Taken from Psychological Abstracts 1981 Vol. 69 abstract number 10803.

15. Merskey, H. (1975) 'Pain'. 'Medicine' No. 10: *Psychiatry and General Medicine*, October.

16. Shontz, F.C. (1977) 'Physical disability and personality' in *Social and Psychological Aspects of Disability*, Stubbins, J. (ed), University Park Press, Baltimore.

17. Rusk, H.A. (1964) *Rehabilitation Medicine*, The C.V. Mosby Company, St Louis.

18. Mumford, J. (1962) *Psychosomatic Yoga*, Thorsons Publications Ltd., London.

19. Le Shan, L. (1979) 'The world of the patient in severe pain of long duration' in *Stress and Survival*, Garfield, C.A. (ed), The C.V. Mosby Company, St Louis.

20. Achterberg-Lawlis, J. (1982) 'The psychological dimensions of arthritis', *Journal of Consulting and Clinical Psychology, 50, 6*, pp. 984–92.

21. Scott, D.L. (1978) 'Hypnosis in Surgery' in *Modern Perspectives in the Psychiatric Aspects of Surgery*, Howells, J.G. (ed), The Macmillan Press, London (see reference 6).

22. Martin, N., Holt, N.B. and Hicks, D. (1981) *Comprehensive Rehabilitation Nursing*, McGraw-Hill, New York.

23. Inglis, B. and West, R. (1983) *The Alternative Health Guide*, Michael Joseph, London.

24. Lewith, G. and Kenyon, J. (1984) 'The physiological and psychological explanations for the mechanisms of acupuncture as a treatment for chronic pain', Special joint edition of the *Journal of Pain and Social Science and Medicine* (1984) 19 (12), pp. 1367–78.

25. Chaitow, L. (1983) *The Acupuncture Treatment of Pain*, 2nd edn., Thorsons Publications Ltd, Wellingborough.

8 STRESS IN SURGERY

Introduction

A chamber of horrors, calculated to arouse the most severe anxieties, would certainly include:

1. Fear of death or mutilation or pain.
2. Uncertainty about the future.
3. Feelings of helplessness and isolation.
4. Anxiety provoked by a strange environment.
5. Relatively impersonal and unresponsive caretakers.
6. Violation of privacy; constant intrusion into the core of one's existence — the body.

Such is the setting of the contemporary surgical service as seen by the patient. All of the above mentioned stressors are potentially pathogenic.[1]

In many ways this chapter is a continuation of the preceding one. Pain and stress are so closely linked that it seems almost artificial to separate them, albeit by a different chapter heading. It would have been almost as pertinent to relate stress to RA as to surgery but this would have been to leave a rich field unexplored. It is possible that the explorations in this chapter may disclose different parts of themes and topics dealt with previously.

The above quotation is a helpful reminder of the feelings that some patients may experience when they undergo surgery. In this chapter Elizabeth — introduced on page 12 — speaks of her feelings following major surgery. They so closely mirror the six points of the above quotation as to be uncanny. And just as many of the points about pain are relevant to stress, so also are the strategies of stress relief. For just as pain and anxiety are bound together in what may become a nightmare, so are stress and anxiety. When pain and anxiety are linked with the stress of surgery, the patient is subjected to what may prove to be an intolerable burden, leading to emotional trauma which may seriously hamper rehabilitation. Therefore, any measure that will lower the level of stress must influence the patient's recovery.

What is Stress?

Wolff[2], following the definition of stress as applied in mechanics, says, '. . . stress is the internal or resisting force brought into action in parts by external forces or loads.' He adds that stress is an effect and not a cause and that the effect is felt only within the individual.

Hans Selye[3] adds to Wolff's definition:

> In its medical sense, stress is essentially the rate of wear and tear in the body. Anyone who feels that whatever he is doing — or whatever is being done to him — is strenuous and wearing, knows vaguely what we mean by stress. The feeling of just being tired, jittery, or ill are subjective sensations of stress.

He goes on to formulate his concept of stress. Stress not only produces signs of damage but the body also produces 'adaptive reactions' as a defence against stress. Selye refers to this as the 'general adaptive syndrome' (GAS). The GAS has three stages:

1. Alarm reaction 2. Resistance 3. Exhaustion

If, as Selye says, it is difficult to arrive at a precise definition of stress, there can be no doubt that such a state does exist. He then goes on to define stress as, 'The state manifested by a specific syndrome which consists of all the nonspecifically induced changes within a biologic system.' It is worth pointing out that Selye did not believe that all stress was harmful (a certain level is necessary for effective daily living) nor that all stress agents were unpleasant. Some events (as we shall see later) are pleasant but at the same time stressful.

Engel[4] (although actually writing before Selye's published work) proposes that, 'A stress may be any influence, whether it arises from the internal environment or the external environment, which interferes with the satisfaction of basic needs or which disturbs or threatens to disturb the stable equilibrium.' Engel thus introduces another element, or rather states clearly, that stress may arise either from external or internal influences. But there is still the very strong suggestion that stress is purely a biological phenomenon.

The view '. . . that stress is a purely biological response' has been challenged by Mason[5] who asserted that a 'single biological response to a wide variety of stimuli is difficult to explain on a physiological basis'.[6] From the literature of those who throw down challenges to the GAS concept, it begins to emerge that stress is — as one would suspect — rather complex.

> The concept of a general stress reaction may be viable, but only if we assume that it represents the sum of a great many psychological and physiological factors rather than a specific all-or-none response to the occurrence of a stressing event.[6]

It will be noted that Bieliauskas, in the above passage, emphasises the psychological before the physiological and he justifies this by saying, '. . . while it is true that psychological characteristics of the organism influence the stress response, stressors can themselves be psychological as well as physical.' Thus far the discussion has moved from considering stress as a physiological response to one which has psychological origins but with physiological manifestations.

Rees[7] adds another dimension — the social. He says,

> My definition of stress will be any stimulus or change in the external or internal environment of such a degree in terms of strength or intensity or direction as to tax the adaptive capacity of the organism to its limit, and which, in certain circumstances, can lead to a disorganisation of behaviour or maladaptation or a dysfunction which may *lead to disease*. [my italics] What may constitute a stress may consist of physical stimuli, infections (bacterial, viral or fungal) or allergic reactions, or may refer to a whole series of stimuli or change in the social or psychological spheres of life.

This passage has been quoted in full, because there is so much in it. What is important is that stress may be so intense and so prolonged that the normal coping mechanisms are swamped (or exhausted, in Selye's term) and disease is likely to result. Rees's definition includes physiological, psychological and sociological factors. It is also interesting to note that definitions so often reflect the basic orientation of the person offering them.

Burchfield[8] says that it is necessary to distinguish between active, chronic and chronic intermittent stress because the organism reacts differently to these states. Acute stress occurs within a given time and may or may not be repeated. Chronic intermittent stress is caused by repeated exposure '. . . over a given time period, for a specified amount of time (usually less than an hour)'.[8] Chronic stress results from continuous exposure to some stressor. But not everyone responds in the same way to identical stimuli. Stress, then, is highly individualised. What produces stress in one person may have no effect whatsoever on another person. Rees[7] tells an amusing story of how one man felt subjected to intolerable stress by the constant demand of having to sort oranges into large or small grades. The constant decision-making pushed his stress beyond 'safety' level. In Burchfield's terms this was chronic stress.

In moving away from the physiological definition of stress we ended up with what was a comprehensive, if long, definition by Rees. So, taking all the definitions together, the following definition is the one to which the remainder of this chapter will refer.

> *Stress is the adverse internal and behavioural responses experienced by an individual, to one or more influences which have physical, emotional or social origins.*

This definition takes account of the accepted fact that there are many influences which arise from physical, emotional or social sources, but not all of them will be perceived as stressors by the individual.

The remainder of this chapter will be based on the following model (Figure 8.1).

Stressors

A stressor, according to Selye[3], is '. . . that which produces stress . . . it is also self-evident that any one agent is more or less a stressor in proportion to the degree of its ability to produce stress . . ..' In other words, only when something is perceived as hostile does it have the power to act as a stressor; adverse effects are then produced.

Before moving on to a detailed examination of the model, two points are worthy of mention. The first is that one cannot make assumptions about what is not 'distressing' for another person.[9] Neither is one able to predict that in a given 'stressful' situation someone will experience stress. The second point is that the action of a stressor is not specific to any one part of the body; stress acts in a general way on the body. Selye[3] says, 'Virtually every organ and every chemical constituent of the human body are involved in the general stress-reaction.' Later in this chapter we shall discuss some of the effects of stress on the body.

Life Events as Stressors

Possibly the earliest work done on the importance of life events, as potential stressors, was carried out by Adolf Meyer (1866–1950), a Swiss-American psychiatrist. In 1921 he said, 'The study of life problems always concerns itself with the interaction of an individual organism with life situations.'[10] And in 1925, in a paper entitled, 'Suggestions of modern science concerning education' he said,

Figure 8.1: A Model of Stress

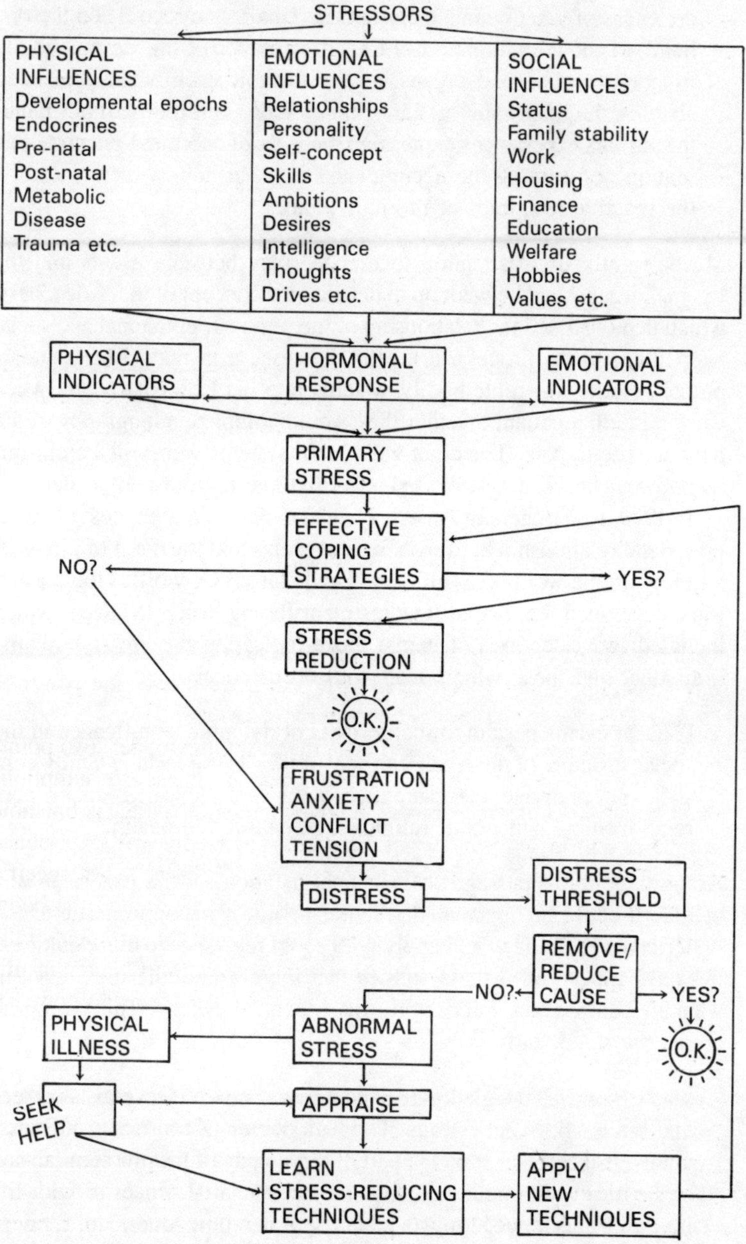

> No words of mine can give you a more graphic picture of the concreteness of what counts than the Life Chart — a record, on the one hand, of the condition and of the performance of the various bodily functions and special organs, and of the role each of these plays in shaping the biography or life of the person; and on the other hand, the various experiences expressing the lines of habit-and-resource formation constituting the accumulated mass of habits, memories and the reactive resources of the individual.[10]

Meyer rightly drew attention to the interplay between events and the 'special organs' and he went on to develop his concept of the 'Life Chart' which demonstrated the relationship of the physical, emotional and social happenings to the process of health and disease in man. Meyer incorporated eight vulnerable bodily systems into his Life Chart, and when working with a patient together they would complete a biography of the patient's life to date. The eight vulnerable systems were: the cerebrum, respiratory, heart, digestive, kidneys, thymus, thyroid and sexual.

In 1949, researchers in America began to devote a great deal of attention to the relationship between stressful events and the onset of illness,[11] building on the work of Adolf Meyer and Harold G. Wolff. Holmes and Rahe developed the 'Social Readjustment Rating Scale' (SSRS)[12] which included two categories of items: those indicating the life style of the individual and those which dealt with occurrences.

> [These] events pertain to major areas of dynamic significance in the social structure of the American way of life. These include family constellation, marriage, occupation, economics, residence, group and peer relationships, education, religion, recreation and health.[12]

A point about this passage bears special mention — 'the American way of life'. It could be questioned whether or not items appropriate to the American way of life would apply with equal relevance to other cultures. It would appear from these studies that there are similarities between what are considered significant in America and elsewhere. This was borne out in the same study

> where there was a high degree of consensus between Orientals, Negroes and foreign born Americans. The high degree of consensus indicated a universal agreement on the part of the subjects about the significance of the life events under study that transcended differences in age, sex, marital status, education, social class, generation American, religion and race.[12]

This may indicate greater commonality than difference. In another study,[13] which compared Americans and Japanese, the results, '. . . indicated essential similarities in their attitudes towards life events, but with interesting differences which reflect cultural variation.'

From these various 'Life Events' studies the researchers developed a scale of 43 'Life Change Units' (LCU) where each event, as a result of being submitted to over 5000 people,[12] was ranked and given a 'score'. Out of maximum score of 100 for each item, the top 7 were:

1.	Death of spouse	110
2.	Divorce	73
3.	Marital separation	65
4.	Jail term	63
5.	Death of close family member	63
6.	Personal injury or illness	53
7.	Marriage	50

The researchers drew attention to what has already been mentioned, that not all stressful events would be classified as 'negative'; the top six listed above are negative; but although most people would agree that marriage is far from negative it achieved a high stress score. Many stressful events are considered desirable in cultures where achievement is highly regarded. The practical value of LCUs lies in that it has been demonstrated that people who accrue 200 or more points at any one time, over a period of about a year, are prone to physical disease or psychiatric disorder.

The foregoing discussion has paved the way for a more detailed examination of the model presented on page 152. It is necessary, however, to point out, as with all human behaviour models, that although certain factors are put into boxes, the boxes should not be regarded as watertight. Indeed, in reality, it is the opposite. No one factor can remain insulated from all other factors which influence the individual's behaviour. In the box labelled 'physical influences', the primary influence arises within the body but what has happened, or is happening, to the individual also exerts a secondary (though not less important) influence on the emotions and social behaviour. It is not the intention to discuss every one of the influences listed in the three boxes, only to select factors that seem to have the most relevance for a continuation of the discussion of stress related to the central theme of this book.

Early Life Events

A point that does not appear to have been covered, in any of the more recent 'life events' studies mentioned, concerns the long-standing effects of some event (or events) in the individual's early history. If Meyer and other researchers are correct, there are many events that are beyond our conscious memory but which still exert their influence upon our present lives. Indeed, some researchers suggest that in early traumata — too painful to be borne — lie the foundations of neuroses and psychoses. It has been suggested that such trauma can occur pre-natally,[14,15] at birth[14,16,17] within the first six months of life (the object relations school of Melanie Klein),[18] about one year old[19] or at about three years of age.[20] It would thus appear that there is little agreement on the issue of how important it is to be able to date a specific trauma in its relation to psychiatric illness. But as Rowan[21] reminds us,

> It doesn't seem to matter very much what we believe about this, it is what the client believes that matters. As long as we as therapists keep an open mind, we can go with the client to wherever the client needs to go. The important thing is that crises in the person's life tend to re-activate the defences which were used before. This means that we have to go back down the chain of crises to find the original traumatic situation.

Rowan here brings out an important point, that we tend to respond to current events as we did to similar events in the past. These responses, while appropriate for a young child, are inappropriate for an adult. But it seems that we become 'hooked in' to responding in certain ways and it may require a great deal of concentrated in-depth psychotherapy to effect any substantial change in our responses. Later on, however, we shall see that even though we may respond in the same way to a given stimulus, we can apply techniques or strategies which will cut short any harmful effect arising from a particular response.

I would like to suggest that far from limiting the study of life events to the very recent past, it is necessary — as Meyer did — to take account of all events that the person considers to be significant. But not all people would readily count all events as significant; this is where the person may need guidance which will come from a discussion of the life history. It may not be sufficient to give a client a blank sheet of paper on which to write his biography. Breaking it down into years may seem tedious, but doing this helps to focus the client's attention. When the biography is complete, then is an appropriate stage to discuss the significance of various events *as the client perceives them*. Even if the event is dimmed by time, the emotions attached to the event may still be surprisingly vivid.

It was commented on earlier that if a person accrues 200+ LCUs he is heading for a crisis. Contrary to what has already been stated — that the critical period is the twelve months or so prior to the onset of illness — I believe that the person's whole life span is critical. If it is possible to accumulate stress factors over a period of one year, it seems equally possible to accumulate them over a lifetime (bearing in mind the point made about the age at which significant trauma is experienced); that is unless the individual has been able to cope successfully with stressful events without being left emotionally damaged. People who have been emotionally damaged are likely to require very skilled psychological help. Life events which damage, and which remain unresolved, add up to what becomes an intolerable burden. It only requires some 'last straw' to push the burdened person into physical or emotional illness, or both. So while the study of current life events is pertinent, it must not be separated from the person's historical life events. Stressful events of the past, together with recent stressful events, may all contribute to stress-related illness.

Developmental Epochs

Pre-natal. In the foregoing discussion attention was drawn to the importance of very early life events, it being argued by some authorities that significant trauma may happen at birth or even pre-natally. In addition to these early events, humans undergo some quite dramatic bodily changes involving massive hormonal alterations. These have startling emotional implications as well as social overtones.

Puberty and Adolescence. Puberty and adolescence, with their psychosexual development, are two epochs — or two parts of the same epoch — that most people would agree to be stressful. The stress arises from the conflict the young person feels between rapidly rising sexual feelings on the one side, and on the other, the social constraints imposed by society; constraints which may be both moral and economic. The young person is biologically capable of being a parent, but economically this is very difficult and socially is unacceptable. The biological changes that are taking place within the young person create some emotional upheaval, even in the most stable. The biological drive, which is pushing the young person toward maturity, only serves to emphasise to him the constraints laid upon him and often leads him into conflict with parents and others in authority whom he sees as responsible for thwarting his desire for independence. Intellectually he may accept that the constraints are reasonable, but emotionally he may not. This state of acceptance/non-acceptance leads to confusion, causing many young people to seek counselling to help them through this bewildering stage of their lives.

Pregnancy. The next major developmental epoch I wish to consider is pregnancy. This is usually one of life's happy events yet, according to the SRRS it rates fairly high — 40 — as a stressor. In the SRRS there was no indication if the score related to the woman or to the man. Yet for both there is stress, of a different sort and intensity, but definitely present for both. For a couple who enjoy a loving relationship, what affects one partner, in some way affects the other. The sickness and discomfort affecting the woman is often felt by the man. Women have to accommodate to a changing body-image, and some — those whose emotions are tied to their bodies — may experience extreme disgust at the visible changes taking place. Husbands who carry around with them an inner picture of their wives as slim, supple and active, may find difficulty accommodating the new inner picture. These conflicts can be stressful, as may the changes of mood that so often accompany pregnancy.

Birth. The stress of nine months, coupled with the physical and emotional stress of the birth, often sour what should be a happy event. The joy at the new member of the family is often muted by the subsequent stress caused by worry, uncertainty and disturbed sleep. The marriage may be subjected to stress as both partners have to accommodate the third member. So, another life event, although basically happy and exciting, has its own in-built stress factor. A study[22] of women toward the end of pregnancy, showed that certain of them — those with high life change scores, but with low social support systems — are more at risk of having complications with their pregnancy and delivery than are other women who have equally high life change scores but who also have high social scores. Effective support systems, therefore, seem to act as buffers against adverse life events.

Miscarriage. Other stressors connected with pregnancy are miscarriage, the very difficult pregnancy, and those instances where the course of a particular disease is worsened by the pregnancy. The trauma of a miscarriage is not, as some uninformed people would argue, 'over as soon as it happens'. The biological trauma of a terminated pregnancy is quite profound and it may take the woman many months before her body adjusts to what has happened. It may take a great deal longer for her to adjust psychologically. Repeated miscarriages are repeated psychological traumata. If pregnancy scores 40 on the SRRS, I would suggest that for some people, miscarriage should be scored significantly higher; for it has connotations of death and not — as a full-term pregnancy — of life.

Infertility. Of particular significance are those couples who suffer the trauma of being told, after having a barrage of tests, that one of them is sterile. Many marriages never recover from this blow to womanhood or manhood. The wounds experienced by a man who is sterile are very different from those experienced by a woman. Many such women feel unfulfilled while men who are sterile feel that they have not proved themselves as 'men'. While such feelings may seem illogical and difficult to understand, this sort of comment may not help:

> It's plain daft to allow yourself to become so obsessed with infertility that you let it come between you and all the good living there is to be done. To yearn hopelessly for what you can't have is to be like a baby crying for the moon. I have much sympathy with those who are disappointed but cope with the disappointment; very little with those who grizzle for the rest of their lives over it, or who allow themselves to become hard and bitter, or who seek pity for ever because they couldn't get everything they wanted.[23]

People whose emotions are deeply wounded know, intellectually, that they are behaving 'childishly' but seem unable to make themselves act like adults. Those who do act like adults can manage without counselling help. Those who cannot, need it. They are the ones who, if their life history is accurately traced, will, in all probability, have experienced some psychological trauma at an earlier stage to which this new trauma has become attached. The re-activated feelings from the past refuse to let go of the present hurt feelings. The double burden thus weighs them down. No amount of 'pull yourself together' will avail unless, and until, the person concerned has the opportunity to express the pain of the past and present. If people cannot do this they may well retreat behind the defences of resentment and bitterness. But these defences are usually brittle and liable to shatter under future traumatic events which in themselves may not seem to be earth-shattering, but whose cumulative effect may be. Counselling should aim at defusing this cumulative effect.

Now it is time to move on to discuss some of the influences within the 'emotional' section of the model. Any one of the factors listed could have been used as a basis for a discussion of emotional stress. But there is one factor on which I wish to concentrate — personality.

Personality and Stress

Personality is defined as '. . . that which constitutes, distinguishes, and characterizes a person as an entity over a period of time; the total reaction of a person to his environment.'[24] Some personality characteristics make it comparatively easy for people who possess them to get on well with themselves and with others. Other people possess characteristics that make them, in certain circumstances, difficult to get along with. Some people possess personalities which make them respond stressfully to certain life events. Some people can experience events of great trauma from which they emerge very much as they were before. Other people become so stressed by events that they emerge psychological cripples in whom some form of stress-induced disease permanently resides.

From a study of personality factors, it would appear that people who cope well with stress are those who: do not avoid dealing with the problem; do not act impulsively but consider the problem from all angles; are optimistic about the chances of success; are not too bothered about their own aggressive feelings; have a strong self-esteem; and are willing to act on their own convictions.[25]

Garrity, Somes and Marx[25], building upon the 14 factors of the Omnibus Personality Inventory (OPI) of Heist and Yonge, Form F[26] added the three dimensions of:

> Social conformity. '. . . the tendency to behave in conventionally approved ways and to espouse attitudes strongly approved in the respondent's social milieu.'[25]
> Liberal intellectualism. '. . . interest in academic, cognitive and intellectual issues . . . and behaviours generally identified with non-authoritarian and liberalism such as flexibility, acceptance of individual differences and independent thinking and action.'[25]
> Emotional sensitivity. '. . . the willingness to express and accept the expression of emotional feelings and concerns . . . [and] the appreciation of the fine arts.'[25]

The authors cautiously state, 'The introduction of personality factors into the life change model adds significantly, though modestly, to the predictability of health change.' From their research it would appear that people who are social conformists are more resistant to illness after life change. People who score high on intellectualism and sensitivity seem to be more at risk. The authors point out that certain characteristics of a person's personality (while difficult to measure) may predispose that person to life change stress. The person who cannot settle in one job, or in one location, and constantly seeks for 'greener pastures' may be creating self-induced stress because of a predisposition to be always on the move.

This view is supported by Jones[27] who suggests that aggressive and impulsive personality traits — often observable when the person is quite young — frequently lead the adult male into risk-taking behaviour in later life, associated with drinking and driving. Rees[7] states that as compared with control groups, people suffering from certain psychosomatic conditions exhibit personality traits of general instability, timidity, lack of self-assertion, anxiety-proneness, marked sensitivity and obsessional attributes. But, he qualifies, there is no evidence that any set of traits is the cause of any particular disorder. 'The important fact is that all these traits of personality are in different ways conducive to development of states of emotional tension in response to environmental difficulties and these in turn may precipitate attacks of psychosomatic disorders.'[7]

Friedman and Rosenman, in another personality study,[28] categorised people in 'A' and 'B' personality groups. They proposed that 'A' type people, because of their personality characteristics, would be more prone to premature coronary heart disease. The main characteristics of type 'A' are:

1. Multiple behaviour patterns — undertaking more than one job at any one time resulting in poorly done work.
2. Time restriction — trying to cram too much work into a given time — a race against the clock.
3. Inappropriate competitiveness with hostility and aggression. The competitive element pervades most activities. This is coupled with a persistent desire for recognition and advancement.
4. An intense, sustained drive to achieve self-selected but usually poorly-defined goals, coupled with extraordinary mental alertness.

Type 'B' people do not show many of the above characteristics. This study, of 3411 men between the ages of 39 and 59 years, showed that a very high proportion of those who developed coronary heart disease were originally diagnosed as having type 'A' personalities. It would thus appear that the cardiovascular system is particularly sensitive to the behaviours which characterise the 'A' type. Although coronary heart disease is probably the best recognised stress-related disease, hypertension, tension headaches and migraine, asthma, allergies of all kinds, peptic ulcers, ulcerative colitis, sexual disorders and skin conditions have all been investigated as stress-related diseases.[6,7,29,30]

Whatever the relevance of stress to disease, the authors quoted in this section, and many others whose works have not been quoted, are cautious in making any specific claims of just how personality factors do contribute to disease. But the weight of evidence does point to there being some link, though it is difficult to be clear what is cause and what is effect. When the life styles of men who have suffered myocardial infarct are studied, it would appear that multiple stress factors have been present for a considerable time. Statistically significant were '. . . a higher incidence of divorce, loneliness, excessive working hours, fluid consumption, night eating, sleep disturbances, nervousness, anxiety and depression'.[31] If these findings are related to the discussion on 'A' and 'B' type personalities, it is posssible to trace a link. There is one factor in the above list — work — which will form the basis for a discussion of social stressors.

Work and Stress

Some aspects of work as a stressor have already been touched on, in the type 'A' personality, for whom competition and excessive hours present a constant challenge. Work provides income, which enables us to buy goods and services, physical and mental activity, self-esteem — a recognised place in society, and social contacts. Occupational stressors have been categorised into four main groupings: problems of work load; problems of occupational frustration; occupational change; and other sources. Within these broad groups 17 sub-groups have been included. For a more detailed account, the reader is referred to Beech, Burns and Sheffield's work.[29] Only occupational change will be considered here.

Change is everywhere present, and rapid change is a feature in the working life of most people. Change seems inevitable, almost as if it were pre-determined, and most of us are caught up in it. If we are able to see the relevance and the benefits of the proposed change, generally we will accept it more readily. But even if we do appreciate the benefits, the change may still be stressful. 'Change can be distressful because it disrupts behavioural, physiological and cognitive patterns of functioning and because it requires adaptation.'[29]

An aspect of rapid occupational change is the stress of uncertainty about the future. If the only way a person can ensure that he retains a certain standard of living throughout his working life is by running ever faster on the occupational treadmill of long hours, intensive study, promotion, and relocation (usually with increased financial commitments), there is little doubt that this stress level will increase. 'Many young executives have their behaviours shaped into the type 'A' pattern as they feel that these are the ones necessary to success in the business world.'[29] But as Peter Nixon says, speaking of what has become known as 'adrenalin addiction', '. . . addiction of work-and-tension may be the chief impediment to cardiac rehabilitation.'[32] He goes on to say that most people live within normal, healthy adrenalin arousal limits

> but once you start deteriorating, then a set of vicious circles sets up. The tendency is to fight harder and work longer hours to keep up. This leads to greater exhaustion, and greater effort to compensate. This goes on until ill-health, and finally breakdown occurs.

The answer is to stay physically and psychologically fit and actively to seek ways of relieving stress.

There are many other occupational stressors that could have been considered, but space permits only a mention of a few, such as the physical environment — temperature, lighting, noise, fumes, desk or bench height and the proximity to, or isolation from, other people. In addition to the physical environment, there is the emotional climate which is created by the people who work together. Some people, by the very nature of their work, are exposed to a great deal of stress. Health care professionals are among such people. That is why it is important to be able to recognise indications of stress in oneself, and in others, and to be able to find ways to relieve it.

This draws to a close the discussion on stressors. The next stage in the model deals with the physical and emotional indicators of the body's response to a stress or stressors.

Hormonal Response

When an individual is confronted by a stressor, changes take place in the body as a result of the action of the adrenals and other endocrine glands. This increased activity prepares the body to take some form of action, either to attack the stressor or to escape from it. This is known as the 'flight or fight' reaction. The feelings most associated with these physiological and biochemical changes are fear or anger — the basic feelings that give rise to flight or fight. Most people have experienced these feelings — taking an examination, being involved in a road traffic accident or hearing bad news. In such situations one may become aware that one's limbs are trembling, that the colour has drained from the face and that there is sweat on the upper lip or on the hands. One may feel angry and realise that the hands are clenched as if to strike someone, and that one's face is suffused with colour. In both instances the heart rate will be increased and palpitations may be experienced.

If action is taken, the excess adrenalin and the sugar and fats, which the hormones have released, are used up. If no action is taken, it may take several hours before the excess adrenalin disappears. All the while the adrenalin level remains high, the physical and emotional indicators will remain, even though the stressor has long since been removed. In other words, the body remains keyed up and ready for action.

Primary Stress — Coping Strategies

What I have been describing is primary stress, and mostly people have developed successful coping strategies to deal with stress at this level. Some of those strategies are less valid than others because they bring with them other forms of stress. Among these would be drugs (which might include an increase in smoking or alcohol), loss of temper, hitting out at people, the cat or objects, perpetual tears and taking sick time. More valid strategies would be to use a problem-solving approach, to engage in 'time out' activity — take a walk, go for a run — work at a hobby, to talk it over with someone else; 'get it off your chest' or a period of relaxation. If the coping has been successful, stress will be reduced and the body will return to its pre-stress 'OK' state.

Sometimes there is little or no escape from a stressor. The young wife whose husband has been disabled as a result of an accident at work; the mother who has given birth to a mentally handicapped child; the employee who, by force of circumstance, cannot change his job to escape from a boss who tyrannises him; the teenager who cannot escape from a home where his parents are constantly at war with each other, are a few examples. If the person is unable to turn primary stress into an 'OK' state, he will experience

Frustration	F	increased emotional tension.
Anxiety	A	feelings of uneasiness, apprehension or dread.
Conflict	C	a painful state of consciousness caused by pressure of opposing emotional forces or desires and failure to resolve them.
Tension	T	the feeling of strain.

Added to this combination, acronymically referred to as FACT, the person continues to experience the physical and emotional indicators of stress which at this stage, if unresolved, begin to assume characteristics of an acute anxiety state.

Anxiety and Stress

According to one study,[33] people with anxiety suffer from a change in thinking and physiological activity. The change in thinking includes worry and dread and reduced concentration, forgetfulness, irritability and mood change i.e. depression and insomnia with nightmares. The fact that depression may accompany anxiety should not be overlooked; for if only the depression is treated, the underlying anxiety — and the stress which contributed to it — will remain untreated. The symptoms of anxiety above are fairly well known, but there is one which warrants special mention, that is insomnia and general sleep disturbance. Healey *et al.*[34] found that people who suffered from chronic insomnia had undergone more life stress during the year in which their insomnia started. Such people had a poor concept of self and suffered from frequent health complaints. The researchers suggest that '. . . poor sleepers internalise their reactions to stressful events rather than externalise their responses through overt behaviour.'[34] Sleep, and disturbed sleep, have been singled out for attention in this chapter because many people become quite anxious when just one night's sleep is disturbed: disturbed sleep — for whatever reason — may thus act as an additional stressor to a person already under stress.

Distress

Stress, if prolonged — because the individual has not developed effective coping strategies, or because there is no escape from it — will turn to distress. Rees[7] defines distress as '. . . an unpleasant emotional experience which may arise in response to environmental influences or to changes in some internal environment, or as a reaction to disease or disability'. Implied in this definition, and in the model that accompanies it in Rees's paper, is that disease may both account for distress and result from it. The discussion here will centre on the latter — that stress, if unresolved, will lead to distress which may then result in disease.

The Distress Threshold

Most of the studies referred to in this chapter consider the importance of stress related to disease; that is when stress becomes distress. Stress has become more than the individual can tolerate. A useful analogy is to think of each person as having a 'stress tank'. Mostly the stress we encounter is contained within the tank because there are numerous outlets by which the stress that is poured in is allowed to escape. But supposing the stress pouring in is greater than the outlets will accommodate, it is logical to assume that the stress will build up in the tank and eventually flow over the top as distress in the form of altered behaviour or in some physical or emotional illness. The point at which the stress becomes distress could be called the 'distress threshold'. The solution may appear simple; turn off the stress 'tap', or, alternatively, provide more outlets. The second may be easier than the first. It is not always easy to identify the stress factor, or if it is, as we saw earlier, it may not be so simple to do anything about removing it or to escape from it. It must not be assumed that people who respond to excessive distress by becoming physically or emotionally ill are weaklings. The strongest of us have a point at which we will crack. It may just be that some of us have not yet reached that point. Wolff,[2] speaking of war experiences — possibly that most dramatic of stress conditions — says,

> it may be inferred that *everyone* has a breaking point, that there are stressors that no man can withstand. Conflict in excess of an individual's current integrative capacity may increase the possibility of an individual being overwhelmed by frustration and conflicts, hitherto managed successfully.

A person overwhelmed is prone to stress-induced disease unless he finds ways to cope succcessfully.

Stress-reducing Techniques

If it is not possible to remove the cause of the stress, it may be possible to reduce the effects the stressor has by providing additional outlets. Counselling may help to unblock some of those outlets that have ceased to be effective. All of this is likely to involve the person in learning and applying stress-reducing strategies. The techniques for pain relief, mentioned in the preceding chapter, also have a place in the relief of stress and on page 164 of this chapter a few more strategies were suggested. But by the time the person has reached the stage of distress, the prospect of jogging or a game of badminton may not appeal. These would be distractions rather than getting at the fundamental problems. The most effective strategies are those which have a direct influence on the stress mechanism itself. These include relaxation, meditation, massage, the laying on of hands,[36] breathing exercises, controlled exercises such as tai-chi, the body work mentioned by Rowan[21] and the use of imagery. A most helpful exercise is to get the person to visualise the stress tank and to watch the stress pouring in, and as it fills up to visualise what the stresses are. The next stage would be to get him to visualise how the stress could be dissipated or neutralised. A combination of relaxation and imagery will work simultaneously on the body and on the emotions. A body brought under the calming influence of meditation or relaxation will, in turn, have a profoundly calming effect on the disturbed emotions which accompany stress. A body that has become habituated to living under stress may not respond immediately to a new technique. But if persevered in, the technique will work.

Stress and Illness

In one study of patients admitted to a medical ward, the patients' 'anxiety and depression' scores were higher in the first 24 hours than at any other time throughout their stay in hospital.[37] In another report,[38] nine stressors were isolated. Only the first four are included in this chapter. Out of 81 patients 58 (71.6 per cent) feared pain and discomfort, 53 (65.4 per cent) feared the unknown, 22 (27.1 per cent) feared destruction of body-image, 20 (24.6 per cent) feared separation from normal environment.

Strain and Grossman[39] listed seven categories of psychological stress to which the sick, hospitalised patient is vulnerable.

1. The basic threat to narcissistic integrity.
2. Fear of strangers.
3. Separation anxiety.
4. Fear of the loss of love and approval.
5. Fear of the loss of control.
6. Fear of loss of or injury to body parts.
7. Reactivation of feelings of guilt and shame, and accompanying fears of retaliation for previous transgressions.

These seven categories link very closely with the six severe anxieties, likely to be experienced by a patient who is admitted to hospital for surgery, listed at the start of this chapter.

Volicer *et al.*[40] identify nine factors which contribute to how the person responds to hospitalisation. Their 'Stress Scale Events' scale covers 49 different items. Some of those items that produced the highest scores were those that reflected uncertainty — of what the exact diagnosis was or what the outcome might be. This supported the findings of other researchers. It would appear that lack of information accounts for a great deal of the stress felt by patients. This stress is heightened by ineffective communication between care staff and the patient.[37,39] Results from various studies show that the more effectively the patient is prepared for surgery, the better the prospect is for a good recovery. The more anxiety a patient experiences, before the operation, the more stormy the recovery is likely to be. If patients do not know what is to happen, they cannot prepare themselves. Inadequate preparation gets in the way of rehabilitation. Wilson-Barnett[37] points out that 'The value of reducing anxiety pre- and post-operatively to adaptive levels is two-fold. Apart from helping the patient to be less depressed, it is aimed at reducing biological stress processes, which have been demonstrated to interrupt healing processes.' Patients who, prior to surgery, were taught how to relax and how to breathe and how to move, experienced less pain, required half the amount of narcotics and were ready for discharge earlier than a comparable group of patients who had not been so prepared.[41]

The foregoing has prepared the way for Elizabeth's story.

Elizabeth — A Case Study

Social History

Elizabeth, aged 59, has been employed for the past twelve years as an information officer in a large industrial library in the South East of England. She has a staff of six. Her basic degree at Oxford was in modern languages; her second degree, in information science, was taken at Bristol. For several years she worked in various countries in Europe.

She lives with her two cats in a spacious, detached house in a much sought-after suburb of the town. Her house is not mortgaged and she has no financial worries. Her job pays well and she enjoys a comfortable style of living. Her parents died some thirty years ago; three sisters and a brother, now in their eighties, live in various parts of England: none lives near her. Elizabeth is a devout Roman Catholic and is active in church activities and local politics. She uses her considerable language ability as a freelance translator and interpreter. She also coaches up to 'A' level in modern languages. She is on the editorial board of a renowned scientific journal and has written many articles and tape slide programmes and a book. She is often in demand as a speaker at national and international conferences. France is her favourite holiday country; she visits it several times a year.

Clinical History

Elizabeth is a wiry, active lady who had been very fit until the onset of the illness which led up to her having major surgery in September 1983. She dates the onset of her trouble to 1972. She had moved to her present post in the spring of that year and in the autumn had bought her house with firm plans that she and her sister (older by eighteen years) would live together. They had barely moved in when her sister died, one day while Elizabeth was at work.

In 1980 her beloved cat, Topsy, died after a long illness. Elizabeth quickly took in a cat from the RSPCA. Within a week Lucy had produced four kittens. Elizabeth kept two of the four, Dandy and Rosie. When the twins were seven months old, Elizabeth came in from work one evening in November to find that Dandy had been killed by a car.

Elizabeth reacted badly to the death of her two cats. All the feelings associated with her sister's death were resurrected. She very quickly developed shingles. The doctor she attended did not seem to understand the depth of her grief reaction, and told her to 'pull yourself together or you'll break down completely'. She did 'pull herself together' and very quickly became involved once more in various activities. She adopted a second cat as company for Rosie. In May 1981, while on a lecture engagement in Strasbourg, she was taken ill with abdominal pain. The pain persisted when she came back to England. It was now waking her up at night. Her GP told her, 'It's all in the mind. You've gone over the top about your cats. Go away for a holiday. Keep a glass of milk on your bed-side table.' She trusted the GP, and thinking that it must be all in her mind, she went away for a holiday, but the pain went with her. She was not offered any medication. Over the weeks the pain worsened and she began to experience nausea and there was evidence of some rectal bleeding. She was suffering from lack of sleep, depression and self-doubt. 'I began to believe that I was neurotic. I just couldn't take myself in hand.'

In the early weeks of 1982 a pyloric duodenal ulcer was diagnosed. She was started on a 10 week course of cimetidine. Almost immediately she stopped the medication she had a crisis, with semi-perforation. This resulted in her being admitted to hospital and recommencing medication. From then on '. . . it was a miserable existence. I had to avoid every food I really enjoyed.'

In September 1983, when returning by car from a holiday in the North, she was attacked by 'agonising pain'. She completed the drive and was seen the following day by the consultant surgeon who had been involved with her case from the beginning. He arranged for an emergency operation the following day; it was to be a selective vagotomy and pyloroplasty.

Elizabeth Speaks

'Questions wanted to pour from me but some of them sounded so silly and juvenile. All I asked was "What will the effect be?" He told me that I would feel much, much better; there would be no more pain; that I would be able to eat normally again. He said all that the operation involved was a snipping of some of the fibres of the vagus nerve, to control the acid secretion. I felt relieved. I had imagined it would be a truly major operation. I had never had an operation in my life. Oh, yes, I did ask him if there was any risk. What I really was asking him was, "Am I going to die?" A question I couldn't ask was, "How long will I be away from home?" There was my home, my cats, the garden and of course my staff. There were so many worries I wanted to share and there was so little time to arrange anything. As I lived alone, the surgeon said he would arrange for me to have some convalescence. I didn't realise that I would need intensive nursing care, following the operation. I was so naive.

'I thought I was dying. Something had gone wrong and I reacted quite badly to the anaesthetic. I lost three days in the intensive care unit. That was a shock, particularly as the surgeon had told me I would be back in my room in a matter of hours. Hours, certainly, but 72! How did I feel? Indescribable! There is a hazy recollection of being forced to get out of bed, trying to hold my stitches with one hand and my drains and things with the other. Oh yes, I can laugh about it now, but at the time I felt humiliated and yes, betrayed, and totally unprepared. My stomach felt like a giant football filled to bursting point with wind that would shift neither way. I asked the surgeon how long it would be before I felt better. He said I would be over the operation in four to six months but it might be two to three years before I felt really physically fit again. "Mentally, that's entirely up to you." I could cheerfully have hit him. I was so angry. He didn't seem to care. Neither did anyone else, or so it seemed. I was twelve days in hospital. Twelve days! and I had thought, "Oh, just snipping a few fibres, a couple of days." Is everyone so simple? I couldn't eat; swallowing was so difficult and the wind kept threatening to choke me. Frankly I was terrified. I spent a great deal of the time in tears. My days were brightened by the flowers and gifts from my colleagues and friends. I did find the nursing staff very impatient. The whole hospital affair made me feel degraded. I was not a person any more.

'Then I went to the convalescent home, where I had the doubtful "privilege" of a small flat of my own. A super view — at the top of forty-three steps! I was like the Grand Old Duke of York; when I was up I was up and when I was down I was down! And down I certainly was. Depression overwhelmed me. This didn't exactly endear me to the staff. "What a lucky person you are. You have a nice flat, lots of visitors, et cetera. Why should you be so miserable?" I suppose I was lucky. Many of the other people there were cancer victims and went for treatment every day. But it seemed totally outside of my power to do anything about my misery. I was treated as a three-year-old. I loathed the convalescent home. I had been forced to become dependent. Everything was automatically taken out of my hands. An example? "Here drink this" (a nursing auxiliary). "What is it?" "Never you mind, just drink it." It was a thoroughly wretched week. It was supposed to have been two weeks, but in no way could I have stayed a second week. Yes, I suppose I was a difficult patient. There was no daily treatment. I wasn't dying (although I often wished I had) and now I was insisting on going home. There was a total lack of understanding of my physical and mental condition. Someone wanted to take me to Mass on Sunday but the staff refused to allow me to go. The priest came but I was in no state to make confession. He talked, and as he did, healing came. I think he saved my sanity.

'There was almost a stand up fight when I told them I was going home. When they saw that I was determined, the only reply was, "Can you make your own arrangements?" I said I could, and did. There was no preparation for my going home; no advice, no guidance, no indication of what I should or should not do. Rehabilitation? I don't think it ever crossed their minds.

'A friend came for me. Then my troubles really started. I was totally unprepared (it seems that I'm totally unprepared for lots of things, doesn't it!) for how weak I felt. I couldn't do anything, no strength to even wash up or make my bed. Eating was difficult anyway and I suppose I just went downhill. Oh yes, I was depressed. I've never minded being on my own but the solitude, coupled with a mountain of fear, made my life quite unbearable. How did the depression affect me? I felt that I had reached the end of the line, useless; I would be forced to retire. My memory went completely, even to the stage that I couldn't remember my sister's phone number. I couldn't concentrate to read or write; I did listen to my music and did jigsaw after jigsaw. That was the level of my concentration. Emotionally I felt to be wandering in an endless desert.

'Oh yes, there was Rosemary; well-meaning but so undermining of my confidence. An example; one day I just fancied some wine gums. When she came back from the shop, what had she bought? boiled sweets! "I thought these might be better for you," she said. I was so deflated, having my intelligence challenged like that.

'The turning point came at my birthday, when I'd been home seven weeks. I think I'd got to rock bottom. There was a picture in my mind. I was locked in a house, staring through a window; people were going past but not taking any notice of me. The predominant colour was blue. Then my family came for the weekend. They brought me back to life. Richard encouraged me to take the car out. I had wondered if I would ever drive again. Things began to improve after that. Now I do feel so much better. But you know, people can be so thoughtless. When the Health

Visitor came she said, "Oh you'll throw this off after a month. It's quite common with your operation." When I didn't 'throw it off' I asked her specifically what had been involved. "The vagus nerve? I haven't a clue, really." I challenged her over her previous statement. "Oh that was just to give you some sort of confidence. I'd never met your operation before." My trust in her vanished instantly. Follow up? None! Not from the hospital nor from my GP. I had a picture of the inside of my body, as if it were an electric cable that had been severed in several places; power was trying to get through, but couldn't. My lower half felt quite separate from my upper half. I just knew that I wouldn't feel right until I could feel that my parts were re-united.'

Elizabeth's story was told with a mild humour that is difficult to convey and by the time the story was told, much healing — physical and emotional — had already taken place. But what she said highlights many of the points made earlier in the chapter. She had been totally ill-prepared for what was to happen. While it is true that her operation was something of an emergency, the surgeon had made light of the after-effects. He had not mentioned the severe discomfort or that several months would elapse before she would begin to feel well. The pain had been intense, but again this had not been mentioned as a possibility. A few weeks after she returned to work, she was taken ill; a doctor neighbour, knowing how little 'rehabilitation' she was receiving, and, therefore, not being afraid of treading on the toes of any other professional, diagnosed 'dumping syndrome'. His explanation, that this was something that frequently occurred in such surgery, both reassured Elizabeth and annoyed her. The reassurance came in that she was not suffering from something so dreadful that no one had dared mention it. The annoyance, mixed with a degree of resentment, came from the fact that here was a bit of information she could have been given which would have saved a great deal of worry. If the surgeon had explained to Elizabeth that dumping syndrome was nausea, weakness, sweating, palpitation and syncope, occurring after a meal, and that the symptoms are similar to a mild hypoglycaemia, I am quite certain she would have understood. Woodward[42] maintains that '. . . the majority of all these patients [partial gastrectomies and allied operations] can be spared the morbidity and discomfort of the dumping syndrome by proper post-operative management.' This advice is neither new nor revolutionary. Woodward was writing about this over twenty years ago.

Elizabeth's recovery was certainly influenced by how little she was told before the operation and afterwards. The point of this case study is not to slate the surgeon or the nursing staff, nor any one else, but to draw attention to how stress may both influence disease, and at the same time be an accompaniment to surgery, the aim of which is to relieve distressing symptoms. Elizabeth had been subjected to three bereavements — her sister and her two furry friends. Rees[7] says, 'There is strong epidemiological evidence that grief reactions are associated with an increased morbidity, including myocardial infarction and other psychosomatic and physical disorders.'

Elizabeth is probably more of a type 'A' than type 'B' personality and her highly technical work is also quite stressful. None of the factors leading up to the crisis, and the resulting surgery, appears to have been noted. Neither does there seem to have been any thought given to rehabilitation. Perhaps the need for rehabilitation after surgery is not considered important by those who carry it out. But Elizabeth's case demonstrates just how important it is. That Elizabeth's recovery was as good as it has been could be attributed to a sound personality that helped her to rise above the assault on her body. Coupled with this was the support she received from her wide circle of friends and colleagues. Another person, not so fortunate, whose emotional life was less stable, and who did not have an effective support system, might well have crumbled under the weight of the stress which could have led to further physical or emotional illness.

Summary

> Stress is the adverse internal and behavioural responses experienced by an individual, to one or more influences which have physical, emotional or social origins. (page 153)

Stress is a state which most people have experienced.[43] It could be argued that a certain amount of stress is unavoidable in daily living. This is true and provided we have been successful in developing strategies for dealing with what has been referred to as 'primary stress', no great harm will ensue. Sometimes, however, primary stress is dealt with inappropriately or inadequately; this then leads to frustration, anxiety, conflict and tension which, if not relieved will, in turn, lead to distress. Every person has a 'distress threshold' above which stress will seek an outlet, either in aberrant behaviour or in illness. The aim of counselling in conditions of stress is to help the individual develop viable strategies to relieve stress before the stage of overflow or 'flash point' is reached.

Three categories of stressors, physical, emotional and social, were identified. It would be erroneous to suggest that any stressor could be identified as operating only within one area of a person's experience. Life is too complex for such over-simplification. What is more likely is that all areas of the person's life will be affected. While a search for the main cause of the stress should not be abandoned, it is likely to prove more fruitful, in the first instance, to concentrate on developing stress-relieving strategies.

Several studies quoted in this chapter deal with the importance of life events as stressors. It was shown that people who accumulate 200+ Life Change Units, over the space of one year, are particularly prone to heart disease. It was suggested that events over a life time were also significant. Heart disease and other stress-related illnesses were related to the type 'A' personality — the type of individual who has become adrenalin addicted. Stress can often be the initiator of the vicious circle of illness, hospitalisation and more stress. Admission to hospital is often a very stressful experience. The stay in hospital, the treatment and subsequent recovery are all influenced by the degree of stress to which the patient is subjected. It was shown that the patients who are involved with their treatment experience less stress and are more able to respond positively to their treatment regimen. It could be argued — with conviction — that the patient has a right to be involved in his treatment. If he is to be involved he needs to be informed, and information, when given needs to be understood in all its aspects. Information, even if it is appropriate, when given inappropriately, will only serve to increase stress, not relieve it. Patients who are helped to understand what is happening, and are given ample opportunity to explore how they feel, are more able to accept the situation and respond positively to what is expected of them. But, it must also be borne in mind that some patients — either because of intellectual or emotional limitations — do not wish to know the details of what is involved in their treatment. It is equally stressful for such patients to be given information they cannot handle, as it is to withhold information from those who can.

A high stress level, often the result of mismanagement, seriously impedes recovery and rehabilitation. The stress experienced by patients in hospital can be effectively reduced by an active programme of education and counselling, the aim of which is to help the patient understand what is happening and to marshal his resources to help him cope with it.

Patients who, while they have been in hospital, have been helped to develop stress-relieving strategies, will take away with them something of inestimable value, which will exert a powerful and lasting influence on their lives by helping them deal with stress in such a way that it can be relieved before it becomes distress.

Notes

1. Baudry, F.D. and Wiener, A. (1975) 'The surgical patient', in Strain, J.J. and Grossman, S. (eds), *Psychological Care of the Medically Ill*, Appleton-Century-Crofts, New York.

2. Wolff, H.G. (1953) *Stress and Disease*, Charles C. Thomas Publishers, Springfield, Illinois.

3. Selye, H. (1957) *The Stress of Life*, Longman Green and Co. Ltd, London.

4. Engel, G.L. (1953) 'Homeostasis, behavioural adjustment and the concept of health and disease', in *Mid-century Psychiatry*, Grinker, R.R. (ed.), Charles C. Thomas Publishers, Springfield, Illinois.

5. Mason, J.W. (1971) 'A re-evaluation of the concept of non-specificity in stress theory', *Journal of Psychiatric Research, 8*: pp. 323–33.

6. Bieliauskas, LA. (1982) *Stress and its Relationship to Health and Illness*, Westview Press Inc., Boulder, Colorado.

7. Rees, W.L. (1976) 'Stress, distress and disease', *British Journal of Psychiatry, 128*, pp. 3–18.

8. Burchfield, S. (1979) 'The stress response', *Psychosomatic Medicine, 41, 8*, pp. 661–72.

9. Katz, J.L., Weiner, H., Gallagher, T.F. and Hellman, L. (1970) 'Stress, distress and ego defenses. Psychoendocrine responses to impending breast tumour biopsy', *Archives of General Psychiatry, 23*, pp. 131–42.

10. Winters, E.E. (ed.) (1952) *The Collected Papers of Adolf Meyer*, Vol. IV, The Johns Hopkins University Press, Baltimore.

11. Rahe, R.H., Meyer, M., Smith, M., Kjaer, G. and Holmes, T.H. (1964) 'Social stress illness onset', *Journal of Psychosomatic Research, 8*, p. 35.

12. Holmes, T.H. and Rahe, R.H. (1967) 'The Social Readjustment Rating Scale', *Journal of Psychosomatic Research, 11*, pp. 213–18.

13. Masuda, M. and Holmes, T.H. (1967) 'The Social Readjustment Rating Scale; a cross-cultural study of Japanese and Americans', *Journal of Psychosomatic Research, 11*, pp. 227–37.

14. Lake, F. (1966) *Clinical Theology*, Darton, Longman and Todd, London.

15. Feher, L. (1980) *The Psychology of Birth*, Souvenir Press, London.

16. Rank, O. (1929) *The Trauma of Birth*, K. Paul Tench, Trubner & Co., London. (Also R. Brunner, New York, 1952.)

17. Grof, S. (1975) *Realms of the Human Unconscious*, The Viking Press, New York.

18. Segal, H. (1979) *Klein*, Fontana, London.

19. Mahler, M. (1975) *The Psychological Birth of the Human Infant*, Hutchinson, London.

20. Duval, S. and Wicklund, R.A. (1972) *A Theory of Objective Self-awareness*, Academic Press, New York.

21. Rowan, J. (1983) *The Reality Game*, Routledge & Kegan Paul, London and Boston.

22. Nicholls, K., Cassel, J. and Kaplan, B. (1972) 'Psychosocial assets, life crisis and the prognosis of pregnancy', *American Journal of Epidemiology, 95*, p. 431.

23. Rayner, C. (1980) *Lifeguide: A Commonsense Approach to Modern Living*, New English Library, London.

24. Miller, B.F. and Keane, C.B. (1978) *Encyclopaedia and Dictionary of Medicine, Nursing and Allied Health*, W.B. Saunders Co., Philadelphia and London.

25. Garrity, T.F., Somes, G.W. and Marx, M.B. (1977) 'Personality factors in resistance to illness after recent life changes', *Journal of Psychosomatic Research, 21*, pp. 23–32.

26. Heist, P. and Yonge, G. (1962) *Omnibus Personality Inventory, Form 'F'*, Psychological Corporation, New York.

27. Jones, M.C. (1968) 'Personality correlates and antecedents of driving patterns in adult males', *Journal of Consulting Clinical Psychology, 32 (2)*, p. 2.

28. Friedman, M. and Rosenman, R. (1974) *Type 'A' Behaviour and Your Heart*, Knopf, New York.

29. Beech, H.R., Burns, L.E. and Sheffield, B.F. (1982) *A Behavioural Approach to the Management of Stress*, John Wiley and Sons Ltd, New York.

30. Glass, D.C. and Carver, C.S. (1980) 'Helplessness and the coronary-prone personality', in Garber, J. and Seligman, E.P. (eds), *Human Helplessness*, Academic Press, New York.

31. Thiel, H.G., Parker, D. and Bruce, T.A. (1973) 'Stress factors and the risk of myocardial infarction', *Journal of Psychosomatic Research, 17*, pp. 43–57.

32. Nixon, D. (1976) 'The human function curve', *The Practitioner, 217*, pp. 765–70 and 935–44.

33. Aitken, R.C.B. and Zealley, A.K. (1970) 'Measurement of mood', *British Journal of Hospital Medicine* (August), pp. 215–24.

34. Healey, E.S. *et al.* (1981) 'Onset of insomnia: role of life stress events', *Psychosomatic Medicine, 43, 5* (October), 439–51.

35. Selye, H. (1978) 'Stress without distress' in Garfield, C.A. (ed.), *Stress and Survival*, The C.V. Mosby Co., St Louis.

36. Krieger, D. (1975) 'Therapeutic touch: the imprimatur of nursing', in Garfield, C.A. (ed.), *Stress and Survival*.

37. Wilson-Barnett, J. (1979) *Stress in Hospital*, Churchill Livingstone, Edinburgh.

38. Carnevalie, D.L. (1966) 'Preoperative anxiety', *American Journal of Nursing* (July), pp. 1536–8.

39. Strain, J.J. and Grossman, S. 'Psychological reactions to medical illness and hospitalization'. See (1).

40. Volicer, B.J., Isenberg, M.A. and Burns, M.W. (1977) 'Medical, surgical differences in hospital stress factors', *Journal of Human Stress, 3*, pp. 3–13.

41. Egbert, L.D., Battit, G.E., Welch, C.E. and Bartlett, M.K. (1964) 'Reduction of postoperative pain by encouragement and instruction of patients', *New England Journal of Medicine, 270*, pp. 825–7.

42. Woodward, E.R. (1963) *The Post-gastrectomy Syndromes*, Charles C. Thomas, Springfield, Illinois.

43. Selye, H. (1974) *Stress without Distress*, Hodder and Stoughton, London.

9 THE TRAUMA OF SENSORY LOSS

Introduction

Many traumatic life events could have been the focus for this chapter. Surgery is traumatic, as is being stricken down with a paralysing disease such as poliomyelitis. A severe accident, which brings permanent disability in its wake, is trauma of yet another kind. Then there are emotional traumata such as bereavements or the birth of a child who is deformed or handicapped. In fact many of the topics that were covered in the previous chapter on stress are traumata. Every one of the events mentioned above is likely to produce its own particular emotional consequences.

I have chosen to concentrate on sensory loss — related to blindness and deafness — as trauma because of the important place both sight and hearing play in everyday communication between people. But I also wanted to draw attention to some of the difficulties that therapists may encounter when they are involved with people who are visually- or hearing-impaired. While the problems of children with visual or hearing defects will be mentioned, the discussion will not centre on them. I have decided on this because the needs of deaf or blind children are very specialised. It would be impossible to discuss the problems of blind and deaf children without also considering family relationships, education and training. While therapists may encounter children who have suffered the trauma of sensory loss, it is more likely that they will be called upon to deal with adults. Nevertheless, some reference to children is both appropriate and essential, for much of what applies to them also applies to adults who are deprived of hearing or sight.

The Stigma of Disability

Goffman, in the introduction to his now classic essay, says that stigma is 'a spoiled identity'. The term arises from the Greeks who burned or cut signs into the bodies of people to denote something bad about the moral status of the person. These signs drew attention to the fact that the bearer was a slave, a criminal, a traitor; 'a blemished person ritually polluted, to be avoided, especially in public places'.[1] Stigmatisation is an attitude. The stigmatised person is considered to be different from others, tainted, and not a whole person.

People with handicaps are often on the receiving end of the stigmatising attitudes of others. If one reflects on the origins of stigma it is easy to see how people would wish to separate themselves from, and not be associated with, stigmata. If those bearing these marks were criminals, or morally depraved, or in the case of the leper with his bell, 'unclean', it is understandable that people not so distinguished would regard these people as different from themselves. They may well have feared that contact with the tainted would have tarred them with the same. It is possibly significant that the only people who did not fear such contact (or if they did experience fear they did not let it act as a barrier) were those devoted to charitable works. Perhaps they did not fear contamination because they were secure in their identity and knew that the stigmata of others would in no way compromise it.

People of our own day who are disabled are often recipients of the stigmatising attitudes of the rest of us; attitudes which have been passed down to us just as surely as we have inherited many of our racial, national and familial characteristics. Coupled with this is the fact that certain people in our society have adopted the role of carer, caring for the individual whatever his stigma. In our generation we may no longer brand people with stigmatising marks, nor are they required to carry a bell and declare themselves 'unclean'. But just as indelibly we stigmatise physically and mentally handicapped people, people with psychiatric illness, people who are blind or deaf and many others who do not conform to the norms of society. Their presence threatens our identity. When we feel threatened we very often isolate the person or group by highlighting some difference that we call a defect which we ourselves do not possess. This makes us feel superior: by implication they are inferior. And while the stigmata are not visible — as they once were — they are no less felt by the people who are subjected to the same feelings that the outcasts experienced when they were branded as slaves, criminals or lepers.

Reactions to Disabled People

The reactions of non-disabled people are quite often to ascribe a low level of intelligence to the disabled person or to regard him as deficient in every faculty. 'He's a cripple but he's quite intelligent.'[2] Blind people are often shouted at and treated as if they were crippled. People who are not disabled react in different ways toward those who are. Some shower pity on them, some scorn them, some ignore them as if they (and their disability) did not exist. Many people who are disabled say how isolated they feel. Many try very hard not to let this isolation get at them; some of them succeed. Some disabilities evoke more constructive responses than do others. A person, who, with the aid of crutches is struggling to board a bus, will generally be given a helping hand. A blind person, pausing at the kerb will generally receive some assistance. A person whose movements are obviously spastic may not receive the same degree of willing assistance as he attempts to negotiate a difficult road-crossing. A person who is deaf, or suffers from a speech defect, or a person with no speech at all, does not evoke the same feelings of helpfulness in others as, for example, someone who is blind.

Some disabilities evoke the emotion of powerful helplessness and it is this that makes us turn away from people who are profoundly handicapped. If there is something we feel we *can* do, we are more likely to offer a positive response.

Goffman, while not actually spelling it out, hints at something else. Some people, it would seem, make capital out of their disability. It may be used to play on people's sympathy, to create a situation of helpless dependence and so manipulate people into satisfying their needs. Though this may be true for some it is by no means applicable to all. Some people have a fear that by helping someone, they run the risk of creating a dependent relationship. So to avoid this they do not become involved at all. While there are such people who shun any involvement, there are others who react in the opposite way. They foster dependence and engulf the disability and make it part of themselves. Unfortunately this attitude does little for the independence of the person with the disability.

Stereotypes of Disability

Sutherland[3] draws attention to the stereotypes of disabilities and the depersonalising reactions based upon these assumptions.

> visually repulsive; helpless; pathetic; dependent; too independent; plucky; brave and courageous; bitter, with a chip on our shoulders; evil (the twisted mind in a twisted body); mentally retarded; endowed with mystical powers; and much else. The fact that many of these characteristics are quite incompatible is an indication of how unreasoning such stereotypes are.

Attitudes towards people with disabilities are important. Provision of services and aids, as well as employment and grants, are all influenced by attitudes. If the attitude is one of pity, what the disabled are given is charity: they want to receive what is their right. The majority of those who control local and national spending are not themselves disabled; so perhaps it is understandable when they lack the vision for providing for those who are. Nevertheless, they should listen to people who themselves are disabled; perhaps then appropriate services will be provided. This point is an echo of the discussion on page 9 where constraints and conflicts were considered. Constraints and conflicts must always be considered alongside 'rights'. As long as people react in stereotyped ways towards people with disabilities, rights will not be recognised, neither will needs be met.

Reactions of Disabled People

Some people, as has already been mentioned, make emotional capital out of their disability; others fight it and live life as fully as possible. Some, because they refuse to compromise and cover up their disability, are often accused of making other people feel uncomfortable. But no one can make another feel anything. The fact that person 'B' does feel something as a result of what person 'A' is or what he does, cannot be denied. Person 'A', however, may not be held responsible for the feelings of person 'B'. This does not mean that we should be insensible to the feelings of others, but it would be more positive and would be more likely to lead to mutual understanding if person 'B' were to say something like, 'When we have contact I feel . . .' This puts the emphasis where it should be — with the person who experiences the feelings; it does not seek to put blame on person 'A'. There is no doubt that disability does create uncomfortable feelings in some people. Perhaps what they see is a stark reminder that, for them, disability could also be a painful reality. A similar point is made by Sutherland who says, 'This reverence for "normality" has little to do with our genuine needs. We have it thrust upon us because many able-bodied people have a great need to be reassured that there is nothing wrong with their bodies.'[2]

Goffman again draws attention to something which he calls 'passing'. This is where the person with the disability attempts to pass as 'normal'. Examples are; the partially sighted person who by not carrying a white cane refuses to draw attention to his disability; the hard-of-hearing person who, although he has difficulty hearing, will not wear a hearing aid. Some disabilities are more difficult than others to conceal. But 'passing' often creates acute awkwardness and strain. Brace,[4] blinded following a firework accident when he was a boy, records,

> I was flattered that I had 'passed' for five hours as normal, but at the same time angry with myself for putting myself in such a situation. *I* had worried about his sensibilities [a traveller who had not realised that Brace was blind] at the cost of my own. Yet if I was honest I had

to admit that I had been projecting my embarrassment of owning up to being blind.

Brace was not 'caught out' and he was able to laugh at himself afterward. George, too, could laugh at his effort not to disclose that he was very deaf. He hated the glass partitions in banks. Getting as near as he could, without actually poking his head through the gap, he leaned on the counter and fixed his eyes intently on the cashier. The cashier kept gesticulating at George and was saying something. George kept saying 'Yes, yes'. But his affirmations did nothing to soothe the cashier who was now becoming almost frantic. The background noise in the bank competed with the indistinct hum of the busy high street traffic.

> By this time [said George] the cashier was jumping up and down and he kept pointing at me. Suddenly my wife prodded me in the back and her lips said, "Your elbow". I nearly collapsed. I'd had my elbow on the bell all the time. The poor cashier. The whole bank must have been in an uproar. I can laugh about it now. I couldn't at the time. So much for my independence!

Most people who have disabilities complain of loneliness, isolation and frustration. These feelings are not lessened by the feelings they pick up from non-disabled people. Battye[5] says, 'The cripple is an object of Christian charity, a socio-medical problem . . . a vocation for saints, a livelihood for the manufacturer of wheelchairs . . . a means by which prosperous citizens assuage their consciences.' This may seem a harsh condemnation, but it expresses how many people with disabilities feel about stigma.

Robert Glanville,[6] a sufferer from rheumatoid arthritis, relates his experience of total inability to raise a mortgage-protection insurance policy from his house. He could secure one were he prepared to pay a premium many times the going rate. Margeret Gill[7] also draws attention to how disabled people are discriminated against.

> But when it comes to deciding who is to make the opening speech, take a chair at an important meeting, propose a toast at a dinner party, then often the disabled person finds that 'normal society' is ashamed of him. The reaction is usually, "Good Lord! Couldn't they find anyone better than a *cripple* to represent them?"

Let Hunt have the final word. 'One reason why we must resist prejudice, injustice, oppression, is that they not only tend to diminish us, but far more to diminish our oppressors.'[2]

Sensory Deprivation

Sensory Deficit/Sensory Deprivation. 'The born-deaf child has a sensory deficit which interferes with all aspects of his development — cognitive, intellectual, emotional and social — while the person who is suddenly deafened in adult life suffers an acute sensory deprivation which may affect his whole life style and call for many readjustments.'[8] Much of the above quotation from Denmark applies equally to blindness as to deafness.

The Need for Sensory Stimulation. Spitz[9] investigated the sensory deprivation suffered by children reared in institutions where there was little contact with other humans. Sheets were hung on the cot sides which meant that the baby could see little of what was going on. The children so reared experienced both social isolation and sensory deprivation. These children, when compared with another group raised in a stimulating environment, suffered more from infection and their mortality rate was higher. They talked less and were older before they walked. They showed signs of low intelligence, passivity and dependence.

Studies on animals showed that when reared in isolation they are more prone to react unfavourably to stress. As with isolation, when they are deprived of visual input during development, they are liable to suffer physiological damage. If the deprivation lasts long enough this damage may become irreversible.[10]

The sensory deprivation experiments on adults are well known and have been well documented. The results of some experiments, at times, conflict with the results of others but there is little doubt that most people react badly to being suddenly deprived of sensory stimulation.

To test sensory deprivation, subjects have been confined in rooms, in respirators and in water tanks; sitting, lying down or floating; in total darkness, diffused or subdued light; in silence, with reduced sound, or with white noise; for minutes or weeks; allowed some or no movement; with apparatus attached or unencumbered; and so on.[10] In such conditions, stimulation of all the senses is virtually non-existent. It would be difficult to say with any degree of certainty just what the influence of contact for feeding and elimination purposes would be; these procedures must constitute a break in the deprivation and thus help to keep the subject in touch with reality. Notwithstanding, most studies do show quite conclusively that even a few hours of deprivation produces startling and at times bizarre experiences. Several subjects in one study could not tolerate more than a few hours and were released via the 'panic button'. The following sensations have been reported.

Hallucinations and Images. Although subjects started off being amused or fascinated by these hallucinations and images, which varied from flashing lights and geometrical patterns to dreamlike actions, they very quickly became irritated by them, especially when they interfered with sleep.

Intellectual Difficulties. Subjects experienced inability to do problem-solving and arithmetical tasks. Prior to the experiment some subjects were determined to use the time constructively, but they found that concentrated thought very quickly gave way to random and free-floating thought.[11]

After-effects. The effects of being deprived of sensory stimulation persisted for several days after the experiment ended. It seems that subjects had difficulty readjusting to the real world. An interesting observation was that during the period of deprivation many of them felt a great desire to talk. This raises an intriguing question. Was this desire to talk related to the sensory deprivation or to the isolation imposed on them by the experiment? It would be too easy to draw conclusions from this; but if sensory deprivation — of those who have lost hearing or sight — does increase isolation, perhaps the desire to communicate is all the stronger. For the deaf, perhaps talking becomes easier than listening.

Patients in Hospital. Whether the desire to talk is influenced more by isolation than by sensory deprivation is debatable. It is accepted, however, that 'Too much rest, silence, solitude, and darkness loosen the patients' hold on reality and make them prey to fantasy.'[10] Does this give a possible clue to the sensorily deprived person who talks a lot? Is he striving to prevent himself from floating off into a world of fantasy? The writer goes on, '*Arthritics and chronic invalids too carefully protected from environmental stimulation may be affected similarly*.' [my italics]. This has an important bearing on many aspects of patient care. Premature babies, for example, are nursed on sheepskin to provide tactile stimulation. Other patients who need compensatory stimulation are those with eye disorders, and patients whose movements are restricted by heavy plasters, traction or respirators. Also included are those who are isolated from others because of some susceptibility to catch disease, those who have communicable diseases, and patients who have had mouth or throat surgery and are not allowed to talk. Sensory stimulation aims at keeping the person in touch with reality.

Several studies of patients in hospital demonstrate the vital importance of sensory stimulation. In one study[12] the authors reported that patients nursed in an intensive care unit that had no windows were twice as prone to delirium as those nursed in units with windows. Ashworth[13] says, 'The provision of a change of scenery for the patient . . . so that he can see through a window . . . is one means of increasing visual stimulation.' Visual stimulation is one way of reducing the risk of delirium and disorientation. It would seem from these two studies that patients, even when unconscious, or minimally conscious, benefit from visual stimulation via window light. Someone once said, 'There's more to a window than glass.' In symbolic form, a window is the meeting place — as is a wall or a door — between the outside and the inside worlds. In a way different from a door, a window permits communication, albeit vicariously, with what is taking place in the world from which the window separates us physically. A windowless room speaks of non-communication, a shutting out of the most powerful of all stimuli — the sun; and with the sun, some awareness of time, albeit perhaps only of night and day. A windowless room must give the impression of endless night. Too little is known of what exactly the conscious, or near conscious, patient perceives by way of his senses. Many nurses have been caught out by patients repeating what they have overheard as they lay 'unconscious'. The studies quoted stress how important it is to maintain appropriate levels of sensory stimulation for patients who so easily could be deprived of it.

When people undergo surgery for the removal of cataracts, they frequently experience what has become known as 'black patch delirium'; delirium and confusion caused by the total exclusion of light to both eyes. There are some very well documented studies, from as far back as 1894, where patients have suffered auditory and visual hallucinations, disorientation and behavioural disturbances associated with eye surgery. Many patients have attempted — and some have succeeded — to pull off their bandages, sometimes with sad results. These symptoms are more prominent at night, which is not surprising, when one considers that the normal noises of the ward are then hushed. In the strange environment of the ward, and deprived as he is of sight, the patient is placed in a world in which nightmares can take place. Weisman and Hackett[14] say that delirium is more likely to occur in the elderly than in the young. They also noted that 'private' patients were less likely to develop delirium. From their study, three factors emerge as being important in preventing postoperative delirium. They are:

1. The relationship between therapist and patient.
2. Adequate and repeated explanations.
3. Keeping the patient in touch with reality by discussing some important event or events of the patient's past.

They compensated for the patient's lack of visual stimulation by stimulating other senses. For example, they shared an Italian meal with one patient and encouraged another to recount tales of her childhood in Ireland. They concluded their study with these words, 'It has long been recognised that a friendly nursing staff, the presence of the family and the understanding support of the doctor will forestall delirium.'

It must not be thought that the three factors of Weisman and Hackett's study relate only to the prevention of a state as extreme as delirium. The mild confusion and disorientation experienced by many patients could so easily be forestalled by the quality of the relationship which the staff develop, keeping the patient in touch with the present through careful explanation of what is happening and lastly by encouraging the patient to link the present to some significant event from the past. These three points re-emphasise certain aspects of what takes place in counselling. Therapists who actively seek ways to minimise sensory deprivation, or help to compensate for the loss of one sense by stimulating others, will be helping to establish the sort of relationship in which counselling may take place.

The Stress of Disability

In the Life Events studies to which I have already referred on page 155, the death of a relative was given the highest rating. 'Personal injury or illness' was given a rating of 53. I would suggest that severe disability carries with it a substantial measure of stress of the kind normally associated with bereavement. Jack Ashley put it thus,

> I thought I had known despair, but now I felt a chill and deeper sadness, as if a part of me were dead . . .. At that moment [when he returned to the Chamber of the House of Commons and watched the Members as if they were miming] I felt in my heart that I had begun a lifetime of tomb-like silence.[15]

Kathleen Bowman, a nurse blinded as a result of an accident at work, says, 'There is an initial period of anger, fear, frustration and desperation

. . . which I now recognise as "mourning". Unfailingly this is usually seen as self-pity. This is nonsense. Why should we not mourn the loss of precious faculties . . .'[16] The opinion, that profound sensory loss is akin to mourning, is supported by Fitzgerald's study[17] of people who had become blind. Speaking of mourning, he says, 'The turning point was associated with increased self-esteem from attempting and mastering self-sufficient acts, and with the establishment of important inter-personal relationships with care-givers and other blind persons.' Readers who have experienced the death of a loved one will recognise in that quote similarities to their own period of mourning and subsequently picking up the threads of their life. Not everyone survives the trauma of disability. As I was preparing the material for this chapter there appeared a brief newspaper report which said, 'Keep-fit fanatic . . . hanged himself after doctor said he would never play squash again because of an eye injury.'[18] For that man, taking his own life was the only satisfactory resolution to his loss. That was his way of dealing with the stress of disability.

There are many factors which influence the way a person manages disability. Stubbins[19] puts forward the idea that certain personality types do not cope well with the stress of disability. They are:

1. The Adolescent — because he has not yet acquired stability of personality.
2. The Authoritarian Personality — because he sees everything in black or white terms and cannot tolerate ambiguity. The course of his disabled life is uncertain, and he lacks the ability to deal with uncertainty.

The person who does cope best with disability is the one who has a clear self-concept, is capable of tolerating ambiguity, whose values are more or less stable. Although Stubbins was speaking of the person with the disability, it must not be overlooked that relatives are also caught up in the stress of disability. How they cope must be dependent on how well they can tolerate ambiguity and uncertainty and how clearly defined is their self-concept.

The Self-concept

People with disabilities have suffered trauma of their self-concept. The self-concept is the cluster of feelings we have about ourselves — in every part — warts and all! Body image is a part of that concept. 'Negative evaluations about the body are associated not only with low self esteem and feelings of insecurity, but also with anxiety over pain, disease and bodily injury.'[20] The evaluation of self (for men) is often tied up with occupation and many women (though whether this will change as a result of women's liberation remains to be seen) define themselves in terms of roles within the family — wife, daughter, mother. Of equal importance are the whole range of complicated attitudes and fantasies an individual has about his identity, his life role and his appearance (refer to page 111).

To help a person assess his self concept it is useful to have a few 'coat-hangers' on which to hang the exploration. A useful approach is to identify what the person regards as the positive (the idea about what he is really like) and the negative aspects (the idea of what he is not like).[21] Here are some points:

Positive	*Negative*
Decisiveness	Conceitedness
Logical consistency	Lack of self-control
Self-confidence	Enviousness
Emotional vulnerability	Insincerity
Sincerity	Distrustfulness
Self-criticism	Inner insecurity
Nervousness	Spitefulness
Independence	Lack of self-criticism
Excitability	A tendency to being sarcastic

These are not intended to be 'opposites'; they were certain qualities that blind students identified as being important.[21]

A negative self-concept is not necessarily related to disability however crippling that may be. Severe and sudden disability produces 'shock waves' that rock the self-concept. Most people recover and their concept of self, although altered, is not permanently warped, however warped their body might be. This was borne out in a study of 14 paraplegic men where no significant difference was revealed between them and a control group. In contrast was a third group. These were patients suffering from tuberculosis who did show a marked reduction of self-esteem. The researchers suggested that this finding could have been influenced by the stigma of tuberculosis. 'One of the social implications is that tuberculosis is a dirty disease because it involves a great deal of coughing and expectorating. The TB patient may feel personally undesirable, unloved by his or her spouse and family and, in general, ostracised.'[22] The authors of the above article also suggest that the maintenance of self-esteem is due to pre-injury personality, economic security and present stability of relationships. They conclude, 'Rehabilitation counsellors need not automatically expect loss of self-esteem in their physically disabled clients, and if poor self-esteem is evident, it may be more advantageous to look elsewhere for the etiology.' A word of caution is necessary. While it may be true that a loss of self-esteem is not necessarily present *in the long run*, it would not be surprising that even the most well-adjusted individual would experience such feelings as an immediate reaction to physical disability. And if what the above writers say is true, then permanent loss of self-esteem may be forestalled by helping the person explore his feelings, maintain relationships and by aiding other people as they seek to support that newly disabled person.

Body-image and the Self-concept. In the above study, body-image and the concept of self are closely related. There is always the possibility, though by no means is it certain, that crippling illness or disability will produce changes in both body-image and the self-concept. On the other hand, Fisher[23] says that the majority of studies have found that disabled people 'do have lower self-esteem than the non-disabled'. While it may be difficult to state with any certainty which of these two studies[(22, 23)] is more correct, what is important is that we must always be prepared to hear what the patient is saying about his body and how he regards himself. And we must resist making assumptions based on the observations of other people. Fisher[23] says 'One cannot but be surprised by the capacity of the average person to assimilate gross body distortion and to come to terms with it. In this there is agreement with the study of paraplegics.[22] Nevertheless, it must always be borne in mind that however well the patient does eventually adjust, in the initial stages he is likely to experience a disruption of self-confidence, feelings of panic, confusion, depersonalisation, and anxiety or depression.

In chapter 6 (page 118) I drew attention to a study in which it was proposed that '. . . a relatively intact body-image is an anchor point or foundation necessary for the performance of certain judgements and skills.'[24] An inference which may be drawn from this is that people who have suffered a distortion of their body-image, as a result of some trauma, may then have difficulty learning new skills, particularly skills which involve fine judgement. The implications for rehabilitation are important. A patient who has had a traumatic amputation of a leg has to cope with the whole gamut of emotions associated with the loss. In addition he experiences tactile sensory deprivation coupled with decreased mobility. Alongside these, his body-image has to: accommodate a part that is no longer there and accommodate a 'foreign' part — the prosthesis. Accompanying these physical and emotional adjustments, he is almost certain to have to make a personal and social adjustment which may include learning a new skill or trade. If the hypothesis suggested above is correct — that a person with a damaged body-image may experience difficulty learning new skills — therapists may need to help such a person at the level of body-image and self-concept before he can be adequately motivated to press on to learning a new skill. In other words, a damaged body-image may act as an effective stumbling block to rehabilitation.

The Stigma of Sensory Loss

People who are deaf or blind, in common with people with other disabilities, experience the stigmatising attitude of society. The merry-go-round of life is geared to people who are sound of mind and limb and who can see and hear. Partially deaf or blind people are tolerated, provided they can manage without troubling the rest of us too much. Somehow there appears less stigma attached to blindness or deafness when the person is old. It is possible that the blind or deaf young person poses a greater threat to the rest of us than does a similarly disabled old person. Most people, as they get older, do experience a fall-off in hearing and sight. Impairment is then regarded as 'normal'. The attitude toward disabled people probably has its roots in the religious belief that such 'afflictions' resulted from past sins.[25] In this context, the attitudes toward blindness and deafness are similar but in other ways they are different.

Several writers have drawn attention to the fact that in the world of the theatre, blindness is of the tragic, while deafness is of the comic. Blind people were often treated as objects of pity and lived on charity. People who were deaf, in particular those who were both deaf and dumb, were treated as daft. People who poke fun at the disabled strike at those who are already stricken. There is still the tendency to treat deaf and blind people as if they lack intelligence and often they are not afforded opportunities which other people are offered. This point is made forcibly by Scott who says, '. . . the fact that blindness is a stigma leads them [other people] to regard blind men as their physical, psychological, moral and emotional inferiors. Blindness, is therefore, a trait that discredits a man by spoiling both his identity and his respectability.'[26]

From what various people say and have written, it seems that not only does stigma arise from society at large; the professionals also play a part in the process. Scott[26] says that blind people adopt the attitudes which professional blindness workers believe the blind person should have. When they refuse to 'conform' they are often accused of 'not facing up to reality', or some other controlling remark. Minton[27] also makes this point. In his book, 'Blind Man's Buff' he criticises professionals for trying to force blind people into pre-determined patterns of behaviour, particularly where the blind person is thinking about future occupation. The person who asserts, 'I'm not going to make mops for the rest of my life', is likely to be labelled 'difficult' and 'lacking in insight'. Yet it is this self-same desire not to conform, not to be lumped together as 'the disabled', that has enabled so many profoundly deaf and totally blind people to defy society's expectations and prove that they need not be objects of pity, destined to live the rest of their lives on charity.

Reactions to Loss of Sight, Gradual or Sudden

The adjustments to gradual or sudden loss of sight are different. The person who loses sight over a period does have an opportunity to get used to the idea, or so one could imagine. But in reality the fading sight produces its own hazards and stresses. 'If the loss of vision is degenerative, then it is often frightening even to go to sleep.'[16] A person with fading sight is likely to engage in the process of denial: 'It's not as bad as it was.' 'It could be worse.' 'I'm no worse today than I was this time last year.' The stress the partially sighted person experiences influences relatives and work-mates, as the visually handicapped person desperately insists on proving that he doesn't need the services that would help him live more independently.[28] Another difficulty of those with partial or failing sight is that acceptance of the loss is more difficult. All the while some sight is there, there is hope. A false hope gets in the way of rehabilitation. These false hopes are often unwittingly supported by care-givers who say things such as, 'Well it's possible that . . .' 'There's a one-in-a-million chance that . . .' 'Miracles can happen.' The study by Diamond and Ross[29] showed that soldiers remembered these phrases, even when they forgot many other things. These false assurances are, without doubt, offered by people who cannot face reality. If they cannot face reality, they are in no position to help the patient. Far better that the patient is engaged in frank discussion and is given the facts, sooner rather than later.

Klemz,[30] speaking of the problems of the partially sighted — as distinct from the totally blind — says, 'They must live permanently in a world of limited and distorted vision, and have the constant strain and frustration of trying to make sense of it.' This 'trying to make sense' is very real to many people with partial sight. And because they have some sight, their plight is not always recognised by other people. Some of the common, everyday difficulties are: shopping; reading directions and labels on goods (often in tiny print); mobility; reading street names and bus numbers; crossing the road. Some of the practical things that people with visual handicap worry over are: 'Am I wearing a pair of socks?' 'Is there a hole in my tights?' 'Is my make-up on properly?' 'Are there stains on my clothes?' Then there is the constant fear of misplacing something and not being able to find it. Some people are so neat and orderly that they have little difficulty keeping things in order. Others, because they are basically untidy, experience great difficulty with routine daily tasks.

Some people experience distortion of vision. Typical distortions are being able to read only parts of words, or as if looking through frosted glass or into a thick mist. When objects are recognised, they may appear twisted. Even when shapes are distinguishable, they may disappear when the light changes. Double vision and colour distortions are often present and emphasise the sense of unreality. Some people complain of parts missing from the picture they can see, as if it were peppered with gun-shot. Others complain of black patches in the picture. Thus, for some people, the world of partial sight may be more terrifying and confusing than the other world of total blindness. In total blindness, '. . . the mechanisms for coping with lack of sight may be brought successfully into play.'[17]

However long a person has had to get used to the idea that total or almost total blindness is just around the corner, where the shutters finally come down, he is then in the same position as another person for whom loss of sight has been sudden and dramatic. Fitzgerald's study[17] (see p. 186) in one region of London, of 35 men and 31 women who had been registered blind in the year preceding the study, showed the following:

Gradual loss of vision over one year or more	40%
Loss over two weeks to one year	25%
Loss over one day to 14 days	20%
Sudden loss over 24 hours	15%

Fitzgerald says, '. . . the intensity of the initial reactions to the loss seemed unaffected by either the rapidity of the loss or the amount of previous sight in all but a few of the individuals.'

Four reactive phases were identified: disbelief; protest and distress; depression; recovery. These phases are similar to those identified by Kubler Ross (p. 138) in people who have been bereaved, as well as in children suffering from maternal deprivation, amputation and deafness.[17] The reactions which scored 50% or above are listed:

Depressive affect	80%+	Anger	60%	
Anxiety	70%+	Weight change	60%	(increase 31 decrease 5)
Crying	60%+	Lowered self esteem	60%	
Withdrawal	60%+	Suicidal ideation	60%	
Somatic complaints	60%	Insomnia	60%	

This would seem to support the hypothesis that loss of vision is similar to bereavement. There the feelings of loss may be present for up to two years without becoming pathological. As Fitzgerald's study was of people who had become blind within a year, they had not been able to work fully through their grief. This showed in the affective reactions listed above. It is obvious that much more attention needs to be paid to the feelings of people who suffer sensory loss.

Another significant issue raised by the above study was how at risk certain people are of becoming blind.

> The single, widowed and divorced have a higher incidence of the diseases leading to blindness and they become blind more often as a complication of these same diseases. Two cases suggestive of this were men who had retinal detachments within weeks of their wives' deaths.[17]

While one would hesitate to draw conclusions from just two cases, caregivers should be alert to the effects on the body of the stress of bereavement.

Mobility. The skill and confidence with which blind people use the white cane often belies their feelings as they venture out on to the street. Most of them will agree that it is an emotional experience. Roy said, 'The first time I used it I felt starkly naked, knowing that I was broadcasting the fact that I could no longer see.' Brace[4] draws attention to how vulnerable visually handicapped people are, even when they are skilled white cane users. It is possible, as he discovered to his cost, to collide with scaffolding bars, and nearly fall into holes in the road, or to be tripped up by objects left lying around. He emphasises just how much the everyday world is geared to sighted people. On the other hand, many visually handicapped people do enjoy very active and full mobility which includes participating in sports of all kinds.[4,31] But the sport they once enjoyed may no longer hold pleasure. The fact that Alex could still play a game of golf gave him no satisfaction. Now he has to rely on someone else to guide his shot and tell him where the ball fell. Some people react in one way, some in another. While the majority of people who lose sight do adapt, others do not. Many spend a great deal of their lives fighting the blindness they cannot accept. Fitzgerald[17] says that the use of the white cane is a reliable indicator of how well the person has adjusted to his loss of sight.

Pathological Reactions. Loss of sight is a violent threat to a person's identity. He may feel that he is no longer the person he was, that he is maimed, damaged and deformed. He may be ashamed of his handicap and feel that others will see him as being different from, and less worthy than, themselves. He may interpret offers of help as manifestations of pity.[30] Any of the normal reactions to handicap may become pathological — exaggerated or continued for too long. Klemz gives the following pathological reactions:

refusal to admit to the blindness,
delusions about possessing supernatural powers,
obsessions to avoid having time to think about the blindness,
behavioural — getting drunk (in Fitzgerald's study[17] approximately 10 per cent of the subjects reported an increased intake of alcohol),
depression which does not lift,
suicide or attempted suicide,
extremes of frustrations/anger,
paranoid delusions,
manipulation of other people. 'Their blindness becomes for them a badge of office which entitles them to become eternally deferred to and waited upon.'[30]

Helplessness, which becomes a part of manipulation, places a strain on relatives and friends. As a result, the blind person becomes more than visually handicapped: he becomes socially handicapped and isolated. His pathological reactions deepen for his delusions are given a firm basis of fact: people do isolate him. But they avoid him not because he is blind but because he *is* difficult and suspicious, and they can no longer relate easily to him.

Family and friends need to be supportive and encouraging without becoming permanent leaning posts. But they may collude with and condone any of the blind person's reactions, and so contribute to their becoming pathological. Depression and anxiety — to mention but two of the affective reactions — are 'contagious'. Relatives may thus 'suffer' with the blind person and may themselves require medical and/or psychological treatment. 'Relatives may hinder the blind person's coming to terms with his blindness by themselves not accepting the handicap. The blind person's bid for independence may be seriously impaired by relatives who are over-protective.'[30]

Acceptance must precede rehabilitation.

Rehabilitation

If acceptance must precede rehabilitation, it follows that non-acceptance will obstruct rehabilitation. For rehabilitation to be effective, and for it to be effective as quickly as possible, the individual may need a great deal of help to explore his feelings. His feelings will determine whether, and how quickly, he reaches the stage of acceptance. Acceptance, in this sense, *does not* mean accepting the role in which society so often wishes to place the blind person — the role of the helpless, dependent person who has a limited place in society. Rather it is,

> OK, I'm blind. I can no longer live life as I did previously. I have to make changes. But I am determined to live, not just exist. I'll learn to cope. I want to be given the same opportunities I had when I was sighted. I want to take my turn at the washing up at the wives' club.[32]

However much blind people may want to be treated the same as other people, there is ample evidence that they are not. Perhaps this has something to do with blind people themselves, or at least some of them. It is all too easy to point to those who are difficult, suspicious and depressed, and to attribute these characteristics to all blind people. It is easy to forget that among sighted people there are those who are difficult, suspicious and depressed. It is very likely that the person who develops pathological reactions to blindness displayed these characteristics in his personality, to some degree, before he became blind. Tragedy may ignoble a person, but it will only do so if the raw material of personality traits was there before tragedy struck. This raises a question: Is there any relationship between the 'pre-morbid' personality and a good prospect for rehabilitation? Diamond and Ross,[29] admittedly speaking of soldiers blinded in action, say, 'The soldier of sound personality structure, free from pre-existing neurotic or psychopathic traits . . . is fully capable of making an adequate emotional adjustment to his disability *provided adequate orientation and rehabilitation facilities are available*.' (my italics). The authors go on to say, however, that adjustment to blindness may be influenced by the circumstances in which the blindness occurred. So once again, it is vital to take account of the emotional world of the individual. Guilt over what has happened may interfere with adjustment and therefore with rehabilitation.

One of the principal features of rehabilitation is to enable the person to resume normal activities as quickly as possible. These activities may include employment, or in the case of some, work at home. The needs of blinded housewives are special, but perhaps their needs are often overlooked. This applies with equal force to all women who are disabled.[33] Many blinded people will not be able to continue with the work in which they were previously engaged. Being employed is a mark of one's financial independence.

Not being able to continue with one's trade or profession is a shattering blow. The blindness itself, as we have discussed, is a loss of a precious faculty. Added to this, loss of job is a double bereavement. Then starts the frustrating and often futile round of questions: 'What *can* I do?' People who have been made redundant suffer from a serious lack of confidence, but generally they have all their faculties. The blinded person starts the job-hunting race with a severe handicap. But even before he can start, he has to learn how to cope in a near sightless or totally sightless world. Therapists working with the visually handicapped must have a conviction that even total blindness need not be totally incapacitating. Jackson, speaking of working with blind children says, 'If not warmly enveloped by love, if not encouraged to grow by a variety of interesting experiences, he may retreat within himself.'[34] If this applies to children it applies equally to adults. They, too, need to feel loved and supported; for it is love and support that will provide a firm base from which rehabilitation will take place. People who are suddenly deprived of sight need to develop the other senses to compensate for the deprivation. It has already been discussed just how important the sense of touch is, not only in helping to focus feeling, but to provide a positive link with the world which the blind person can no longer see. Establishing and maintaining contact with the world from which they are separated by sightless eyes is of vital importance when employment is considered.

In Fitzgerald's study,[17] 45 per cent were unemployed at the time of interview. The majority of people, as a consequence of blindness, suffer an occupational downgrading. Tony had recently qualified as an architect. One night, driving home on his scooter, he ran into the back of a lorry parked without lights. His blindness was sudden and total. He re-trained as an audio-typist. He wasn't bitter or resentful that he could not pursue his career. But the fact was plain. His standard of living had been affected. It would have been impossible for Tony to have continued as an architect. Klemz says, '. . . blind people are seldom allowed to perform even those tasks that they can do without difficulty. Society constantly undervalues their assets, their achievements and their potentialities.'[30] Klemz also places the responsibility for the successful integration of the blind person on sighted people with whom they come into contact.

Mehta[35] in a study of blind students in India, structures the results of her study into 22 different headings. These show quite definitely that blind people have to work harder to achieve a status equivalent to their sighted colleagues. They are more likely to spend time with other blind people than with sighted people. Communication between blind and sighted people is low. When considering employment, Mehta says that employers were satisfied with blind employees on account of the: relative independence of their mobility, high standard of their work, attention they paid to punctuality, and few demands they made. The conclusions of Mehta's study were that integration of blind persons with sighted people may be facilitated by encouraging blind people to study more, helping them to get employment with sighted people and to intermix more frequently on a variety of occasions. Both blind and sighted people need to communicate more in order to understand how they both feel about each other.

A final word on rehabilitation comes from Ryeron's study.[36] Drawing on his own experiences, the author argues that rehabilitation of newly blinded people should emphasise the development of remembered and created visual experiences. His rationale is that memory and imagination are important in helping the person learn new skills and to be able to move about freely in the world and remember it. He says that many blinded people actively suppress visual images and remembered experiences. Active visualisation of the kind that has been mentioned several times in this book, and in this chapter dealing with black-patch delirium, will help keep the person in touch with reality and help to bridge the gap between past and present, a gap that loss of sight has created and across which it is impossible to reach in any other way.

The Clients Speak

The following comments have been gleaned from a number of sources, from the written word and from personal accounts. '. . . when the eye consultant found out that I was pregnant he was horrified to think that a blind person should be having a baby and in fact it was suggested that I should have an abortion but again this thought horrified me.'[32]

Gordon, a manager in a large organisation, began to lose his sight at the age of 52, following a blow to the eye by a squash ball and a second knock to the temple with a squash racquet. He said, 'My confidence was knocked for six. I felt I could no longer compete. For the first time I began to think of my age and about retirement. For a time I struggled, trying to keep up with all the activities, driving, squash and sailing. I was determined not to give in. It was the stress of it all that brought on my coronary. My fear is of losing my sight completely. The other eye is starting to play up; it must be the strain. My pride took a blow. I'd always been superbly fit. I now feel less than a human being, less complete. I'm not so independent as I was. Night driving is very tiring. Our social life has been affected. Now I have to make a deliberate choice to go somewhere or not go. Jessica doesn't like driving. We stay in more often. I get easily tired. All this paper work to wade through. Reading and writing are getting more difficult. My colleagues are kind, but I sense they get impatient. Would I rather be blind or deaf? Blind, I think. There are so many beautiful sounds I would be cut off from. I don't know that I could bear the isolation of deafness. Tell them in your book of how I felt following eye surgery, will you? Terrified and very, very isolated. I needed someone to talk to, but they didn't come and sit. You're the first person in nine months I've really talked to about how I feel. Jessica's too involved, she'd get upset. Why can't the doctors and nurses listen? I tried. "Nurse," I would call, "come and look at my bandage, has it slipped?" I knew it hadn't but I thought it would give her a chance to hear what I was really trying to say. But as soon as she'd checked the bandage she was off. Honestly, I don't think they know how to talk to people who have become disabled.'

Rose is a lady of 63 who was born with cataracts in both eyes. She was registered as 'partially sighted' at the age of 28; and as 'blind' at the age of 49. Until the age of 55 she worked as a helper in a school for mentally handicapped children. 'No, I don't carry a white stick. I think it would get in the way and be a nuisance. Yes, I suppose it would tell other people that I'm visually handicapped, but of course I'm not really blind. Yes, I do watch the TV but I think I listen more than I watch. My one real regret is that I was never able to learn to drive a car. I would have loved that.'

Mike is 21, totally blinded following a motor cycle accident one year previously. He had just completed his apprenticeship as a heavy plater in the shipyard. Following the accident he was unconscious for eleven weeks. It was four months before he realised that he was blind. He lives with his parents and older sister. 'It's too soon to think about the future. I just don't know. My only interests were motor cycles, engines and football. I can't do any of them now. I'm not getting much help at the Centre. "Sit there, Mike. I'll get somebody to come and show you what to do," but they never come. So I just sit there — bored. The only lad who does me any good is Joe, a lad from the Sixth Form College. He comes once a week for experience. We have a talk and a good laugh. I'm getting stronger every day but I still get very tired. I eat too much and don't get enough exercise. Look at my pot-belly! And I used to be fit. I feel cut off. My mates don't come round now, at least not much. Perhaps they don't know how to talk to a blind chap. Ron, his father's blind, takes a crowd of us to football. He's our commentator. I really look forward to that. It keeps me in touch. I'm starting to get around with the white cane, not quite able to manage on my own, but nearly there. Dad or Mum take me out. I feel terrified when I first go out. I think everything is closing in on me. I want to work, but all they've suggested so far is telephonist or computer operator. They would both drive me mad. Something will turn up, though.'

Mike's Parents and Sister. 'Yes, of course we are grateful that Mike's alive. The care he received in the Intensive Care Unit was superb, and the understanding we received was great. They didn't hide anything from us. Our troubles really began when Mike was transferred to the orthopaedic ward. They didn't seem to know how to handle Mike when he was in his aggressive moods. They didn't seem to realise that it was his head injury. I think they were out of their depth. They told us he would never walk again but Mike was determined that he would — and he did. The doctors never came near us and when they did they hurried past and obviously didn't want to meet us. Then one evening, on our way out, a junior nurse passed us in the corridor and said, "Oh, by the way, did you know that Mike will never see again. He's blind. His optic nerve has been damaged." We knew that he couldn't see, but we never dreamed that it was for ever. It was the casual way we were told. We were shot to the very core. The almost callous way we were told shocked us. They weren't as honest with us there as they had been when Mike was so ill. We felt betrayed. Yes, it was difficult for us, but we think it was impossible for them to handle our feelings. We felt helpless and kept saying, "How do we cope with this? How do we help Mike cope?" We needed practical advice at that time: how to lead Mike when he started getting around; how to put food on his plate, and so on. It wasn't until he finally came home in November [7 months after the accident], when the Mobility Officer called, that we began to see a ray of hope. Tell doctors and nurses to be honest with relatives. What they have to hear may be hard and painful, but they can take it. What they can't take is being kept in the dark; always hoping, with no real grounds for hope.

A Mobility Officer. 'Sighted people have a lot to learn about visually handicapped people. Ask a blind person if he needs help, don't assume he wants to cross the road. Don't grab hold of him or shout at him, unless the shout is meant to stop him in his tracks because of some danger. Let him hold your arm, not hold his. In that way you will be in front, and can help your companion negotiate obstacles more easily. And don't just say, "A step", say if it's up or down, and whether they are broad steps. Some people find their way around remarkably well; others have great difficulty and never seem to be able to place themselves. For them, walking must be a great strain. It can be quite embarrassing at times. I'll be walking arm in arm with a blind person, someone will approach and say, "Hello, how are you? And how is he/she?" Talking to, and not at, a blind person seems a great hurdle many people have to overcome. If only they would remember that the blind live in the world of someone else's eyes.

Reactions to Loss of Hearing

The deaf person is cut off from his fellows by a communication barrier. He cannot hear the spoken word. Conversation is difficult while lip-reading can so easily lead to misunderstanding. Many, as a result of their deafness, feel a profound sense of isolation. The fact that deaf people are cut off from many of the pleasant sounds and activities of life — theatres, concerts, bird-song, radio — is readily understood, but one activity from which they are also cut off is religious worship.[37] Hilary Blank makes the same point. 'Language is not only a powerful means of communication with others but also with oneself. Language is essential to the expression of our faith.'[38] The force of the argument of the last two writers is that not enough attention is paid to providing alternative means of communicating with deaf people when in Church. If worship has been an important event in a person's life, to be suddenly deprived of joining in the prayers, hymns and responses, is a definite trauma. Someone once said, . . . 'deaf people suffer from intellectual malnutrition, social deprivation, educational retardation, emotional frustration, economic limitation, aesthetic impoverishment *and* moral and spiritual starvation.' While the author of those words was no doubt speaking of the profoundly deaf from birth (and there is evidence that when deaf children leave school, educationally they are, on average, eight years behind their hearing peers[39]), there is little doubt that deaf people do suffer many deprivations.

It could be thought that deafness from birth would cause an impairment to the personality of the child. Bolton[40] refutes this. If there are problems, they are more likely to arise from the child growing up in a sheltered and over-protective environment. On the other hand, hearing loss in adults, of whatever age, whether partial or profound, '. . . influences a personality that is already formed; the sequelae depend for the most part on how well integrated the individual was before the accident, illness or other cause of loss.'[41] This may not came as a startling revelation, but it is worth being reminded that most people do cope with life's knocks and traumata, provided their emotional life has a secure base. There are those, as Denmark[8] reminds us, whose lives can be so affected by loss of hearing that severe psychiatric illness results. But as with personality problems, psychiatric breakdown is likely to occur more as a result of the stress of coping with the deafness than with the deafness itself. Altshuler states that schizophrenia occurs with no greater frequency in people who are deaf than in people with normal hearing.[42] Bolton[40] challenges several myths surrounding people who are deaf.

1. Few deaf people can speech-read (lip-read) with any degree of proficiency.
2. Their thought processes are not impaired.
3. They do not possess superior visual memory.

The majority of deaf people have to struggle to make sense of conversations they cannot properly hear, and for a lot of their day they are imprisoned within a world of total silence or muted sound. 'Oh, he can hear when he wants to', is a remark often cast at the hard of hearing, but this shows a lack of understanding. They may be able to hear sounds of certain frequencies, but others they cannot. This may lead to misunderstanding and give an impression of stupidity. The presence of a deaf person is often an embarrassment. Group conversation is difficult for most deaf people and as a consequence, they are often ignored. It is a strain always to have to make certain that Aunt Jane has heard precisely what has been said, and this may require several repetitions. Frustration is more likely in a group — a family, for example — with a deaf person than with someone who is blind. Many people with normal hearing give up the struggle to communicate with those who are deaf.[43] Communication would be made easier if those with hearing would remember that

> The deaf person cannot lip-read through walls, or round corners — his eyes can only be in one place at a time. Family decisions are often unintentionally made at a meal table when the deaf person has looked down to butter his bread. He was not part of that decision-making, and the family have not known how to make him a part.[44]

Lysons[45] speaks of the need for the deaf person to develop empathy with other people he meets.

> Empathy leads to the realisation that even the most patient husband or wife [or working colleague (author)] will also experience strain from having to act as a second pair of ears for a partner with defective hearing. It is all too easy for a hard-of-hearing person to become so full of self pity that he is oblivious to the needs, difficulties and rights of others.

While this caution is appropriate, if the deaf person is constantly ignored, his feelings of isolation will almost certainly turn into feelings of inferiority. Lysons discusses four factors that will help to lessen these feelings of isolation and inferiority:

1. Emotional security — the knowledge that he is loved, respected and accepted.
2. Positive self-concept — he needs to be a full and active partner in various activities.
3. Communication skills — a determined effort by both the hearing and the hearing-impaired to make communication effective.
4. Communication aids — to supply a hearing aid is not a short cut to rehabilitation: it is but the beginning.

Many people will not wear an aid because it is uncomfortable. Others find that it increases noise but not clarity. Others, like the blind person with the white stick, feel that a hearing aid is announcing to the world that the wearer is a deviant from what is normal and he wishes to 'pass' as normal. In other words, he tries to bluff his way around. Some people go to what seem to be extraordinary lengths to bluff their way out of their deafness: divert attention, create noise, wear ear muffling clothes, pretend to be preoccupied. But as with the blind person, bluffing produces its own stress and anxiety. Continued bluffing makes it more difficult to accept the handicap.

Rehabilitation

Wright[46] says that the main purpose of rehabilitation of the deaf is to overcome the handicap. For the partially deaf, the hearing aid is the first step toward rehabilitation. How well the person takes to the aid is governed, to a large extent, by the instruction he receives about his disability, how the environment can influence his hearing, the care of the aid and the ear mould, the use of the controls, and so on.[47] Mrs Young came to work one day in a distressed state. She was having trouble with her hearing aid. She had worn one for a number of years and had recently had a new mould fitted. 'I can't get used to it, it's so uncomfortable, it hurts my ear so.' Her friend, who knew a little about hearing aids, when she had a look, said, 'I think the loop is too long. It needs to be much shorter.' A quick snip with scissors and the hearing aid fitted snugly behind Mrs Young's ear, and she was happy. A few minutes of personal attention by the girl at the hearing aid department, to ensure that the aid did fit, would have saved Mrs Young several days of distress. More than that, if that had been Mrs Young's introduction to the hearing aid, it is very possible that she would have been so disheartened that she would have given up the struggle and the aid would have lain unused in its box.

Successful rehabilitation of a deaf person is influenced by two sets of attitudes. The person's own attitude toward his deafness and other people's toward him. On the one hand the deafened person has lost a vital faculty but on the other he has acquired what Ashley[15] calls 'a badge of shame' which, unlike other badges, he cannot remove and hide in his pocket if he so wishes. Bolton says that deaf people devalue deafness more than do hearing persons. They also believe that hearing people hold more negative attitudes toward deafness than they actually do.[40]

An essential part of rehabilitation is work. Many hard-of-hearing people find promotion blocked. 'Few get the chance to prove themselves worthy, so there develops a self-fulfilling prophecy that the deaf do not make good supervisors.'[48] Profoundly deaf people, possessing suitable educational qualifications, find themselves particularly handicapped in the work market. In some jobs, hearing is essential, lack of it may be a safety hazard. Deaf people may be excluded on grounds of safety. Lysons,[45] when at the age of 18 it was discovered that he was rapidly going deaf, was told, 'It is difficult to suggest an occupation in which he will not be handicapped although farming should be a suitable calling for a deaf person.' While opportunities have increased since then, there are still many careers that are closed to someone who cannot hear. Jack Ashley tells of the awful periods of self-doubt as he struggled to cope with life as a Member of Parliament. But for every Jack Ashley there are dozens of others who are not able to battle against the indifference, apathy and rejection they experience in the labour market. While it would be uncharitable to draw comparisons between the blind and the deaf, Jack Ashley makes the point that (at the time he was writing) annual donations to the blind were £2m as against £20,000 to the deaf. Although these amounts will have altered, it is highly probable that there still exists a gap; an indication of how blindness and deafness are perceived by those who donate their money. If more money were available, perhaps more could be done to develop aids to help deaf people function in a wider range of occupations than at present. A drowning man doesn't need sympathy; he needs someone to throw him a life line. Work can be that life line.

The Clients Speak

'. . . there can be no relaxation in human society, no refined conversation, no mutual confidences. I must live quite alone and may creep into society only as often as sheer necessity demands. I must live like an outcast.'[49] These poignant words of Beethoven may seem too sharp, and speak too critically of a society which did not understand deafness. But deaf people today often express similar feelings, although, as with most people with disabilities, the response is so varied that it would be unfair to generalise and say, 'This is the prevailing attitude.'

Peter. Peter, who has had a hearing loss since birth, feels that one of the most useful things for fully hearing people to remember when talking to a deaf person is 'Put the light on, I can't hear you'. People who depend on lip-reading need to be placed so that they can see the other person clearly. 'What I find most difficult', he said, 'is when at the office I'm holding a telephone conversation and someone comes up and tries to over-ride. I can only listen to one person at a time. Background noises often get in the way of hearing what people are saying.'

Mrs Parker. Mrs Parker, in her mid-seventies, had worn a hearing aid for about twenty years. One morning she awoke to find that her hearing had completely gone. 'I was terrified. All I could hear were faint sounds. Then the tinnitus started. That nearly drove me quite mad. There is a cow bell, a door bell, a tune, a noise like rushing water and a roaring like traffic in a tunnel — all at once. Six months after, my husband died. That was just too much. I wanted to end it all. My deafness had isolated me before, but at least Sam was there. What do I miss most? The TV. It's only half a set now. I'd like to have one of those sets that print the words, but I can't afford one. We don't get any concessions, you know. I miss not hearing the birds and my grandchildren and great-grandchild. Even if they shout I can't hear. They must find it frustrating too. I do enjoy the Bingo. The numbers come up on the screen. I must get out and meet people or I'd go mad. People tell me I shout: that makes me feel guilty. I can't tell the difference between a whisper and a shout. They sent Sam and me away to the Link Centre [described below] for two weeks. What a lot I learned there. I couldn't go back without Sam. They taught me how to relax. That helps the tinnitus. Still, I don't want to give the impression that I'm miserable all the time. I'm not. I try not to think about the future. I push it firmly out of my mind.'

Counselling Deaf People

The above conversation with Mrs Parker was carried out by means of written questions, lip-reading and sign language. A neighbour, who has a great deal of contact and rapport with Mrs Parker, also acted as interpreter when I got stuck. Active counselling with a person who is profoundly deaf is profoundly difficult. Feelings transcend words and we must discover ways to understand feelings when we cannot rely on words. Most deaf people to whom I have talked unanimously agree that their loss of hearing has cut them off from normal social activities. The strain of trying to listen produces high levels of stress which, as Mrs Parker said, is helped by relaxation. When stress is prevented from developing, or is relieved when it has built up, the person is more able to cope with the events of daily living.

Conclusion

Helen Keller said,

> The problems of deafness are deeper and more complex, if not more important, than those of blindness. Deafness is a much worse misfortune. For it means the loss of the most vital stimulus — the sound of the voice that brings language, sets thoughts astir and keeps us in the intellectual company of man.[50]

These words are thought-provoking and it is possible to gain some insight from them. This chapter did not set out to draw comparisons between those who are deaf and those who are blind. Nor do I attempt to say that loss of one sense is less of a misfortune than loss of the other. I have attempted to draw attention to some of the work that has been done with disabilities and at the same time to highlight how some blind or deaf people feel about their disabilities so that therapists may have a little more knowledge and feeling for people with hearing or sight problems. Counselling both the deaf and the blind is as specialised a work as is, for example, working with the bereaved. In fact, there are many similarities between bereavement counselling and counselling those with sensory loss.

In the initial stages of sensory loss, most people feel in need of practical help; how to perform the simple tasks that have depended, hitherto, on sight or hearing. The blind are likely to need advice and guidance on how to become mobile in and outside of the home: the deaf will appreciate guidance on how to communicate with people whom they can no longer hear. How a blind person copes with early mobility, or how a deaf person copes with the frustration of lip-reading will provide adequate opportunity for getting at their feelings.

I end this chapter with a short poem. Although it is written by a deaf person, and refers to deaf people, the feelings behind the words apply with equal force to those who have become blind.

'For One Who is Going Deaf' A Prayer

O God,
The trouble about being deaf is that most people find deaf people just a nuisance.
They sympathise with people who are blind and lame.
But they just get irritated and annoyed with people who are deaf.
And the result of this is that deaf people are apt to avoid company, and get more and more lonely, and more and more shut in.
Help me now that my hearing has begun to go.
Help me face the situation and to realise that it is no good trying to hide it, for that will make it worse and worse.
Help me to be grateful for all that can be done for deaf people like me.
If I have got to wear a hearing aid, help me to do it quite naturally and not be shy or embarrassed about it.
Give me the perseverance not to let this trouble get me down, and not to let it cut me off from others.
And help me to remember that, whatever happens, there is nothing can stop me hearing your voice.

Even if I cannot hear the voices of men, let me remember Samuel and say, 'Speak, for thy servant hears.'

(1 Samuel 3:10)

Notes

1. Goffman, E. (1973) *Stigma*, Penguin Books, Harmondsworth. Original American Edition (1963) Prentice-Hall, Englewood Cliffs, New Jersey.
2. Ford, R. (1966) 'Quite intelligent', in Hunt, P. (ed.), *Stigma: the Experience of Handicap*, Geoffrey Chapman, London.
3. Sutherland, A.J. (1981) *Disabled We Stand*, Souvenir Press, London.
4. Brace, M. (1980) *Where There's a Will*, Souvenir Press, London.
5. Battye, R. (1966) 'The Chatterlye Syndrome' in Hunt (ed), *Stigma*.
6. Glanville, R. (1966) 'When the box doesn't fit', in Hunt (ed), *Stigma*.
7. Gill, M. (1966) 'No small miracle', in Hunt (ed), *Stigma*.
8. Denmark, J.C. (1978) 'The psycho-social implications of deafness', in Howells, J.G. (ed) *Modern Perspectives in the Psychiatric Aspects of Surgery*, The Macmillan Press Ltd., London.
9. Spitz, R.A. (1958) *'Hospitalism' The Psychoanalytic Study of the Child*, vol. 1 (3rd ed), International University Press, New York.
10. Solomon, P. and Leeman, K. (1975) 'Sensory deprivation' in Freedman, A.M., Kaplan, H.I. and Sadock, B.J. (eds) *A Comprehensive Textbook of Psychiatry*, Williams and Wilkins Co., Baltimore.
11. Zubek, J.P. (1969) *Sensory Deprivation: Fifteen Years of Research*, Appleton-Century-Crofts, New York.
12. Wilson, L.M. (1972) 'Intensive care delirium', *Archives of Internal Medicine, 130*, p. 225.
13. Ashworth, P. (1979) 'Sensory deprivation: the acutely ill', *Nursing Times* (15 Feb), pp. 290–4.
14. Weisman, D.A. and Hackett, T.P. (1958) 'Psychoses after eye surgery', *New England Journal of Medicine, 258*, pp. 1284–9.
15. Ashley, J. (1973) *Journey into Silence*, The Bodley Head Ltd., London.
16. Bowman, K. (1983) 'Blindness following a fall at work', *Nursing Times* (10 August).
17. Fitzgerald, R.G. (1970) 'Reactions to blindness', *Archives of General Psychiatry, 22*, pp. 370–9.
18. *Daily Express*, 9 May 1984.
19. Stubbins, J. (1977) 'Stress and disability' in Stubbins, J. (ed) *Social and Psychosocial Aspects of Disability*, University Park Press, Baltimore.
20. Adamson, J.D., Hershberg, D. and Shane, F. (1978) 'The psychic significance of parts of the body in surgery', in Howells, J.G. (ed) *Modern Perspectives in the Psychiatric Aspects of Surgery*, The Macmillan Press Ltd., London.
21. Calek, O. (1980) 'Some aspects of self-concept in blind students', *International Journal of Rehabilitation Research, 3 (2)*, pp. 248–50.
22. Nelson, M. and Gruver, G.G. (1978) 'Self esteem and body-image concept in paraplegics', *Rehabilitation Counselling Bulletin* (Dec), pp. 108–13.
23. Fisher, S. (1970) *Body Experience in Fantasy and Behaviour*, Appleton-Century-Crofts, New York.
24. Fisher, S. and Cleveland, S.F. (1958) *Body-image and Personality*, Van Nostrand Co. Inc., New York.
25. Advani, L. (1972) 'Attitudes toward the blind in Asian countries', *Proceedings of the 12th World Congress of Rehabilitation International*, 1972, pp. 617–19.

26. Scott, R.A. (1969) *The Making of Blind Men*, Russell Sage Foundation, New York.

27. Minton, H.G. (1974) *Blind Man's Buff*, Paul Elek, London.

28. Evans, R.L. and Janrequy, B.M. (1981) 'Telephone counselling with visually impaired adults', *International Journal of Rehabilitation Research, 4(4)*, pp. 550–2.

29. Diamond, B.L. and Ross, A. (1945) 'Emotional adjustment of newly blinded soldiers', *American Journal of Psychiatry, 102*, pp. 367–71.

30. Klemz, A. (1977) *Blindness and Partial Sight*, Woodhead-Faulkner Ltd., Cambridge.

31. Fawcett, L. (1965) 'Sports for the Blind: St. Dunstan's', *Physiotherapy, 51*, pp. 284–5.

32..Brechin, A. and Liddiard, P. (1981) *Look at it this Way*, Open University Press, Milton Keynes.

33. United Nations Department of International, Economic and Social Affairs, Centre for Social Development and Humanitarian Affairs. (1981) S.T./E.S.A./111 'Integration of disabled persons into community life'.

34. Jackson, C.L. (1961) 'Blind children', *American Journal of Nursing, 61, 2*, pp. 52–5.

35. Mehta, S. (1980) 'A study of integration of the blind person with sighted', *International Journal of Rehabilitation Research, 3 (2)*, pp. 246–8.

36. Ryeron, N. (1982) 'Using and creating visual images: a new task for rehabilitation?', *Journal of Visual Impairment and Blindness, 76 (10)*, pp. 421–3.

37. Rohe, H.W. (1977) 'Deaf segregation — integration in the church', *Journal of Rehabilitation for the Deaf, 11, 2.*

38. Blank, H. (1977) 'When you can't hear the word of God', *Journal of Rehabilitation for the Deaf, 11, 2.*

39. Thomas, A.J. (1981) 'Acquired deafness and mental health', *British Journal of Medical Psychology, 54*, pp. 219–29.

40. Bolton, B. (1976) *Psychology of Deafness for Rehabilitation Counsellors*, University Park Press, Baltimore.

41. Altshuler, K.Z. 'Personality and deafness', in Bolton (ed), *Psychology of Deafness*.

42. Altshuler, K.Z. (1971) 'Studies of the deaf: relevance to psychiatric theory', *American Journal of Psychiatry, 127; 11*, pp. 97–102.

43. *Social Work Today, 10, 21* (23 Jan 1979).

44. *Communication*, Breakthrough Trust, Feb. 1979, No. 8.

45. Lysons, K. (1978) *How to Cope with Hearing Loss*. Published originally by David and Charles (Holdings) Ltd and re-published 1980 by Granada Publishing Ltd, London.

46. Wright, D. (1969) *Deafness: A Personal Account*, Allen Lane/Penguin Press, London.

47. Brotherwood, J. (1975) 'Rehabilitation of the deafened adult', *Proceedings of the Royal Society of Medicine, 68.*

48. Sydenham, R. (1972) 'Employment and deaf people', *Proceedings of the 12th World Congress of Rehabilitation International*, 1972, pp. 763–4.

49. Beethoven Ludwig Van from the *Heiliganstadt Document* and quoted in Thomas, *Acquired Deafness* (ref. 39).

50. Keller, H. (1933) *Helen Keller in Scotland*, Methuen, London.

51. Breakthrough Trust, Feb. 1979, No. 8.

The Link Centre for Deafened People. The Centre aims to help rehabilitate those, who in adult life, have to face the experience of total or severe deafness. The object of Link is to invite deaf people (with a friend or member of their family) to stay in Eastbourne in the company of those who understand their problems and have the professional ability to assist. Because of the age range, stage of adjustment and degree of deafness, each person's programme is tailor-made. Guests stay with local families or, in the case of someone with normal hearing, in a small hostel. (The above details were taken from information supplied by 'Help for Health' an information service provided by Wessex Regional Library Unit, Southampton General Hospital.)

10 RELATIVES AS CARERS

Introduction

A rehabilitation programme that ignores the client's relatives will fail. The therapist who ensures co-operation of the relatives has laid the foundations of a workable programme. This opinion has been expressed several times already in this book. Now it is time to expand the theme and to consider disability through the eyes of those most closely involved — the relatives. No one disability is singled out and no attempt is made to deal comprehensively with any of the issues that emerge. Rather, the chapter considers some of the emotional, social and practical consequences experienced by families who care for a disabled person. For convenience, the chapter is divided into two: children and adults. This division is, to some extent, artificial; many of the subjects considered apply to all ages. The discussion will concentrate on physical disability.

Caring for Children with Disabilities

'The News'. It is trite to say that the birth of a handicapped baby places great stress on the parents. No words can ever plumb the parents' depths of feelings as they struggle to receive the full impact of the news they have been given. The intellectual understanding — so necessary for successful adjustment — is likely to be overshadowed and swamped by strong emotions which shriek 'reject', 'reject', 'I don't want to know'. Jenny and Alan, re-calling the moment they were told that Tim had spina bifida, said,

> We felt only an aching void. All emotion had gone. It was not until some time later, just as hands numbed with the cold revive painfully to warmth, that our feelings returned. But with them pain, so intense that it threatened to tear us apart and destroy us. All manner of feelings flooded in: fear, anger, anxiety for the future, and guilt. At the same time, we knew that this emotional turmoil must not be allowed to get in the way of caring for our baby.

Jenny's and Alan's feelings were given a practical focus. As parents cope with the physical care, their own emotional needs are pushed into second place. Indeed it would appear that many professionals judge the coping capacity of parents by how well they satisfy the infant's physical needs. Yet the emotional needs of the parents must be met if the handicapped infant is to receive more than adequate physical care.

Hope and Reality. The first two months following the birth of a baby who is handicapped are critical, and the resultant trauma requires emergency treatment.[1] Part of this emergency treatment is concerned with striking a balance between hope and stark reality. The harsh realistic view, presented by some people who believe that the 'short sharp shock' is best, if delivered in the early stages, can lead to despair which may seriously get in the way of any thought of rehabilitation. On the other hand, hope founded on evasion does not reassure. 'Coating reality with hope does not mean living in a world of unreality. Accepting a disability does not mean banishing hope.'[2] No one may ever say with certainty that a child with a disability will do this or that, any more than one may predict what any child will achieve in later life. But if parents are supported through the 'bad news weeks' they, themselves, will begin to seek for realistic rays of hope.

Adjustment to Disability. A study by a schools medical officer, of 50 handicapped children from one day school, identified in the children: over-anxiety, depression and over-protection on the one hand and rejection, friction and aggression on the other.[3] It seems that the way a child adapts to his handicap is directly related to how the parents themselves cope. The feelings identified in the above study very probably reflect the feelings within the family. The factors which exert the strongest influence on how the parents respond are: the severity of the handicap, the prognosis and the degree of hopelessness or hope which the parents feel.

That the child reflects the feelings and attitudes of the parents is not a new finding. Allen and Pearson,[4] writing in 1928, say

> The child seems to adopt the same attitude to the disability that his parents do. If they worry about it, so does he. If they are ashamed of it, he will be sensitive also. If they regard it in an objective manner, he will accept it as a fact and will not allow it to interfere with his adjustment.

McMichael[3] says that if the parents reject the handicap, the child may feel that it is he who is being rejected. This is almost certain to lead to problems of adjustment.

Mothers' Influence. In all the studies of children with handicap or serious illness, the central figure is the mother; women, traditionally, are the 'carers', men, the 'providers'. It is alleged that present day society is less willing to care for its handicapped members than were previous generations. But this is not so, and it is generally the closest female relative to whom the task of caring falls.[5] It is not surprising, therefore, that mothers powerfully influence the development of the attitudes of their children with disabilities. Mothers are normally more involved with their children, for many more hours of most days, than are fathers. So it should not evoke surprise that the mother's influence is so powerful. Where there are other children in the family, the father is more likely to be involved with them than with the handicapped child.[6] It is reported that handicapped children spoke more of their mothers and less of their fathers and siblings, whereas the reverse was true of non-handicapped children who talked more of father and other relatives and less of mother.[7, 8]

We see that the mother is the centrally important person in caring for the child with a handicap, while the father '. . . remained in a psychologically, physically and financially, peripheral position'.[9] How the mother adapts and copes is a crucial factor in developing positive attitudes in the child. And, although it has not been mentioned specifically in the studies quoted, how the mother adapts must have a bearing on how the other members of the family also adapt. For the remainder of this section I will concentrate on the mothers' feelings and how mothers cope.

'Tell Me How You Feel'. There is evidence that mothers who express grief in the early stages, following the discovery of handicap, adapt more quickly to the child and find ways of providing for the child's needs.[6] Mothers who talk about the handicap, and face up to the reality of the problem, cope better than those who did not admit to the seriousness of the handicap. Expression of feelings, then, is an important factor in helping the mother to accept her child's handicap. Feelings she may want to express are: panic, self-blame, guilt, rationalisation and worry about the future. These may be coupled with disorganisation, busyness and overwork.[9] None of these feelings or experiences is 'wrong' but mothers who feel them also say that they feel shame, guilt and worry *that they do feel them*. Women who, up to this time, have been 'copers' are liable to feel swamped by such powerful feelings. If they cannot express how they feel, they are likely to reject or disown their feelings. The dangers associated with rejecting feelings is that they will turn inwards and cause deeper emotional problems of anxiety and depression. Coupled with the rejection of the feelings, the source of the conflict — the handicap — may

also be rejected. And because the handicap is located in the child, he, too, may be rejected. That is why it is vital for parents of handicapped children to be given repeated opportunities to explore and express how they feel.

Guilt. Although it is essential that adequate opportunity be given for exploration of feelings, it is not necessary, and indeed could be counter-productive, for the mother to be subjected to a full-blown analysis of her guilt feelings, to take one feeling that has received much attention. Wakefield[10] says,

> So much has been written about guilt feelings of parents that one can spend the whole time ascribing all their feelings and reactions to their guilt feelings and that is that. Unless they are making the mother ill, why not say 'OK, you have guilt feelings, so what? So have I . . .' From my experience, the guilt issue is heavily over-subscribed; many parents react in what would seem to be an irrational manner not from guilt but from frustration and a sense that they must cope alone. This leads to feelings of inadequacy and despair.

Few of us are free from feelings of guilt, so Wakefield's point — that unless the feelings are making the mother ill, why not accept them? — is relevant. But, as has already been mentioned, guilt may cause a person to act irrationally and irrational behaviour may lead to rejection of the child, even though the mother may not be 'ill'. So, in spite of the fact that guilt may be an overworked idea, it should not be ignored. As with all other aspects of counselling, the therapist must be alert to the feelings that are being expressed, albeit hesitantly.

Wright[11] draws attention to how necessary it is for the counsellor to recognise that the mother is over-burdened with stresses of various sorts, and that the conflict and associated guilt arise from the attempt to come to terms with the problem. She goes on,

> Such an emphasis, being directed toward the growth potential of the parent in the wake of enmeshing, undermining factors, is one of the best guarantees that the counsellor will look with an attitude of acceptance essential in constructing counsellor–client relationships.

Thus, how the counsellor views the client-mother will influence attitudes toward her. Seeing her as torn with conflict, and wanting to resolve it, will engender a more positive attitude than seeing her only as a rejecting parent.

Over-protection. A factor in caring for a handicapped child is over-protection. One indication of over-protection is doing something for someone which he is capable of doing for himself; of giving assistance where no assistance is needed.[2] For some people the drive toward independence for their children may prove to be a gigantic stumbling-block. Parents of children with handicaps have to strive for a realistic balance between dependence and independence. Independence forced upon any young person, not yet sufficiently mature to handle it, can be a frightening experience. It may also lead to difficulties later in life in accepting dependence of someone else, possibly of his own child. In a sense, trying to push a child too quickly into independence (held by some cultures as a virtue) may be perceived by the child as non-nurturing and rejecting. Being dependent is a feature of many relationships. When one person asks another for assistance, dependence is being acknowledged. A relationship in which dependency moves easily and naturally from one to the other, is more likely to endure than a relationship in which both are so fiercely independent that neither can get emotionally near the other. The very independent person is less likely to want to show his emotions, and be less able to recognise other people's feelings. The child — handicapped or non-handicapped — who has experienced physical and emotional dependence and who has been gently encouraged to explore the boundaries of that dependence and push them out when he feels ready, is enjoying a rich experience. Not all handicapped children have had such an experience. The mother's own emotional needs very often prevent the child pushing out the boundaries of his independence. A non-handicapped child has many avenues in which he can explore his independence; a handicapped child is vulnerable to protracted dependence and over-protection. Genuine love and concern on the part of the mother become overshadowed by anxiety and fear. Guilt may provoke compensatory behaviour which leads to indulgence and protection from danger — real or imaginary. All this is understandable and the mother's feelings must not be brushed aside as 'wrong' or 'silly'.

Women are not suddenly endowed with superhuman or supernatural gifts merely because children are born to them. Mothers of handicapped children must feel doubly vulnerable and doubtful of their ability to rear their child with sensitivity while still coping with their own feelings of shock and dismay.

In spite of their own vulnerability, many mothers do manage to raise their handicapped children in such a way that there is relative balance between dependence and independence. If some succeed less well than others, let those who offer help, through counselling, remember that what has been done has not been done through malice. Rather, it has come about because the mother has not been able to 'let go' at the appropriate time. Her own emotional needs, and her vulnerability that makes her think with her heart,[10] have prevented her from learning to do for her child only when and what he is unable to do for himself. Counselling may help such a mother release some of her feelings that still hold her child in an over-dependent and over-protected relationship.

Disability and the Family. An over-protected and over-dependent relationship can have a profound effect on other relationships within the family. If the handicapped child is to receive the care he needs, it is natural that the time the mother can devote to other family members will be lessened. This can lead to jealousy, from both the husband and the other children. Normal jealousies are intensified and the handicapped child is then regarded as 'favourite'. Where there are brothers and sisters, they and the father are often thrown together more. This may then lead to schisms — mother and handicapped child on one side; father and other siblings on the other. Fathers are thus able to gain some benefit from more contact with the other children: where there are no other children, the father is likely to feel a deep sense of rejection. McMichael[3] reports that in 21 per cent of the 37 cases studied, there was a moderate or severe degree of failure to adjust on the part of the siblings. Harvey and Greenway[6] say that while the presence of a handicapped child need not handicap the whole family, the handicap is a constant source of stress upon everyone. Although the stress should not be denied, it need not cripple the family. Where the handicap is dealt with constructively, siblings have developed greater maturity, tolerance, patience and responsibility than is common among children of their age.[12,13] Parents who themselves enjoy a rewarding, satisfying relationship are the ones most likely to be able to deal constructively with handicap and to help their children to do likewise. Where the parental relationship is not maturely grounded, the stress of a handicap may prove to be a wedge that drives the parents apart.[10] A genuine acceptance of one's partner's differences is vital for the success of any relationship. Parents who are unable to accept each other may well experience difficulty accepting the child and his handicap. Acceptance will lead to constructive adaptation; resignation, to over-dependence with the danger of rejection. How well a family deal with the stress of handicap depends, to a great extent, on how psychologically adjusted the parents are and how secure the marriage is. But '. . . we should consider that any parents, no matter how psychologically adjusted, would face such doubt, insecurity, and considerable tension if they had to manage a physically ill child.'[8] Sooner or later a physical handicap will become an emotional challenge for the child and his family.[1] This is when counselling is appropriate.

Not all disabilities are congenital. Parents who have coped with a congenital disability in one of their children, it is hoped, have been given adequate support which includes counselling. Parents who, later on, are faced with caring for a child with a handicap, have a different cluster of difficulties for which counselling help may be appropriate. They have already started to make plans; their expectations for their child have not been constrained by disablement. It would be neither appropriate nor helpful to discuss which would be the greater blow; to be told at birth or to realise some time later — at adolescence, for example — that one's child was handicapped. It is natural for parents to expect that their children will be born healthy[14] and remain so throughout their lives. Most parents will acknowledge that illness may strike, and that their child may be less than perfectly healthy. Nevertheless, when disability is the legacy of accident or illness, there are many adjustments to be made both by the parents and by their child; they must all readjust their sights and their expectations. Plans that have been firmly laid may need to be re-cast when it becomes obvious that a particular goal, if not unattainable, in its attainment may produce unwelcome and unbearable stress. The relinquishing of cherished hopes may lead to resentment and bitterness. These negative barriers are almost certain to interfere with satisfactory readjustment. Satisfactory readjustment is necessary if energy is to be directed into creating new plans and seeing them through. Parents, disabled child and siblings may all become caught up in the struggle to overcome the distress of disappointed hopes. They experience what has been called 'family pain'.[15]

> This is the hurt experienced by the entire group in response to this misfortune in one of its members. The family members may feel fear and anger. They may feel powerless in face of the disease . . .. Sometimes, 'family pain' appears not only as anger but also as bitterness, lack of caring and insensitivity.[16]

This extract, taken from a study of people with multiple sclerosis, offers the therapist another concept to understand the impact, on the feelings, of illness and disability. If illness is the 'night side of life',[16] counselling may help to bring some light that will make the night journey less wearisome.

The aim of counselling would be to help the parents '. . . accept their child's projected limitations as a fact, and they must begin to discover the ways by which his medical, educational and social-recreational needs can be met.'[17] To return to an earlier theme; parents need to be helped to face reality, but with hope, not stark reality with despair. The need to help these parents does not ease when the particular crisis is passed. Disability does not go away: neither should help, assistance and support. They should be available to ensure that difficult happenings do not become crises that threaten the stability of the family and place at risk the child with the disability.

Caring for Adults with Disability

So far the discussion has been concerned with how disability in children influences parents and other members of the family. Now I want to concentrate on the effects of disability in adult life.

The Stress of Caring. In preceding chapters reference has been made to stress: stress as a concept (p. 150), the stress of illness, (p. 167) and the stress of disability (p. 185). In this section I want to deal with another source of stress — caring, over a long period, for a person who is disabled. Although the discussion centres on adults, passing reference will be made to the carers of children.

The following story by Edwin, aged 49, caring for his wife, Pam, who has had brain damage, highlights numerous points that many other people mention as problems.

> I have been looking after my wife for three years. It is 24 hour care. I didn't go to bed for two years. I do everything for her, wash, bake, iron, shop, cook. I wash her, she is incontinent and there is washing every day. It sounds impossible, I think I have done too much. I've been told that there would have been more help forthcoming if I hadn't put myself about. It's destroyed my life absolutely because Pam and I have always gone about together. My normal life has finished.
>
> I have extra washing costs, my biggest help would be help with the washing and ironing. It would be very expensive if I didn't take great care. I never buy anything for myself. I receive Invalid Care Allowance, and I was told I could have help with the electric bills, but it was only as a loan. I can't do with the fussing about. I would have had a Home Help if I was prepared to pay £1 an hour. I think there should be some sort of Community Centre for people to go to get information, and I don't mean where everyone can hear. I did try and get some assistance when we moved and got nowhere with the

authorities.

> If I wasn't caring I'd be at work. I don't sleep very well, for two years I slept on the floor, now we have twin beds. It's very hard as you lose friends. They offer to do things, but now they avoid us. Even my best friend, we were inseparable, he just rings up occasionally. I feel that even if I go out for a drink, I have no conversation. We've never had any holidays, this is the first year we have tried. I almost wish I hadn't got involved. It's been suggested that she goes into hospital while I take a holiday, but it would be too hard to take up the responsibility again. I have always been a worrier, I wonder if I can carry on.[5]

Edwin's experience is not uncommon. He does not use the word 'stress', but that he does experience it could not be denied. Topliss[18] makes it clear that most physically disabled people under retirement age (in the Southampton study) are cared for within the family. 'The presence of such heavily dependent persons in a private household puts a heavy burden of care on the families concerned.'[18] Stubbins[19] says, 'If any threat to the organism constitutes stress, then certainly disability itself is a source of stress'. And, '. . . the course of a disease is not only determined by its causes but by the individual's reactions to it'. If these comments apply to the person who has the disability, they apply equally to his relatives. For how the person copes with the stress of disability must be influenced by the relatives' reaction to it. Thus there is established a cycle of 'disability, dependence and stress', where each person experiences his own stress and also contributes to the stress experienced by all others.

Who are the Carers? The person who is confronted with the realisation that an adult relative is, or will be, handicapped as a result of disability, and will need constant care, experiences a different cluster of psychological and practical needs than does the parent of a child with a congenital disability, or of a child who acquires a disability. There are many examples that could have been the focus for this discussion; any one of them would present a slightly different picture. It has already been stated that the majority of carers are women,[5,9] so it would seem obvious that many of the studies on disability deal with the needs of female carers. But men do give care and their psychological needs are different from those of female carers. In one study (of families of stroke patients) 27 per cent of the carers were husbands.[20] I shall, therefore, make reference to the needs of both men and women as carers.

Wright, speaking of women disabled by arthritis, says that psychologically their concerns are anxiety, frustration, depression, fear of losing their independence and a fear of being a burden.[21] If these feelings were to be tested, they would surely apply to men who were disabled. Most of them, with the exception of the fear of being a burden, do apply. Two studies[21,22] mention explicitly, while others imply, that disabled men do not express undue concern at the burden they place upon their wives. Sainsbury[22] says

> This may have been due to a refusal to acknowledge utter dependence or it may reflect the expectations of submissiveness in a wife on the part of a husband in our culture . . .. Whereas men tended to expect to be cared for by their wives, women did not feel that husbands had the same obligation.

This expectation possibly arises from the traditional type-casting of man as the provider. It would thus seem that while women who are disabled are likely to experience problems with the reversal of their traditionally 'caring' role, men are more likely to experience difficulty with the erosion of their role as provider.

Not every man can accept being thrust into the role of carer. If the female in our society is the 'carer', it would be a natural assumption to make that the characteristics of the carer are more feminine than masculine. Emma Jung,[23] speaking of the difference between the feminine and male mentalities, says,

> In general, it can be said that feminine mentality manifests as undeveloped, childlike, or primitive character; instead of the thirst for knowledge, curiosity; instead of judgement, prejudice; instead of thinking, imagination or dreaming; instead of will, wishing.
>
> Where a man takes up objective problems, a woman contents herself with solving riddles; where he battles for knowledge and understanding, she contents herself with faith or superstitition, or else she makes assumptions.

And in another place in the same book Emma Jung says, 'Being essentially feminine, the anima, like the woman, is predominantly conditioned by eros, that is the principle of union, of relationship, while the man is in general more bound to reason, to logos, the discriminating and regulative principle.' If the '. . . development of relationships is of primary importance in the shaping of life, and this is the real field of feminine creative power'[23] it is not surprising that women take more readily to their caring role than do men. But that women 'care' and men 'provide' does not prove that the characteristics of men and women are inherently different and mutually exclusive. Socialisation plays an important part in shaping what is acceptable for either sex to do and what is expected from them.

If it is more difficult for men than for women to adapt to the caring role, those who take it on are likely to need a great deal of understanding support if they, and the people for whom they care, are to survive emotionally. Many men do adopt the caring role. Perhaps they are those who have not allowed their caring feelings to be socialised out. But, however much some men would want to become care-givers, the expectations of society, and the provisions of the Welfare State, do not actively encourage them to do so.

Finding Meaning in the Caring Role. The psychological stress placed on people who become carers is quite severe. Sally Sainsbury[22] says that men who are disabled very often regard themselves as being 'on the scrap heap'. These feelings are likely to be expressed by people whose earning power is cut off by becoming carers. Yet there must be compensations: if there are not, it is highly probable that the task of caring will become onerous and unrewarding. According to 'Equity Theory',[24] all carers need to receive some psychological reward if they are to continue in the role. A person thrust into caring for someone who is disabled becomes a partner in an unequal relationship. In order to continue 'caring', the carer must equalise the relationship. One way of restoring equity is to find meaning in the new role. 'It must be for some purpose'; 'I'm a better person for having had this experience'; 'I think I'm more understanding'; 'It brings us closer together.'[13] In the study of stroke patients, already referred to,[20] which used Equity Theory as a basis, the writer draws attention to how men find the role of carer too stressful because the relationship is unequal. If meaning cannot be found, equity cannot be restored. She says, 'One would not expect husbands to be better adjusted to caring for a sick family member than wives.' On the other hand, a retired man seemed to have adapted very well — in that study. This may have been because the need to be the 'provider' was no longer as pressing. In some ways, the reversal of roles gave him an opportunity to 'repay' the years of nurture his wife had shown him. This man had found equity.

Effects on the Family

If disability produces physical and psychological stress in the afflicted person, it is inevitable that the other members of the family will also experience stress; or as I shall refer to it in this section — tension. The four main factors that act upon the family to produce tension are: social, finance, work and health.

Social Factors

Relationships. Some people say that caring for a disabled relative brings the family closer together. Many testify to the opposite. Tensions cause divisions.[5] Where the disabled person lives with his family, less of the carers' time and energies will be available for the others. 'I feel torn between one and the other' is not an uncommon feeling. Reference has been made earlier to the balance between dependence and independence (pp. 213–14); it is necessary to reconsider it as it relates to the present discussion. Disability, to some extent, implies dependency. The disabled person must give up (to varying degrees, according to the disability) some of his independence. The carers, in turn, must accept increased dependence and find some meaning in it. People who cannot tolerate the caring role may be those who are unable to accept the dependence of another person. If this is so, the resultant tension may cause a breakdown of the relationship and a rejection of the disabled person. Several writers draw attention to the effect caring for a disabled person has on a marriage.[10,13,18,21,22] Wakefield[10] says that caring for a handicapped child may create a rift in a marriage that is not firmly grounded. The rift could be due to the parents' inability to communicate what they think and feel about the handicapped child and about each other and to ask each other for support.[13] Topliss[18] acknowledges the risk of marriage breakdown where one of the partners is disabled. She goes on to say that there is less risk of breakdown if it is the husband who is disabled. This could be because the man's opportunities for meeting other women may be severely curtailed. But for women who are disabled, the risk of marriage breakdown is greater. Topliss says, '. . . it appears that the limitations on domestic life which result [from disability] seem a factor in driving some husbands to seek other partners, thus compounding the disadvantages of disablement with the distress of a broken marriage.' To apply the Equity Theory, such men have not been able to restore equity to the relationship.

Sainsbury[22] makes a similar point and adds that breakdown is likely to occur soon after the onset of disability, rather than where it had existed for a long period. This is supported by the Leeds study of people suffering from arthritis. In this study Wright says, 'It would seem that if the husband marries the arthritis as well as the woman, the marriage is more likely to succeed than if the rheumatoid disease began after marriage.'[21]

Intrusion. Disability intrudes into the privacy of family life. Intrusion is one of the factors of potential friction between husband and wife; it may also affect other members of the family. Brothers and sisters of a handicapped child may well experience jealousy far in excess of normal. It has been reported[3] that '. . . in 21 per cent of the 37 cases studied, there was a moderate degree of failure to adjust on the part of the siblings'. Caring for a handicapped person demands a great deal of time and energy. Many siblings with a handicapped brother or sister admit to feeling 'pushed out' and of being left to their own devices. Caring for a disabled adult in the home presents different difficulties than when caring for a disabled child. Jealousy may certainly be present, but the main source of friction appears to be intrusion. 'Sometimes I feel the house is not my own. There is someone in the house who wasn't part of the original family unit. I think it has curbed a little of our family life.'[5] (So said a woman who was looking after her mother-in-law who had suffered a stroke.) Caring for an adult means less privacy for everyone else. 'I feel his eyes are on me the whole time. I don't know what he's thinking.' (A woman looking after her aged father, disabled after a fall.) 'We never seem to have any time together alone.' (Woman looking after mother-in-law.)

Isolation. Coupled to intrusion is isolation. Isolation may be 'self-induced', where the people involved are not able to overcome the psychological hurdles; or 'imposed', resulting from inadequate resources and services. It should be noted that although resources may, at times, be adequate, they are not always appropriate to the specific needs of the particular person. Very often adequate resources are not appropriated. In spite of enormous publicity, there are many people with handicaps who are deprived of resources because they are ignorant of their availability. Members of the 'caring professions' need to be more aware of what can be done to reduce isolation of people with disabilities.

People with disabilities often have limited mobility. This means that the 'carer' has the task of acting as the disabled person's legs or wheels. In an earlier chapter we saw that people often feel isolated by their own disabilities. It may not always be easy to ensure that isolation does not happen. The hurdles to be got over — for both carers and cared-for — are many and great. There is the hurdle of time. 'It takes me two hours to get Tim ready', said Jenny (the mother who spoke at the opening of this chapter). There is the hurdle of transport. Jenny said, 'If we hadn't a car I wouldn't be able to get Tim on the bus by myself, would I?' The practical hurdles are numerous; the psychological ones may not be so obvious, nor are they so easily got over. Some carers never get over the embarrassment of taking their handicapped relatives out; the more severe the disability, the more difficult it may be. In chapter 9, in the section dealing with stigma, people with disabilities spoke of how they felt when on the receiving end of people's unthinking remarks and unenlightened attitudes. Carers, too, become involved; they too, become stigmatised. The stares, the remarks, are just as surely directed at them as at the person with the disability. That is one reason why isolation is an ever-present reality. And it is all too easy for therapists to say, 'Now you must get out. Don't stay in or you will become isolated.' While that is true, and the carer knows it, actually getting out may be too great a hurdle to get over.

Isolation may affect the whole family, who may not be willing to bring friends home. 'If my mother is here and friends come, she butts in and makes things unpleasant; they all stopped coming.' It has also been reported[25] that carers often feel tied to the house; outings are not always enjoyed because of the anxiety which will not allow them to leave their caring work behind. Men, as carers, are particularly vulnerable; they are cut off from male contact and have little opportunity to meet up with male friends. An aspect of isolation frequently mentioned, either by people with disabilities or by their carers, is not being able to go away on holiday. 'We haven't had a holiday for 20 years. Oh, no, he wouldn't go and I wouldn't leave him, so we don't go. I would like to but we need all our money for heating and food.'[5] (Woman, aged 63, looking after husband, aged 70, suffering from bronchitis.) There is no doubt that this deprivation may be related to money, but not always so. The sheer effort of taking a disabled person away, on a journey to a strange house, with strangers who may ask, yet once again, the questions that have been asked and answered so many times before, may be too much of an effort. The psychological stress of separate holidays may be too much for carer and cared-for to contemplate. Perhaps the idea of a holiday is, for many, a wishful thought of normality which for them is not within the realms of reality.

Finance and Work

Many people are financially disadvantaged by their disability. Carers, too, are caught in the same trap. Edwin describes his financial trap from which there seems no escape. Most married couples can look forward to an increase in their income on the wife's return to work when the children are independent. A handicapped child in the family means that the mother's opportunities for paid employment to augment the family income are severely limited. 'Women who become disabled after marriage are unlikely to return to paid employment when their family grows up, or to give up work when her disablement makes it difficult for her to find employment as well as run her home.'[18] Topliss[18] argues that disabled people tend not to be in the higher income occupations; and those on State benefits are barely above the poverty line. Husbands whose wives are disabled are less likely to increase their income by working overtime.

Income which may seem adequate is often whittled away, as Edwin says, by having to provide extras for the handicapped person. Laundering of soiled linen and clothes; special diets; tailor-made clothing, for a paralysed child who drags himself along the floor and wears holes in his trousers; transport; adaptations to the house; heating and lighting; a telephone — so essential to escape from the prison of isolation — all cost money that may be difficult to find. The avoidance of isolation is an important factor in the life of any person. Many non-disabled people choose to isolate themselves from contact with other people. Some people, however, are thrust into isolation by being disabled. The quality of their life depends upon reducing isolation to a bearable level.

Health

People frequently report a deterioration in their own health when caring for a disabled person over a long period.[5] Carers are under constant stress. Stress, as we have seen from previous discussion, leads to increased risk of illness. Stubbins[19] puts forward the case that stress lowers the immunological defences against diseases. Stress, coupled to isolation and the reduction in time and opportunity for relief-giving relaxation interests, may very well lower the carer's resistance to disease.

> I know my health has been affected. The constant anxiety and nervous tension leaves me in troughs of depression from time to time and I'm sure it's my emotional state which gives me these endless throat infections. I have felt so exhausted at times that it feels as though I have run a hundred miles . . . it's a bit like running in the dark.[10] [Rose Seward looking after her autistic child.]

A related point is that emotional fatigue lowers a person's tolerance to deal with problems.[13] Part of this emotional fatigue derives from conflict. However desperately the carer wants to care, the physical and emotional demands often produce a wish that the responsibility be taken away. But someone else taking over the caring role, by the disabled person being admitted to hospital, does not necessarily remove all strain upon the relatives; '. . . nor does it allow them to live a life free from emotional ties or concern about their disabled relative'.[25] Yet people who care for others must have respite in order to recharge their physical and emotional batteries.[20] Counselling may afford psychological as well as social respite and help the relative face the future with less reluctance than many of them express.[5]

Counselling the Carers

Therapists need to be as skilled in counselling as they are in dealing with the physical accompaniments of disease and disability. 'The inclusion of the family in the rehabilitation process is important in making sure that the client reaches full potential and that the family itself does not suffer ill consequences due to stress and changes in role.'[20] A counselling approach to relatives is one important factor that could help them to restore equity to the caring relationship *because the counselling relationship is a partnership of equals*. Exploration of feelings may be the first step towards the carer finding meaning in what is happening in the new role. Elsewhere I have said how essential it is that the client is regarded as an active partner in his own rehabilitation. Success in rehabilitation depends not on compliance (indeed it is necessary to distinguish the compliant client from the active partner) but on the client and his carer making the rehabilitation programme their own. Wright[11] says, 'Inner strength and self-respect grow in a relationship in which the person feels that he has an important role in planning his life and that what he says and what he feels are regarded as important.' Most people want to take responsibility for their own lives; they want to plan and carry out those plans. People who care for relatives with disabilities also want to be treated with respect and to feel that they have a part to play. Therapists who relate to relatives as co-managers are recognising that they perform a valuable caring function. Therapists sensitive to the needs of the carers may offer them help to understand their feelings — whenever it is needed. This may be helping them in the early stages to come to terms with the grief, disappointment, guilt and frustration which are commonly experienced in the period following discovery of disability. Counselling may be aimed at supporting the relatives through the years of unremitting care and the discouragement so often associated with it.

It may not be easy for relatives to engage in counselling, which involves exploring their thoughts and feelings. It has already been noted (p. 220) that an inability to communicate to one's marriage partner how one feels, places a strain on the marriage. People who have difficulty communicating their feelings, within their marriage, may experience similar difficulties when engaged in counselling. But an inability to communicate may not be the only reason. People who have carried the burden of caring, for a long time, may have built up strong defences against exposing their feelings, fearing that their ability to care will collapse without these defences. In a sense this is correct. It may be wise to repeat an earlier warning (see p. 26); counselling does not aim at removing a person's defences. The support a relative receives from an understanding therapist may prove to be a relationship of therapeutic value. The worth of this relationship will benefit therapist, relative and the disabled person for whom the relative cares.

Summary

The basic thesis of this chapter is thus: if the client (the person with the disability) is to derive the optimum benefit from rehabilitation, relatives, or whoever the carers are, must be active partners in the rehabilitation programme. This statement makes the assumption that the carer wants to be involved. From the studies discussed, there seems little doubt that most relatives are already so closely involved in the caring, that to ignore their contribution would certainly undermine the most carefully thought-out programme. Relatives, caught up in the day to day caring, need a great deal of understanding support if they are to achieve the degree of objective detachment necessary to be involved in the rehabilitation programme. A counselling approach is one way to support them as they work with the therapist to achieve the client's optimum independence.

One clear fact is demonstrated; the majority of carers are women. It would appear that in Western cultures there is a great deal of socialisation to ensure that women fulfil this role. Men do not usually find the caring role easy to undertake. If people do not find meaning in the caring role, the relationship is unequal; if equity cannot be restored, there is danger of the relationship ending. Disability is likely to affect the whole family. Disability is intrusive and makes demands on time, energy and resources. Disability often acts as a wedge to widen rifts between married people and between the disabled person and children in the family. On the other hand, many people attribute to disability a closer bonding.

It would seem, as with most traumatic life events, that disability (whether congenital or acquired) will find the weak spots or the strengths in people and their relationships. The consequent breakdown, or the strengthening, rests not so much on the disability as on the cement which holds together the bricks of the relationship. Therapists are definitely not marriage guidance counsellors: yet the relationship they establish with the client and his relatives may be equally therapeutic and may do a great deal to avoid family breakdown. Clients and relatives testify to the benefit they derive from counselling. Counselling is time well spent.

Notes

1. Caplan, G. (1961) *An Approach to Community Mental Health*, London, Tavistock.
2. Dembo, T. (1955) 'Suffering and its alleviation: a theoretical analysis'. Report submitted for the Association for the Aid of Crippled Children, New York.
3. McMichael, J.K. (1971) *Handicap*, Staple Press, London.
4. Allen, F.H. and Pearson, G.H. (1928) 'The emotional problems of the physically handicapped child', *British Journal of Medical Psychology, 8*, pp. 212–35.
5. Survey Report (1980) 'The experience of caring for elderly and handicapped dependants', Equal Opportunities Commission, London.
6. Harvey, D. and Greenway, P. (1982) 'How parent attitudes and emotional reactions affect their handicapped child's self-concept', *Psychological Medicine, 12*, pp. 357–70.
7. Richardson, S.A., Hasterof, A.H. and Dornbusch, S.M. (1964) 'Effects of disability on a child's description of himself', *Child Development, 35*, pp. 893–907.
8. Tavormina, J.B., Boll, T.J., Dunn, N.J., Lucomb, R.L. and Taylor, J.R. (1981) 'Psychosocial effects on parents of raising a physically handicapped child', *Journal of Abnormal Child Psychology, 9, 1*, pp. 121–31.
9. Davis, A.J. (1980) 'Disability, home care and the care-taking role in family life', *Journal of Advanced Nursing, 5*, pp. 475–84.
10. Wakefield, T. (1978) *Some Mothers I Know*, Routledge and Kegan Paul, London and Boston.
11. Wright, B.A. (1960) *Physical Disability — A Psychological Approach*, Harper and Row, New York.
12. Schreiber, M. and Feely, M. (1965) *Siblings of the Retarded Children*, November–December 1965 distributed by the National Association for Retarded Citizens, Arlington, Texas, and quoted in Christensen and De Blaissie, *Counselling with Parents*.
13. Christensen, B. and De Blaissie, R.R. (1980) 'Counselling with parents of handicapped adolescents', *Adolescence, XV, 58*.
14. D'Arcy, E. (1968) 'Congenital defects: mothers' reactions to first information', *British Medical Journal, 3*, pp. 796–8.
15. Pavlou, M., Johnson, P., Davis, F.A. and Lefervre, K. (1978) 'A programme of psychologic service delivery in a multiple sclerosis center', *Professional Psychology, 10 (4)*, pp. 503–10.
16. Simons, A.F. (ed) (1984) *Multiple Sclerosis: Psychological and Social Aspects*, William Heinemann Medical Books, London.
17. Menolascino, F.J. and Coleman, R. (1980) 'The pilot parent programme: helping handicapped children through their parents', *Child Psychology and Human Development, 11 (1)*.
18. Topliss, E. (1976) *Survey of physically disabled people under retirement age living in private households in Southampton*, Southampton University.

19. Stubbins, J. (1977) 'Stress and disability' in Stubbins, J. (ed) *Social and Psychological Aspects of Disability*, University Park Press, Baltimore.

20. Stroker, R. (1983) 'Impact of disability on families of stroke patients', *Journal of Neurological Nursing* (December), *15*, pp. 360–5.

21. Wright, V. (1982) 'The epidemiology of disability', *Journal of the Royal College of Physicians, 16, 3.*

22. Sainsbury, S. (1970) 'Registered as disabled', The Social Administration Trust.

23. Jung, E. (1978) *Animus and Anima*, Spring Publications, Dallas.

24. Walster, E., Berscheid, E. and Walster, W. (1976) 'New directions in equity research', in *Advances in Experimental Psychology*, Vol. 9. Berkowitz, L. (ed), Academic Press, New York.

25. Marks, J. (1977) *Young physically disabled dependants and their families: a pilot study in parts of Hampshire*, Southampton University.

11 ANXIETY IN ILLNESS AND DISABILITY

Introduction

This chapter and the next are linked. This chapter deals with anxiety; the next with depression. Both are considered in relation to illness and disability. To consider anxiety and depression separately is, to some extent, artificial. Sufferers of crippling disease or injury very often display a mixture of both. To avoid possible confusion, the two states will be considered separately, though it should be borne in mind that very often they do accompany each other. Anxiety and depression in their more florid states are, in themselves, crippling. Anxiety neuroses and depressive states are two emotional conditions that absorb a large proportion of psychiatric treatment. These chapters will concentrate on these two emotional disturbances as concomitants of physical conditions, rather than considering them as disease entities. People working in rehabilitation need to be aware of how both anxiety and depression, unless dealt with, seriously interfere with recovery.

The Treadmill of Anxiety

This sub-heading has been chosen to indicate that anxiety is both a prison and a punishment. By this I mean that the person who experiences severe anxiety is trapped within a process over which he seems to have no control, in the same way that a prisoner would be subjected to the treadmill. There the pace was set by a gaoler. If he felt particularly vindictive, a turn on the control lever increased the pace at which the prisoner was forced to run. There was no respite; no escape. Exhaustion was inevitable. This is the picture and the outcome of anxiety: a state from which the victim may not escape unless some influence can be brought to bear on the gaoler to slow the rate at which the mill turns and allow the prisoner to step out onto firm ground.

Mild anxiety is a common feeling, experienced by most people at some time in life. It is a feeling of uneasiness or apprehension. Most times, normal anxiety is based on reality. Some actual event is anticipated; an interview for a new job; having to tackle a difficult assignment; an examination; give a speech; admission to hospital. Not all events that produce feelings of anxiety are necessarily unpleasant. Getting married, or being presented with an award, are two events that could be termed 'pleasant'; yet they may also produce feelings of anxiety. When the event has passed, feelings generally return quite quickly to normal, in much the same way as the heart rate, in a healthy individual, returns to normal after exercise. Normal anxiety, in small amounts, is biologically necessary for survival. Anxiety in doses too large for the individual to handle, leads to panic: panic produces irrational behaviour. Panic is more likely to be caused by 'free-floating' anxiety: anxiety that cannot readily be attributed to any specific event or idea. It is there, constantly lurking in the background. When it attacks, the person is once again set a-running in the treadmill. At the 'normal' end of the anxiety scale, the person experiences butterflies in the stomach, restlessness and possibly some sleep disturbance. In more severe anxiety and panic, the physical accompaniments increase with the severity of the psychological disturbance. Anxiety, other than that which comes within the 'normal' range, which produces crippling emotional and physical symptoms, is pathological. People who suffer from such anxiety need expert help.

Anxiety thus operates on three planes: emotional, cognitive and physiological. The more severe the anxiety, the more these three planes will become distorted. Very often it is what is happening within the body that brings the person to the notice of the physician. Such was the case of Andrew.

Andrew Fisher had been treated by his family doctor for about two weeks: he had complained of palpitations and was worried that he might be heading for a coronary. The doctor had prescribed suitable medication but the symptoms persisted. An ECG had revealed nothing abnormal. The night before Andrew was seen by a psychiatrist, Mrs Fisher had called the family doctor in the middle of the night because Andrew had a panic attack in bed, with racing pulse and palpitations. This extract, taken from a case study,[1] demonstrates the point that physical symptoms often become the first focus of psychiatric attention, and emphasises how necessary it is to consider the whole person and not just to treat the presenting symptoms.

Andrew complained mainly of tachycardia and palpitations, although Heber *et al.*[2] list 28 different physiological manifestations of what could be considered pathological anxiety. One of the characteristics of anxiety is that the more severe it is, the more it erodes every aspect of the person's life. The more this happens, the less able is the person to function effectively. His total psychic energy is taken up with his anxious feelings. His thinking becomes unclear, and problem-solving ability is diminished. The inner struggle which he experiences, the constant feeling of pressure, coupled with the feeling of not coping, leads to exhaustion and defeat. The prisoner collapses on the floor of the treadmill, while the gaoler laughs. Who is this gaoler?

There are many theories that attempt to explain the psychopathology of anxiety. The following are the principal ones:[3]

- Behavioural
- Biochemical
- Cognitive
- Communication
- Existential
- Family
- Humanistic
- Interpersonal
- Psychoanalytical
- Statistical
- Systems

Here is not the place to explore any of these in detail. Every one offers something, but none offers the complete answer. Students of human nature must be prepared to accept contributions from many sources. To follow slavishly one model is to close one's mind to the possibility that the model followed may not possess the whole truth. It cannot be emphasised too strongly that we all must search for, and then use, what we feel is appropriate for us; ever remembering, and being humble enough to acknowledge, that at any one time our knowledge is limited; and that lying outside our awareness other truths exist that could, if we examined them, enrich our experience.

I would like to suggest that the gaoler is whatever, or whoever, it is that seeks to drive the individual on to exhaustion. This may be a punitive conscience, guilt, ambition, fear of failure, or any one of a multitude of fears. Less may be achieved by trying to fit the person into a theory than actually helping him identify what or who the gaoler is. It is possible that there are multiple gaolers, each of whom may be at war with the others; the resultant conflict increases the tension felt by the victim. Pathological anxiety is the likely outcome.

In chapter 5 — self-awareness — the idea of the 'self' and 'sub-personalities' was put forward. The foregoing analogy of the gaoler, or gaolers, picks up the same idea. If one, or more, of a person's sub-personalities is victimising him, then that sub-personality needs to be brought under the liberating influence of the central self. It might be opportune to remind ourselves that every person is made up of body, emotions and mind, that these three parts are influenced by energy, warmth and light (p. 98) emanating from the central self. Not all sub-personalities are malevolent. Some exert a benign influence. But many work against the concept of wholeness; their influence is toward disintegration, not integration. I would suggest that pathological anxiety is the person's response to the negative feelings produced by one, or more than one, of his sub-personalities. They are his gaolers; it is they who force him onto the treadmill and keep up the pressure. They will resist all attempts by the central self to modify their punitive influence. They, the sub-personalities, have much to lose by surrendering their power. The fear that drives the person on will be replaced by the peace and wholeness from central self. That is what the sub-personalities fear. They survive on power based on fear. When that fear is replaced by peace, they lose their sting. The person stops running and may then step out onto the firm ground of manageable, rather than pathological anxiety.

Prevalence

Anxiety is widespread and common. It is estimated to be present in 2–5 per cent of the general population, and accounts for 7–16 per cent of all psychiatric admissions.[4] In one study, carried out in Great Britain, anxiety was found to be as high as 20 per cent. Anxiety was found to rise with age, was greater in women than in men, was not significantly different between urban and rural populations and it was more prevalent in the lower socio-economic groups.[4] Another way of looking at the prevalence of anxiety is: about 15 per cent of the patients on a GP's list will consult him, at least once a year, on conditions that are largely psychiatric in nature. The bulk of these (80 per cent) present with symptoms of anxiety or depression of whom about half present with short-lived disorders, which are often stress-related and most of which resolve within four weeks. The other half have more chronic recurring disorders that last for years.[5]

These figures may not paint an accurate picture. They represent only those patients in whom anxiety is recognised. There are many others whose presenting clinical symptoms are treated but in whom the underlying anxiety remains undetected and untreated. Anxiety often accompanies depression and is present in many physical conditions. It is always difficult to assess if the anxiety the person experiences is caused by the condition or if the anxiety causes the condition. Sufficient to bear in mind that anxiety is likely to be present whenever the body, mind, or emotions are put under stress.

Measurement of Anxiety

Before moving on to discuss stress, it is worth looking briefly at the measurement of anxiety. Anxiety is accompanied by alteration in:

physiology (body) thinking (mind) mood (emotions)

The Hamilton Anxiety Rating Scale[6] considers 13 variables:

Anxious mood	Somatic general (muscular and sensory)
Tension	Cardiovascular system
Fears	Respiratory system
Insomnia	Gastro-intestinal system
Intellect	Genito-urinary system
Depressed mood	Autonomic system
	Behaviour at interview

The grades are from 0 to 'very severe, grossly disabling'.

While the administration of such a test was designed to assess anxiety neuroses, and would only be administered by people qualified to do so, a study of the variables and their sub-divisions provides excellent background material for a fuller understanding of the effects of anxiety.

Stress and Life Events

The topic of stress, and life events as contributory factors of stress, was introduced earlier (p. 149). Now is an opportune place to broaden the discussion. The Life Events studies, referred to in chapter 8, demonstrated that breakdown is more likely in people who accumulate 200 Life Change Units over a period of six months. Since the studies by Rahe, in 1964, much attention has been focused on the relationship between events, stress and anxiety. In keeping with most theories, that of Life Events has its critics. Time could be spent, without much profit, trying to unravel the various arguments. One study,[7] which compared the life events of 183 English subjects with 183 Americans, drew a startling and convincing similarity between the two countries. The authors concluded that events that interfere with the life cycle, family relationships, social and work adjustment and the maintenance of psychological and physical integrity, are important contributory factors in psychiatric illness. They also emphasised that it was not necessarily the event itself, but the symbolic meaning the event held for the person, that was significant. This is an important point as we consider what can be done to relieve the anxiety experienced by people who become patients in need of rehabilitation.

In a study by Janis,[8] of fear related to major surgery, three patterns emerged:

1. *Excessive worry before surgery.* Wanted to postpone the operation. More likely than the other two groups to be anxiety-ridden postoperatively.
2. *Moderate worry before surgery.* Asked for realistic information, focused on realistic threats rather than on imaginary fears. Less likely than group one to display emotional disturbance postoperatively.
3. *Little fear before surgery.* Cheerful, optimistic, denied feeling worried. Gave the impression of being totally invulnerable. Their vulnerability showed after the operation. More likely than the other two groups to display anger and resentment toward the staff. They complained and were unco-operative.

This study shows that a moderate degree of anxiety is healthy and affords the person an opportunity to view the future realistically.

People can be helped to face reality by being given opportunity to discuss their fears. In addition to the ideas put forward in chapter 8, it is recommended that therapists look very closely at the support systems available to the patient; for, 'It has been shown that many people may be able to endure more stress if they have another person with them, preferably one who has maintained a close relationship with the patient over some time.'[9] This theme has been repeated many times in previous chapters but it is worth repeating, albeit with a different slant.

The Crisis of Illness

Many people lack the skills necessary to cope with the emotional stresses of daily living; physical and psychological disorders often result from this anxiety. One of the major causes of emotional stress is the sudden onset of an illness or an accidental injury.[10] The other side of the coin is that relatives are also put under stress when their loved ones become patients. As a consequence, the anxiety they experience may show itself in emotional or psychosomatic disorders.[11] Not every person perceives illness in the same way as others do. It has been suggested that *disabling* disease poses more of a threat to men, while *disfiguring* disease is more stressful to women.[12] This is related to the symbolic significance of the part of the body which is under attack.[7,13] That illness and injury are stressful events is borne out by Holmes and Rahe's study[14] in which 'personal injury or illness' was ranked seventh. In a more recent study,[15] which rated 102 events, and studied 2,627 adults, aged 21–64, drawn from all five boroughs of New York City, 'physical illness' was rated third, while 'unable to get treatment' was rated seventh. Only 'death of a child' (rated 1) and 'death of a spouse' were rated higher than illness. Although these two studies[14,15] did not set out to measure anxiety specifically, it could be inferred that the anxiety rating would relate closely to the stress rating. When disability itself is studied, it has been estimated that 85 per cent of the problems of the physically disabled are emotional reactions to the disability.[16] If this is so, one of the major goals in rehabilitation should be therapeutic assistance in emotional readjustment of the person suffering the disablement.

Disease and injury are crises in the lives of many people. How they cope with the anxiety generated is crucial to their rehabilitation. Three factors are important:

1. The presence and attitude of significant others, particularly family members,
2. The socio-cultural environment in which the person lives,
3. The attitude of community members.[17]

These findings are not very profound and are what most care-givers would expect. Indeed, anyone who has been a patient knows how comforting it is to have the support of friends and relatives. So when researchers[10;16;18-23] all emphasise the importance of support, in the process of coping, we should take notice.

Coping with Anxiety

'By coping we refer to the things that people do to avoid being harmed by life strains.'[23] Defence mechanisms have already been discussed on pages 24 and 225. The ones more commonly brought into play in dealing with anxiety are: regression, suppression, repression, denial, and reaction formation.[13] Most people who work to alleviate the anxiety of others feel that the person has a better chance of coping successfully with the anxiety if encouragement is given to express and explore it. It is often a great relief for a person to be given 'permission' to talk about his feelings. Three types of coping have been identified:[23] change the strain; control the meaning of the strain; and manage the strain. Although this study was concerned with the four areas of marriage, parenting, household economics and occupation, and not with health, some findings are relevant to dealing with people who require rehabilitation. These include:

1. The evidence that a positive self-regard assists in coping. This finding is supported by Garrity[18] who says that supportive networks of family and friends may function to strengthen coping and, therefore, resistance by providing validation of self-worth in the face of challenges which tend to lower a person's resistance.
2. Problems arising at work are less likely to be successfully coped with than those that arise within the family. This is attributed to the impersonality of the work place and the lack of intimate support.

   This has important implications for all health care workers. People become patients by virtue of some event. They are then brought into the occupational sphere of the health care workers, be it as in-patients or as out-patients. The hospital is *our* work place and because it is, it is likely that *we* tend not to deal effectively with problems because of *our occupational and professional impersonality*. If this is the way we operate, patients are likely to feel unsupported. Patients who do feel unsupported will not be able to deal effectively with the anxiety caused by the stress. What we must do is to recognise the potential impersonality of our working environment, then take steps to make it less impersonal; to make it a place where feelings are recognised and acknowledged. Then they can be dealt with effectively.
3. There is no one coping mechanism that would ensure a person being able to ward off the stressful consequences of strains. Therapists in rehabilitation may have to help their clients 'manage the strain', rather than 'change the strain'. Patients will get better from some illnesses, but not from all. Most illnesses and accidents that result in rehabilitation leave strain in their wake; strain which they may need help to cope with.
4. Men seem more able than women to employ strategies to deal successfully with stress. 'Men more often possess psychological attributes, or employ responses, that inhibit stressful outcomes of life-problems.'[23] This is attributed to the socialising process that equips women less well than men with effective coping patterns.
5. Successful coping appears to be linked to achieved status and to socio-economic status. 'The less educated and the poorer are more exposed to hardship and, at the same time, less likely to have the means to fend off the stresses resulting from the hardships.'[23]

This study identified three coping mechanisms: self-denigration, mastery and self-esteem. 'The greater the scope and variety of the individual's coping repertoire, the more protection coping affords.'[23]

Many of the findings about coping are substantiated in another study which looked at 170 middle-aged and elderly adults faced with hypertension, diabetes, cancer and rheumatoid arthritis.[22] These researchers produced six coping strategies:

1. Cognitive restructuring	(13 items)	—	finding something positive.
2. Emotional expression	(8 items)	—	anger against others.
3. Wish-fulfilling fantasy	(7 items)	—	pining, hoping.
4. Self-blame	(7 items)	—	'all my fault'.
5. Information-seeking	(5 items)	—	searching for information and advice.
6. Threat minimisation	(11 items)	—	a refusal to dwell on thoughts about the illness and a conscious decision to put distressing thoughts aside.

Cognitive strategies, including information-seeking, are related to positive affect, while emotional strategies, particularly those involving avoidance, blame and emotional ventilation, are related to negative affect, lowered self-esteem and poorer adjustment to illness. This comment is pertinent to counselling in rehabilitation. If, as the researchers suggest, '. . . further deterioration of physical health may be the outcome of a vicious cycle of illness-based stress, ineffective coping and poor emotional adjustment' then the aim of counselling should be to help a person develop more effective coping strategies. This may be done by strengthening those strategies indicated in groupings 1, 5 and 6 and diminishing the impact of items 2, 3 and 4. At the same time, however, it must always be remembered that being able to express one's negative feelings — about one's illness, or one's self — is integral and essential to counselling. But there is a difference between the 'emotional expression' of this study and expressing one's feelings within a therapeutic relationship, where the essential aim is increased understanding and insight to assist in the process of readjustment.

Support and Coping

Speaking on the subject of readjustment, Ben-Sira[24] says that the effect of primary group support is more important in readjustment than the severity of the disability or the length of time since the loss. This study raises an important and interesting issue: that reliance on professional support during readjustment increases the risk of dependence which is detrimental to positive adjustment. The antidote to dependence lies in increasing the involvement of 'significant others' and the support they are able to give. According to Ben-Sira, professionals engage in two types of support:

1. Resource compensation — provision of resources; financial and physical.
2. Resource enhancement — physiotherapy, vocational re-training.

I would add 'counselling' to the list of resource enhancement. Ben-Sira speculatively suggests that there is a '. . . greater propensity for professionals to engage in resource compensation activities rather than resource enhancement'.[24]

The study argues for greater involvement of the primary group, on the premise that its members are supportive. Their support rests on the intimacy of the relationship between themselves and the disabled person. On the other hand, no matter how supportive one's primary group, (this study was of Israeli war widows, bereaved parents and disabled war veterans) unless it is geared up to coping with trauma — and is adequately supported by professionals — help, appropriate to the need, may not be forthcoming. The findings of this study also serve as a reminder to rehabilitation therapists of the necessity always to have realistic expectations of relatives' ability to cope. Most will need a great deal of support and guidance. If relatives do not cope, the patients will not make a satisfactory readjustment or, in Ben-Sira's terminology, homeostasis will not be restored. 'A prolonged failure in restoring homeostasis due to the lack of appropriate coping resources may lead to a further deterioration of their condition, finally resulting in breakdown.'[24]

Antonovsky,[19] also writing about Israel, emphasises that because the Israeli soldier feels an integral part of his unit, he is willing to sacrifice his life for others, because he knows that everyone cares for him. This primary group feeling is also important to foster when considering rehabilitation. Antonovsky also says, 'On the simplest level, a person who has someone to care for him is likely to more adequately resolve tension than one who does not. Even without employing the resources of the other, simply knowing that these are available to one increases one's strength.'[19]

Cobb[21] defines social support as '. . . information leading the subject to believe that he is cared for and loved, esteemed, and a member of a network of mutual obligation.' According to Cobb's study, patients who are not socially isolated, and are well supported, stay in treatment and follow recommended regimens. This, also, has implications for rehabilitation, particularly when patients are discharged from in-patient care. Unless the support the patient experiences while in hospital is maintained when he leaves, his motivation to continue the treatment on his own will suffer a decline. A valid assessment of the support available to him must surely be a high priority when deciding who can and who cannot be discharged. In the same study by Cobb, it was found, when considering men with arthritis, that there was a significant relationship between lack of social support and the number of men with two or more swollen joints: 4 per cent with high support, 41 per cent with low support. It is also worth noting that social support can reduce the amount of medication required by certain patients; social support also accelerates recovery from illness.[21]

Counselling: An Intervention

Wolff[25] maintains that the business of the hospital is more than the physical care of the patient. Care should be psychological and should include helping the relatives cope with the crisis of illness or accident. Relatives whose anxieties are reduced by psychological support are less likely to let their anxieties spill over to the patient. Bunn and Clarke's Australian study,[10] of 40 parents, or immediate relatives, of seriously injured or ill persons, shows how brief periods of counselling help to reduce anxiety. The study considered six dimensions of anxiety: death, mutilation, separation, guilt, shame and non-specific. Counselling of relatives was carried out for 20 minutes, while the relatives were waiting for news of their loved ones: the approach was supportive and empathic. There was significant difference between those who had received counselling and those who had not. The improvement was in the 'non-specific' dimension of anxiety; the other dimensions remained unaltered. Those without counselling had difficulty taking in the traumatic events. Those who had counselling were better able to rally their emotions and control their confusion.

I have said how anxiety can be likened to being on a treadmill, where the person often feels pursued by some fear. Susan was such a person. Susan, in her late 30s, had recently become very afraid of being alone in the house and could not sleep without having a light on. She had lived alone since her divorce and had recently been receiving obscene telephone calls – sometimes in the middle of the night. As we talked, it gradually became clear that the telephone incident had triggered off a deeper, older fear.

When she was in a relaxed state, I asked her to let her imagination take her back to the last time she felt fear. That was related to when someone smashed her front door. A few other incidents took her back to the age of four.

Susan I'm standing at the front door of my Gran's house in Wales. I don't feel afraid, though. I feel quite happy. Why has that image come to me? [Still in her imagination she explored the house, starting at the 'parlour'.] There's a bowl of bulbs on the table. I haven't remembered that room in such detail before. [She moved up the creaking stairs to the bedrooms. When she got to her room and stepped inside, she physically shuddered, but could find no explanation. Then it was time for her to settle down to sleep.]

Dear Lord, I lay me down to sleep,
I pray, O Lord, my soul to keep.
If I should die before I wake,
I pray, O Lord, my soul to take.

Good gracious, I haven't thought of that for years. What a horrid prayer to teach a child. "If I should die before I wake". [She then had a dialogue with her mother.] Mother, leave the light on.

Mother Now don't be silly, Susan.

Susan Mother, leave the light on, please (becoming agitated). [The light was left on. Into her imagination came a white, shiny object which terrified Susan. She took hold of my hand which gave her some reassurance.]

Myself Describe this object.

Susan It's just white and shiny. It doesn't seem to have any definite form to it.

Myself Can you touch it?

Susan I'm terrified, but I'll try. Now it's turned into something white; like a sheet hanging in the air.

Myself What does the sheet want to do?

Susan It's coming towards me; it wants to envelop me.

Myself Let it.

Susan I'm terrified. Don't let go of my hand. It's changed into a wooden chest, the chest that was in my bedroom.

Myself What would you like to do with the chest?

Susan I'll open the drawers. I've got it! (her voice rising with excitement). It's a shroud. Gran kept all her burial clothes in there. I can remember being very puzzled when Grandfather disappeared. He had died and I knew that he had been wrapped in one of Gran's sheets. [As we talked this through, Susan linked the feeling of fear of the dark with the line of the prayer 'If I should die before I wake' and with the mystery of her Grandfather's disappearance.] How could I know the difference between 'going to sleep' and Grandfather 'going to sleep' and being wrapped in a sheet?

This example used the power of imagery to release Susan from her tyrannical gaoler. It is interesting to note how the image changed from something vague 'white and shiny' to the enveloping sheet, then to something solid — the chest. If Susan had not, in her imagination, had the courage to reach out to touch the 'object' and to allow the sheet to envelop her, she might not have been able to identify what her gaoler was and so release herself from its power.

I have included this brief extract, from a number of sessions with Susan, because it demonstrates, in some detail, this particular approach to dealing with anxiety. Not every therapist would feel comfortable using such a technique. Nor may it be appropriate for every person or every situation. But it worked for Susan.

Summary

This chapter has considered anxiety as a normal experience, but in its pathological state the person usually requires psychiatric help. For the purpose of our discussion, anxiety has been considered as a concomitant of some condition that requires the person to have rehabilitation. The treadmill analogy was used to describe anxiety, where the person experiencing it is often pushed to physical, intellectual and emotional exhaustion. The fact that most people would acknowledge that they have experienced some of the normal symptoms of anxiety provides a common base for an examination of a fairly universal phenomenon. For those people whose experience of anxiety has moved from the 'normal' end of the dimension toward the 'pathological', the theory was put forward that they are the victims of antagonistic sub-personalities who are at war with one another. Identifying these sub-personalities may be enough to drain them of the destructive power they hold over the person.

The topic of Life Events and stress was again examined, this time with more specific reference to anxiety. People who become patients experience a life event of some significance. The anxiety they feel is often compounded by the anxiety felt by significant people in their lives. Patients are often helped to deal with their anxiety by the support they receive from the primary group. It has been shown that relatives, and other primary group members themselves, need support if they are to offer effective support to help the patient manage the strain of illness, injury and subsequent rehabilitation. Patients who do not receive adequate support are less likely to deal effectively with rehabilitation. The role of the professional 'supporter' should not be so much 'provider' as 'enhancer'. Counselling — even brief periods — is an enhancement skill that professionals can use with patients and relatives as a support measure. Patients — and their relatives, who are also affected by the stigma of illness — frequently suffer from a battered self-esteem. Counselling support may help to restore self-esteem, so essential to optimum recovery. One study[22] demonstrated that it is possible, by concentrating on cognitive restructuring, information-seeking and threat minimisation, to help the person reduce the anxiety level; this could be an appropriate counselling approach to use.

The chapter closed with a short description of another approach — the use of imagery — not to control the anxiety, but to attempt to identify the gaoler of the treadmill. As with all counselling, it is essential that the therapist uses a broad repertoire of skills. A limited repertoire may prove to be too restricting on the client. While one approach may suit one client, it may not suit all. One technique may suit the personality of one therapist but not of every one. One of the aims of counselling is self-awareness; this applies to both clients and those who counsel. We who counsel need to know why we do it and why we prefer to use the particular approaches we do. If our counselling is to be truly effective, it is our duty to extend our awareness of ourselves as well as the approaches to counselling which other people have developed.

Notes

1. Stewart, W. (1979) 'Hidden conflicts: a case study of the Fisher family', *Occupational Health 31, 12, Dec. 1979*, pp. 568–78, *32 1, Jan. 1980*, pp. 22–9, *32 2, Feb. 1980*, pp. 76–83.
2. Haber, J., Leach, A.M., Schudy, S.M. and Sideleau, B.F. (1982) *Comprehensive Psychiatric Nursing*, McGraw-Hill, New York.
3. Davison, G.C. and Neale, J.M. (1982) *Abnormal Psychology*, John Wiley, New York.

4. Rees, W.L. (1973) (ed) 'Anxiety factors in comprehensive patient care', *Proceedings* of the symposium held at St Lucas Hospital, Amsterdam, The Netherlands, 31 March, Excerpta Medica.

5. Herrington, R.N. (1982) *Anxiety and Depression*, Update Publications Ltd, London.

6. Hamilton, M. (1959) 'The assessment of anxiety states by rating', *British Journal of Medical Psychology, 32*, pp. 50–5.

7. Paykel, E.C., McGuiness, B. and Gomez, J. (1976) 'An Anglo-American comparison of the scaling of life events', *British Journal of Medical Psychology, 49*, pp. 237–47.

8. Janis, I. (1958) *Psychological Stress*, John Wiley, New York.

9. Bovard, E.W. (1959) 'The effects of social stimuli on the response to stress', *Psychological Review 66*, p. 267.

10. Bunn, T.A. and Clarke, A.M. (1979) 'Crisis intervention: an experimental study of the effects of a brief period of counselling on the anxiety of relatives of seriously injured or ill hospital patients', *British Journal of Medical Psychology, 52*, pp. 191–5.

11. Rees, W.L. (1975) 'Stress, distress and disease', *British Journal of Psychology 128*, pp. 3–18.

12. Lloyd, G.G. (1977) 'Psychological reactions to physical illness', *British Journal of Hospital Medicine*, October, pp. 352–8.

13. Howells, J.G. (1978) (ed) *Modern Perspectives in the Psychiatric Aspects of Surgery*, Macmillan Press, London.

14. Holmes, T.H. and Rahe, R.H. (1967) 'The Social Readjustment Rating Scale', *Journal of Psychosomatic Research, 11*, pp. 213–18.

15. Dohrenwend, B.S., Krasnoff, L., Askenasy, A.R. and Dohrenwend, B.P. (1978) 'Exemplification of a method for scaling life events: the PERI Life Event Scale', *Journal of Health and Social Behaviour, 19* (June), pp. 205–29.

16. Ben-Sira, Z. (1981) 'The structure of readjustment of the disabled: an additional perspective on rehabilitation', *Social Science and Medicine, 15A*, pp. 581–8.

17. Bartolucci, G. and Drayer, C.S. (1973) 'An overview of crisis intervention in the emergency rooms of general hospitals', *American Journal of Psychiatry, 130*, pp. 953–60.

18. Garrity, T.F., Somes, G.W. and Marx, M.B. (1976) 'Personality factors in resistance to illness after recent life changes', *Journal of Psychosomatic Research, 21*, pp. 23–32.

19. Antonovsky, A. (1972) 'Breakdown: a needed fourth step in the conceptual armamentarium of modern medicine', *Social Science and Medicine, 6*, pp. 537–44.

20. Lin, N., Simeone, R.S., Ensel, W.M. and Kuo, W. (1979) 'Social support, stressful events, and illness: a model and an empirical test', *Journal of Health and Social Behaviour, 20*, pp. 108–19.

21. Cobb, S. (1976) 'Social support as a moderator of life stress', *Psychosomatic Medicine, 38*, pp. 301–14.

22. Felton, B.J., Revenson, T.A. and Ainrechsen, G.A. (1984) 'Stress and coping in the explanation of psychological adjustment among chronically ill adults', *Social Science and Medicine 18*, 10, pp. 889–96.

23. Pearlin, L.I. and Schooler, C. (1978) 'The structure of coping', *Journal of Health and Social Behaviour, 19*, pp. 2–21.

24. Ben-Sira, Z. (1983) 'Loss, stress and readjustment: the structure of coping with bereavement and disability', *Social Science and Medicine, 17*, pp. 1619–32.

25. Wolff, S. (1974) *Children under Stress*, Penguin Books, Harmondsworth.

12 DEPRESSION IN ILLNESS AND DISABILITY

Introduction

As in the discussion of anxiety, depression will be considered mainly as a concomitant of illness or injury and not as a psychological disorder in its own right. But in order to do this, it is necessary, first of all, to examine the tenets of depression. Some of the ideas that will be introduced are fairly traditional; others do not fit easily into any one 'school' of psychopathology. I have deliberately taken a broad approach to this distressing condition because it needs to be tackled on as wide a front as possible. Our knowledge of depression is great; but like the bottomless pit into which depressives invariably tumble, our understanding of this condition can never be fully satisfied. This chapter attempts to plumb, still further, the depths of the ocean of depression.

The 'Limbo' of Depression

In the previous chapter I suggested the analogy of the treadmill. There the person was constantly driven to exhausting activity. In many ways depression is the opposite: the person is caught in a trap that cuts him off from his environment, so preventing him reacting appropriately to it and with the people in it. This feeling of being cut off — of not being able to make emotional contact — led me to another analogy: the Limbo of depression. Limbo, according to theological belief, is a region on the border of Hell. It is the abode of those who died before the birth of Christ; they died without Salvation. It is also the place of unbaptised infants and of mentally subnormal people. The souls in Limbo are there through no fault of their own. Some theologians maintain that the infants in Limbo are affected by some degree of sadness because of felt deprivation.[1] Without becoming caught up in the vagaries of philosophical and religious discussion, it would be useful to consider the similarity between Limbo and the state of depression.

The Clinical Picture

Symptoms can be grouped under two broad headings:[2]

1. Psychological:
   Sadness. Loss of enjoyment in life.

Guilt and worthlessness.	Disturbed time sense.
Paranoid states.	Suicidal tendencies.
Loss of energy and interest.	Anxiety and obsession.

2. Physical

Disturbance of sleep	Disturbance of sexual function
Disturbance of appetite and weight	Retardation and agitation

Not every item on these two lists will be considered, and the discussion will move from psychological to physical symptoms where appropriate.

Sadness. Sadness is unhappiness brought down a degree. Most people know the feeling of unhappiness. Many know the feelings of sadness. Not everyone understands the deep, lasting, incapacitating sadness of a person depressed to the point where he feels 'like a dried out husk',[2] and where tears — therapeutic in normal sorrow — dry up in the eyes before they can be shed. It has been suggested that the sadness of depression has its genesis in loss of some valued person, possession or status;[3] in the way we attribute meaning to our ideas, feelings, ideals and circumstances, the sense of lack or loss of positive emotions, such as love, self-respect and feelings of satisfaction;[4] in a sense of deprivation, pessimism and self-criticism.[5] While sadness is a normal and healthy response to any misfortune[6] and is common, sorrow that does not lessen with the passage of time is pathological. People who experience normal sadness are usually able to talk about it, to know why they are sad, and still feel hope that the sadness will lift. Depression sets in when normal exchanges are absent or greatly diminished.[6] The words that would express how a depressed person feels are blocked in the well by the dried up tears. Sadness is also referred to as 'psychic pain' — pain that is not physical but mental.

Arieti[4] describes the characteristics of sadness as unpleasant; not rapidly extinguished — unlike anger that normally disappears; and that it slows mental processes. If sadness is psychic pain, is the psyche able to tolerate only so much pain? Is it possible that excess psychic pain is transformed into other feelings — anxiety, anger, rage and psychosomatic manifestations? Arieti suggests that sadness, particularly when it follows a definite event, such as a death, is reparative: but renewal may take a long time. He also proposes that a person who passes from normal sadness to depression is one in whom the reparative work of sorrowing has not taken place; he cannot do 'sorrowing work'. Such a person is psychologically ill-equipped (because life experience has not prepared him) to solve his sorrow or sadness.

Sadness is characteristic of a depressed state. That it is a universal feeling found in many disparate cultures is highlighted in a WHO study[7] in which sadness appeared in 95 per cent of the subjects from the five centres of Basle, Montreal, Nagasaki, Teheran and Tokyo. This study shows that, in spite of some differences between and within different cultures, depressed people are fairly consistent in the way they use figurative language to describe their feelings: the heart may be 'heavy', 'dark', 'constricted', 'sunk'; the patient may feel as if he has a 'stone in the heart': he may feel that he has a 'dark cloud over his head'.

Lader's list of major symptoms (p. 243)[2] does not give any order of priority or weighting. Sadness tops the list in many studies of depression. A close second is 'loss of joy',[2] 'inability to enjoy',[7] 'lack of pleasure'.[8] This particular feeling is so closely related to sadness that it is helpful to consider them together. Lader says that there is an increasing inability for depressed people to enjoy themselves. This affects relationships with their families; hobbies become boring; appreciation of art and music, which they previously enjoyed, lose their appeal; the world of nature and sound is dull and insipid. The fact that life is dull and cheerless causes them concern. They know the joy has gone but they cannot find where or how to recapture it. Not all depressed people are able to express this spontaneously, but when helped to do so, it is obvious that they do experience this loss. In the WHO study,[7] of the 573 patients, 93 per cent of them rated 'joylessness' second. The fact that the person finds no pleasure in things or people has the effect of cutting him off emotionally from activities and people who would normally stimulate him. That such a feeling of joylessness causes problems should come as no surprise. When any mood separates husband from wife; parent from children; working colleague from his mates; neighbour from neighbour; and when all of these relationships are affected *all at once*, the person's emotional world shrinks so much that even he, himself, is reduced to nothing. This is how some people express the depth of their feeling of isolation their depression has brought.

Rowe[9] says that the overwhelming feeling is that of isolation.

> The depressed person finds himself alone, separated from all human contact and in a world which has taken on a hostile appearance. Each person can describe his experience in an image, and all these images have one common feature — the person sees himself as imprisoned in an inescapable isolation.

One of the characteristics of depression is that it is contagious. Therapists may well find themselves 'picking up' the sadness, and reacting to it, by themselves becoming sad and losing some of their own joy. The effect which depressed people have on others is an important factor in their increasing isolation. On the one hand the depressed person desperately needs human contact, yet there is very little that he can offer to establish or maintain affectional relationships.[6] Indeed, it has been said that in depression, the person's ability to love, and be loved, is impaired.[4] A measure of this — which reinforces the feeling of isolation — is a decrease of libido. This was a significant symptom in 67 per cent of the respondents in the WHO study.[7] The decrease may range from 'little desire' to 'total inability' and 'impotence'. For couples who, hitherto, have enjoyed satisfying and fulfilling sex, loss of desire, or inability, may put their relationship under great strain.

Another part of an 'affectional relationship' is communication. Yet the profound feeling of isolation usually makes communication difficult. Communicating becomes a burden.[7] One of the difficulties expressed by depressed people is that the conversations of other people jar; their normal laughter seems totally out of place; their attempts to 'keep things going' become sources of irritation. The wave-bands of communication have become distorted by depressed feelings. Communication — of any meaning — virtually ceases.

Guilt and Worthlessness. Lader[2] makes the point that in a severe case of depression, the person becomes preoccupied with feelings of guilt and worthlessness. 'I am worthless'; 'the world is meaningless'; 'the future is hopeless'.[5] Harrow *et al.*[8], however, found that the depressed women they studied '. . . took a relatively hopeful view of the future. Most believed that they would get well.' This finding conflicts with many other findings and the researchers stress that the difference probably lies between 'thinking' and 'feeling'. They say, 'The affirmation of discouragement and hopelessness may be based on the patients' having *felt* this way. In contrast, their expectations of getting well may be based on their *knowledge* (or belief) that they will get well, despite these blue *feelings*.' This distinction between *thinking* and *feeling* is important. The importance of the way we construct our thinking is crystallised in the following maxim:

> It's not what I think I am, but what I think, that I am.

In the most severe cases of depression, these feelings of guilt and worthlessness assume full-blown delusional proportions. In such cases the belief cannot be reversed by evidence to the contrary despite being out of keeping with the person's social, educational and cultural background.[7] Minor misdemeanours and omissions are blown up into mountainous breaches of morals.

The WHO study[7] separates 'guilt' from 'worthlessness'. In that study 'ideas of insufficiency', inadequacy, worthlessness and lack of confidence (a) are separated from 'feelings of guilt and self-reproach' (b) and from 'delusions of guilt' (c).

(a) was present in 89% of subjects
(b) was present in 62% of subjects
(c) was present in 6% of subjects.

This suggests that a majority of depressed people have feelings of worthlessness (or feelings closely akin to it); a substantial number experience feelings of guilt, but not many have *delusions* of guilt. This last point is substantiated by the findings of a study already referred to,[8] in which the authors commented on a 'remarkable lack of guilt'. They go on to say, 'Reports of 50 years ago indicate that one would see depressives lying about in hospital corridors telling everyone about their terrible guilt. This is a rare phenomenon today, and our data reflect this change.'

Delusional responses may include the firm conviction that the individual is the worst possible sinner; he has committed 'the unforgivable sin'; it is his fault that the world is in the state it is, and so on. It seems that when depressed, our normal feelings of doubt become so exaggerated as to 'take over' and crowd out rational thought and feeling.

Self-esteem. Self-esteem is defined as, 'The degree to which one feels valued, worthwhile or competent.'[10] On page 186 the 'self concept' was discussed; self-esteem is a part of that. Very low self-esteem equates to feeling worthless.[10] In chapter 9 it was suggested that illness and disability alter one's self concept. It is natural, therefore, to further suggest that illness and disability not only may alter self-esteem but may plunge a person possessed of a low self-esteem into a state of depression.

Becker[11] says that lowered self-esteem is accompanied by feelings of unhappiness, anger, sense of threat, fatigue, withdrawal, tension, disorganisation, feelings of constraint, conflict and inhibition. High self-esteem is accompanied by feelings of integration, freedom, positive emotion and availability of energy. The first list equates very directly to the list of symptoms of depression, and one cannot help but speculate as to the place of self-esteem in the onset and course of depression.

According to Coopersmith[12] — who studied 10–12 year old children — positive self-esteem relates to parental warmth, acceptance, respect and clearly defined limit-setting. The study also showed that children who were expected to conform to ambiguous limit-setting standards tended to remain dependent or tended to withdraw. Stewart,[13] speaking of 'authority and counselling' says 'A child reared without boundaries will forever seek to escape from the wilderness of the wide world into which he has prematurely strayed.' Epstein[14] says, 'A person with high self-esteem carries, in effect, a loving parent within him.' It could be inferred that the person with low self-esteem carries a non-loving parent within him. If this is so, such a person becomes one of life's vulnerable personalities, prone to become caught in the quicksands of depression. Parke and Weiss[15] suggest that esteem for others is as necessary as esteem for one's self. They say, 'As long as a person has a reasonable degree of self-esteem, and other esteem, he or she has little grounds for feeling helpless or hopeless in the face of loss.' Brown and Harris[16] also link hopelessness with self-esteem. '. . . hopelessness is the key factor in the genesis of clinical depression, and loss is probably the most likely cause of profound hopelessness. Self-esteem influences the way a person deals with loss; low self-esteem leads to generalised hopelessness.'

Anxiety with Depression. 'Symptoms of anxiety are so common in the more mildly ill, that some practitioners believe depressive and anxiety states are inseparable.'[2] Harrow *et al.*[8] found that anxiety was one of the most common symptoms of the 52 depressed patients they studied; an outstanding feature of the anxiety was the feeling of restlessness. Lader[2] says that anxious, depressed patients are tense, jumpy, irritable and apprehensive, worrying about trivial matters and agonising over decisions. Beaumont[17] believes that although anxiety is frequently the presenting symptom, pure anxiety is rare. He says, 'Providing that the anxiety is not a feature of the personality type, then I believe that further questioning reveals that the majority of our anxious patients are also depressed.'

Anxiety, to recapitulate, is the emotional reaction to the expectation of danger or damage. When the event has taken place — e.g. death of a loved one or loss of job — and the damage has already been done, sadness results. But in many people — according to the studies quoted — the anxiety has become trapped in the feelings of sadness, thus preventing the completion of 'sorrowing work'.

Anxiety featured in 83 per cent of the respondents of the WHO study[7] and was rated third in four out of the five centres and fourth in the other one. Anxiety was linked with tension; the researchers believing that the feeling of tension may also be associated with a feeling of inner restlessness, particularly evident in the inability to relax. If, as these observations suggest, anxiety and depression are twin sisters, and if restlessness and tension contribute to an inability to relax, it would seem logical that one way for the patient to control how he feels, is to be taught — *and to practise regularly* — relaxation.

Sleep. MacDonald[18] presents a useful three pattern matrix of the symptomatology of depression. One of his six variables — 'bodily functioning' — has 'sleep' as a sub-division. In mild depression — pattern 1 — the individual has trouble getting off to sleep. This is a state that most people will have experienced. In more severe states the content and quality of the sleep is altered. The alteration may assume the form of dark and foreboding dreams and nightmares. Some people become tortured by early morning waking, after which they try miserably to get back to sleep. Lader[2] says that the typical sleep disturbance is for it to be lighter throughout the night with less deep sleep than normal. In contrast to 'normal' sleepers, the depressed person is almost constantly on the move while asleep. This is related to the level of sleep. During the stage of light sleep, we move more frequently.

Like sadness, disturbed sleep is one of the principal characteristics of depression. In the WHO study,[7] disturbance of sleep, of one kind or another, was present in just over 66 per cent of subjects. 'Early morning waking' — at least two hours earlier than usual with inability to fall asleep again — was present in 51 per cent of subjects. 'Inability to fall asleep' — within two hours of getting into bed and wanting to sleep — was present in 72 per cent of subjects. 'Fitful or restless sleep' was present in 71 per cent of subjects.

Sleep Deprivation. Sensory deprivation, and some of the disturbances that may result from it, were discussed in chapter 9. In a curious way, being deprived of sleep can produce similar disturbances. There is no doubt that sleep deprivation is a stressful experience. Prolonged deprivation affects muscle-tone, causes a drop in body temperature and interferes with attention. Psychological disturbances include illusions, and sometimes, hallucinations.[19] Closely connected with sleep is the 'biological clock', or 'circadian rhythm' — the daily rhythm with a periodicity of about 24 hours. With strict regularity the body temperature rises and falls; the time for optimum activity is when the temperature is at its highest. Other 'Ultradian' rhythms control the sleep-dream cycle. Disturbing any of these rhythms is like disturbing a delicately balanced clock by putting its hands 'back' instead of 'forward', or by tampering with the pendulum. The biological clock is upset in the well-known phenomenon of 'jet-lag'. But it is also disturbed by the less well recognised effects of severe illness. Sensory deprivation is an example of how the biological clock may be upset. It is also important to remember that disturbing one bodily rhythm may cause disturbance in all — for all rhythms are inter-related. 'Desynchronisation of biological rhythm is related to a loss of health and well-being.'[10]

Sleep is nature's way of ensuring rest and restoration; any disturbance will produce anxious feelings. In sleep, many bodily functions are suspended but during sleeplessness these functions, which should be resting, remain activated. This, plus the anxiety that inevitably accompanies disturbed sleep, leads to increased irritability and tiredness, yet tiredness that does not induce sleep. So, depressed people not only have their depressed mood to contend with, they are caught in a cycle of:

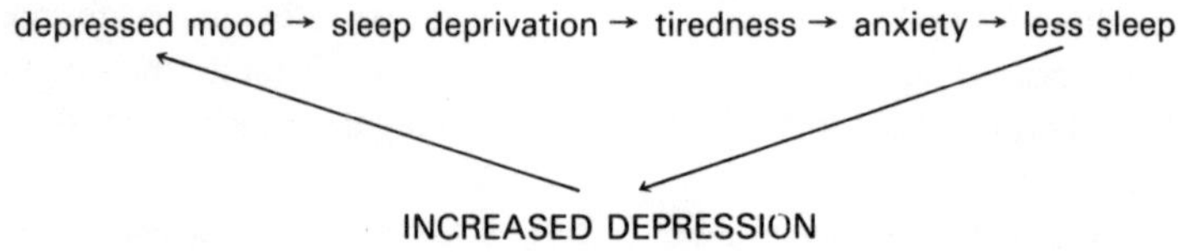

During periods of lying awake, the individual has ample opportunity to ruminate upon many of the darker facets of his emotions. Lying awake for several hours, after getting into bed, or lying waiting for the dawn to set the world astir, are not the best times to fill one's mind with light, positive thoughts. If the person is to climb out of his depression, he needs help to break the vicious cycle. Improved sleep, and with it improved well-being, may be the first step.

Prevalence of Depression

Bibring[20] postulates that, like anxiety, depression is a primary experience, and, as such, is common to everyone. If this is so, then we have all developed ways to deal with such feelings. Many people would argue with Bibring. Not everyone has experienced depression, at least not as the picture has been painted in this chapter. But we all carry the potential within us; and given the right set of circumstances we would become depressed. To imply that every single person is depressed, is fatuous, and it is certain that Bibring did not mean that. But there is abundant evidence that depression is both widespread and crippling. The WHO study[7] estimated that every year at least 100 million people in the world develop clinically recognisable depression. The researchers issue a warning: that many people with depression remain untreated and so run the risk of disablement. The families of such people, and the communities in which they live, are also affected. The 100 million people mentioned is a staggering figure. To make it more significant, it may be helpful to consider a geographical area smaller than 'the world'.

In Manchester, in 1980, it was estimated that 250 in 1000 of the population were at risk of psychiatric illness.[21] If the previous points are resurrected — that anxiety and depression should be considered together (p. 248); and that it is estimated that around 80 per cent of all psychiatric referrals are for anxiety or depression — it is readily understood that depression is a serious mental health problem. Watts[22] speaks of the 'iceberg of depression'. Suicides (0.12 per 1000) represent only the tip. On a much broader base are 12–15 per cent of people whose depression is recognised as such. Beneath them, 15 per cent, *or more*, suffer from undetected depression. Brown and Harris, in their study of depressed women in Camberwell, say, 'There is good reason to believe that depression is not just another problem but a central link between many kinds of problems — those that may lead to depression and those that may follow from it.'[16]

A curious statistic to emerge from several studies,[7,23,24] are examples, is that twice as many women as men are depressed. These are mainly well educated, economically stable, married housewives.[7] Brown and Harris also say that women with three young children under the age of 14, and who do not go out to work, are four times more at risk of developing depression than others.

Theories of Depression

If depression is the common cold of psychopathology, at once familiar and mysterious,[25] then the theories about depression are just as widespread. There is considerable overlap — as one would expect when the link is explored — between theories of anxiety and those of depression. The most common theories are:

Biochemical	Interpersonal
Cognitive	Learning
Communication	Physiological
Existential	Psychoanalytical
Family	Systems

As with anxiety, no single theory will be exclusively used[10,26] but it will be noted that all except interpersonal and learning appear on the list of theories of anxiety on p. 230. Many will be freely drawn from, in the belief that an eclectic approach will provide a deeper understanding.

Limbo Revisited

The picture of the depressed person which I have painted may appear sombre and perhaps depressing. This is precisely the effect depression has. Very often counsellors '. . . discern on the radar screens of their own feelings the shapes of the depressions that others cannot consciously describe.'[27] Kennedy's use of the 'radar screen' picture is apt; for it is with radar-like intuition that we try to pierce the Limbo-gloom that surrounds the depressed person. One of the points about Limbo is that it is a prison: a prison from which the only escape rests in eternity. Nothing the condemned soul can do, no prayers, no oblations — neither by himself nor by others still in this world — may effect an escape. The soul is powerless to escape from the darkness. In Limbo there is no light. Milton, in 'Paradise Lost', contrasts Hell (and with it, Limbo) with Heaven. The one is dark and punishing. The other is perfect.

On page 103 the 'Emotional Awareness Wheel' was presented. The quarters represented the four seasons. The emotional content gets progressively more negative as one moves from 'Pessimism' to 'Optimism'. Many of the feelings that have been described in the preceding pages are to be found in the lower half of the 'wheel'. In my theory I suggest that this is so because of being removed further from the light. When this is linked to the complementary theory of the central self — as the supplier of light, warmth and energy — it is possible to see how people who are trapped in depression do feel cut off from all that is light, and so become exposed to cold. I would suggest that they have been drawn (or pushed) into this state by the negativism of one or more sub-personalities.

Rowe[28] says, '. . . this experience [depression] becomes a ghost whose unbidden presence mars every feast, or worse, whose walls, though invisible, are quite inpenetrable.' The word-pictures painted by Rowe's patients are of dark prison cells; of being in a deep dark hole; of being wrapped in an inpenetrable cloth; in a vast empty desert; of being enclosed by thick soundproof glass. 'The images vary, but the underlying concept is the same. The person is in solitary confinement. And as the days pass, the torture grows worse.'[9] Rowe postulates further, that people become imprisoned in depression by the negative constructs by which they seek to regulate their lives. She proposes two basic philosophies:

1. Outgoing: joy, happiness, freedom, creativity, confidence, optimism, courage, benevolence.
2. Enclosing/restricting: mere existence, diminished, inhibited, helpless, despondent, anguished, pessimistic.

The list of propositions is long, and the inference may be made that we all have a choice of how we shall think of ourselves and others, and how we shall respond to them. None of us is entirely free from negative thoughts about ourselves and others, but when most of our thinking and reacting is negative, we will spend increasingly more time (and emotional energy) in the dark halls of Limbo, represented by the lower half of the 'emotional wheel'. This becomes the prison of depression. Such a view is shared by the cognitive theorists. Beck[5] sees depression, and other mood disorders, as being caused by irrational thinking. The person interprets events, his own self-worth, and the expected outcome of events, in a negative fashion.

If this view is correct (and it would be wise to retain a healthy scepticism that any theory has 'the answer') then it does suggest that the person gains something from such a philosophy. Seligman[25] puts forward the theory of 'learned helplessness'; a term derived from the response of dogs to inescapable stress. The learned helplessness model of depression maintains that when a person is faced with a situation, the outcome of which he has no control over, he learns that response is futile. One may infer that he then becomes a victim of circumstance, and as such he cannot be held responsible for whatever happens. He learns, therefore, to exploit his weakness and complaints, in order to force others to give him his way. But this drives him still deeper into the darkness, and isolates him further from others. Every manipulation that results in increased isolation, reinforces the negative view he holds of himself.

Life Events, Health and Depression

The link between stress and anxiety has already been demonstrated. Part of that discussion was related to life events. It is now time to link stress and illness or disability, as life events, to depression.

Psychic stress has been classified as: situational; social; family; psychosexual; or physical.[7] In the WHO study, 49 per cent of subjects, had experienced continued psychic stress. A study,[29] carried out in Warsaw, of 97 patients suffering from affective disorders, revealed that acute and chronic factors occurred in 90 per cent of the subjects; 33 per cent reported stress related to health (disease, accidents, surgery, poisoning, climacteric, delivery, abortion). Only 'marital' and 'family conflicts' scored higher, but only by 1 per cent. 'Health' as a contributory factor in depression seems as significant as it does in the aetiology of anxiety (p. 232).

In Paykel's study,[30] 53 per cent of patients reported 'health' events (serious personal illness, serious illness of family member, pregnancy, childbirth and stillbirth). In a British study of 63 families containing an adolescent member with spina bifida,[31] as many as 66 per cent of the adolescents were considered to have experienced feelings of misery during the preceding years. Girls experienced more such feelings than boys; girls 61 per cent as against boys 39 per cent. Dorner, who conducted that study, felt that girls were more likely to have these feelings because they had greater mobility problems, and the loneliness that accompanies reduced mobility seemed greater for them than for boys. 31.1 per cent of mothers were depressed. This was probably due to the increased vulnerability of these mothers. Their vulnerability made them more susceptible to stress from other events.

Ben-Sira[32] says, 'A traumatically disabled person may feel unable to cope satisfactorily with his work, to cope with his social relationships due to a sense of stigma, to maintain an affective relationship with his wife or children.' The fact that one does not cope, creates a fertile soil in which the seeds of depression may develop.

From the previous chapter's discussion on 'coping', we saw that how a person copes has a strong bearing on his readjustment and rehabilitation. One factor that emerges from all the studies on depression, linked to illness and disability, is the loss of self-esteem and independence. *Depression is common at the outset of a disabling condition and may recur periodically thereafter*. These periodic bouts of depression are usually caused by feelings of discouragement when rehabilitation seems not to be going as well as was hoped.

On pages 12 and 168, Elizabeth relates her feelings following surgery. There is no doubt that this life event was a stressful one for her and produced feelings of depression. Howells[33] says that patients who face life-threatening surgery often are depressed. These feelings '. . . can be regarded as a grief reaction of severe depletion. However, the majority of patients are not able to make clear to the doctor their depressed feelings and anxieties.' They are grieving for loss of health but also for loss of self-esteem which is linked to:

1. Loss of autonomy.
2. Reduced earning power.
3. Having to give up certain habits.
4. Sexual restriction.
5. Invalidism.
6. Premature old age.

Torrie[34] reported that 83 per cent of women who had undergone mastectomy suffered depression in the year after the operation. The emotional tension and stress following accidental trauma or major surgery, will be high when what has happened produces dramatic changes in body-image. Depression, secondary to loss and combined with grief, may develop or be aggravated and may lead to further impairment of general physical health.[35]

Pain and Depression

Pain is frequently present in illness, and invariably a prominent feature of surgery and trauma. Pain is linked with depression. Bond[36] says that when depression and anxiety are relieved, persistent pain is also reduced. He goes on, 'As a result, the need for specific pain-relieving measures may be removed altogether, or at least the potency of drugs required for relief may be reduced.' He adds that the depression accompanying severe illness is often made worse by the inability to control pain. Emotional support, Bond believes, in the form of discussions which deal with problems raised by illness, establishes confidence in the treatment. This, plus the marshalling of family and social resources, is often more effective than administering antidepressant drugs. Pain sometimes develops after loss — of loved ones, status, occupation. The link between pain and depression is significant. 'When pain precedes depression by months, it is probable that the mood disturbance is a secondary effect but, if both depression and pain begin roughly at the same time, it is more likely that pain is a symptom of depressive illness.'[36]

The pain, that depressed people experience, may affect many parts of the body and may include atypical facial pain or 'neuralgias', vague 'rheumaticky' joint pains and headache.[2] In some instances the preoccupation with the pain becomes hypochondriacal. In a study referred to on p. 139, the authors concluded that of 100 patients being treated for chronic pain, 25 were definitely depressed, 39 were probably depressed and 36 were not depressed. Pain is one more stress which, when added to the other stress of illness or disability, makes the person vulnerable to depression.

Vulnerable Personalities

Before going on to consider 'loss' as a stressful life event that may precipitate depression, it is necessary to spend a little time considering those personalities that are vulnerable to depression. The foregoing discussion on negative constructs (p. 252), and on the position of self — cut off from all that is light and warm — identifies negative thinkers as one potentially vulnerable group. According to Paykel[24] these are the characteristics of personalities vulnerable to develop depression:

1. Breakdown under stress.
2. Lack of energy.
3. Insecurity.
4. Introversion and sensitivity.
5. Tendency to worry.
6. Lack of social adroitness.
7. Unassertiveness.
8. Dependency.
9. Obsessionality.

What is not clear, is which of these characteristics, and which combinations, are crucial in the development of depression. But it is important to remember that when illness or accident come as additional burdens, a person already vulnerable may collapse under the weight.

There can be little doubt but that 'the family' is one significant and dominant force in the creation of a vulnerable personality. Family dynamics are so complex, and their influences so widespread, that it would be impossible to consider them here in any depth. One of the points that comes through in many reported studies, is the central role of the mother in establishing the stability of the family. Depue[37] says that disturbed children are more likely to occur in families where there is a depressed parent. He then goes on to relate this to problem adolescents with depressed mothers, and the mothers' inability to negotiate, to set limits, and display genuine interest. This is attributed to '. . . the mother's conflict between her feelings of deprivation and need to receive support versus her need to cope with heavy maternal role demands'. The conflict experienced by such mothers — a set of circumstances over which they seem to have little or no control — creates an atmosphere in which the 'learned helplessness' theory[25] gains credence. If their lives have been filled with situations in which they were unable to influence the source of their suffering, small wonder that they are depressed. Children reared in an atmosphere dominated by depression, where affectional relationships are neither established nor maintained, where the depressed parent constantly dwells in the underworld of negative thought and feeling are, themselves, likely to respond similarly. They have learned what emotional capital may be gained from being the helpless victims of circumstance. Paykel confirms this viewpoint. 'There is evidence that a disruptive, hostile and generally negative environment in a child's home constitutes a risk factor.'[24] This discussion has echoes of what has already been said about self-esteem on p. 247.

Loss and Depression

The discussion in this section will concentrate mainly, but not exclusively, on illness and disability as symbolic loss. The link between actual loss and symbolic loss has long been recognised, particularly in psychoanalytical theory. Paykel[24] says, 'The psychoanalytic concept of loss is a broad one, including not only deaths and other separations from key inter-personal figures, but also loss of limbs and other bodily parts, loss of self-esteem and of narcissistic gratification.'

There is nothing quite so potent a loss-source as death. There is trauma in death: the trauma of final separation. Loss is sometimes anticipated; very often is totally unexpected. Paykel says that the reaction to unexpected loss is more profound than when there is opportunity partly to work through the grieving before the event takes place. Paykel was speaking about death, but what he says applies with equal force to loss due to illness or accident. Depression, according to Poss, is the stage before the final stage of acceptance; acceptance both for the dying person and for his relatives.[38] Grieving is the natural and usual response to loss. The absence of grief is suggestive of psychopathology.[39] But there is more to bereavement than grieving for the actual physical loss of the person. When a loved one dies, a hole is left somewhere in the emotions, a hole which, according to some accounts, is never filled. It would be understandable to assume that death could be a major event in precipitating depression. A study carried out in St Louis[40] found that 16 per cent of the widows were still depressd 13 months after bereavement. And according to a study carried out in a Welsh community,[41] males who were bereaved had a higher mortality rate — at a ratio of almost 2 to 1 — than females who were bereaved. The first six months were the most crucial.

The feeling of loss when a loved one dies is real and often profound. But the loss may not always be within the conscious memory of the person who still carries the loss around. Brown and Harris[16] say that women who had lost their mothers before the age of 11, and who had been subjected to a severe event or major difficulty, were almost 50 per cent more at risk of developing depression. Such women may well have remembered their mothers, but also they may not.

June and Ian

The two extracts from the case notes of June and Ian show that the feeling of loss transcends memory.

June. When June's sister-in-law (of whom she was very fond) died, the grief she felt seemed exaggerated and prolonged. Gradually it emerged that the recent grief had reawakened the sense of loss she felt about her mother's death, when June was aged two years. Now aged 50, she had no conscious recollection of her mother.

Ian. Ian was in his mid fifties when his father died. His mother had died four years previously. Half seriously he said to me, 'I'm now an orphan, William.' As the truth of these words sunk in, he began to weep. He was not one of life's vulnerable personalities, when judged by the criteria on page 256. But, 'It's the first time in my life I've ever been depressed. I feel as if I'm in a hole in the ground and I'm covered over with a grey blanket. It's very dark and cold.' One of the curious things about sadness is that, as a piece of string dipped into wax will gradually collect more and more wax, one sadness will attract others to it. Too much sadness, expressed all at once, may be too much for the person to bear. Without trying to stop the process at all, it may be necessary to slow it down by helping the grieving person to identify and distinguish the different sources of sadness. In Ian's case, the loss of his father attracted some hitherto unexpressed sadness about the loss of his mother. But that was not all. As we talked, over a number of sessions, it became clear that there were other losses that were not so obvious as the sadness over his parents. A brother had died before Ian was born. Ian had always felt deprived of this brother's love. He had never felt much love for his only other brother, several years older than himself. He lived in America. Another factor was that the death of his parents, and particularly his father's death, had come at a time when he was having to make some personal adjustments to his own 'middle age'. So, all in all, Ian was carrying the accumulated weight of actual and symbolic loss. His depression — which did not require medication — began to lift after a few weeks, though he did find that being brought into contact with the sadness of others reawakened his own for many months afterward.

When a child is born handicapped, the symbolic loss can be quite as severe as actual death. 'I felt I had lost something which I had been looking forward to for at least nine months and probably much longer.'[42] Women who have had abortions — induced or spontaneous — frequently report feelings of deep loss. The loss of hopes, prospects and ambitions may be just as traumatic and as difficult to adjust to as loss of loved ones; for these may be just as precious.

Disability as Loss

The Camberwell study[16,37] dealt with 10 life events: two related to illness and accident, to the subject or to significant others. These two items accounted for 55 per cent of the responses. Death accounted for 62 per cent. There is no doubt that illness exerts a profound influence on most people, for it represents a symbolic loss of health, and heralds decline and eventual death. People tend to think more of death when they are ill than when they are fit. When trauma is considered, particularly where part of the body is actually removed, the resultant depression may be invested with a symbolic significance far beyond reality.[43]

The topic of loss, and the feelings that accompany it, has been discussed in previous chapters. Depression was a feature in surgery, blindness, rheumatoid arthritis, deafness and trauma. If disability increases isolation — as in blindness and deafness, or as a result of reduced mobility — then the depressed person has to carry a double dose of isolation. The impact of loss due to illness or disability is affected by:

1. The function of the part.
2. The symbolic value.
3. Any alteration of appearance.
4. Visibility of the change.
5. The feasibility of rehabilitation.
6. The degree of restoration possible.
7. Altered life style.
8. Whether it is permanent or not.

Health care workers need constantly to remind themselves that the patients for whom they care, whatever the nature of their illness, may experience feelings of loss which, if not dealt with, can lead to depression. The psyche will respond with feelings of loss whenever any part of the body, which it inhabits, is attacked by disease or trauma. That is why any illness or accident, however minor, may act as a precipitator to depression.

Measurement of Depression

The most widely used measurements of depression are:

1. Completed by an observer:
   — Hamilton's Rating Scale for Depression (HRSD).[44] This scale contains 17 items.
   — WHO Schedule for Standardised Assessment of Depressive Disorders.[7] This scale contains 57 items.
2. Completed by the person:
   — Zung's depressive scale,[45] which comprises 20 sentences.
   — Beck's Depressive Inventory (BDI)[46] which consists of 21 categories of symptoms and attitudes.

No space will be devoted to a discussion of these measurements. A perusal of the various items would provide a fuller understanding of what to observe in someone who is at risk of developing depression because of some illness or injury.

Counselling: An Intervention

One of the significant findings of the Camberwell study[16] was the role of confidant — husband or someone else. Women were more vulnerable to depression if they had no one with whom they could share intimacies. An associated finding was that women with young children were more at risk. It could be deduced that this was because women with children are less likely to work away from home. This makes it less likely for them to meet with people with whom they could share intimacies. They were also less likely to attend for treatment on a regular basis. Going out to work halved the risk of depression. This study highlighted the importance and value of intimate and caring relationships. If the lack of such relationships is conducive to developing depression, then everything must be done by care staff to foster an atmosphere in which intimate feelings may be shared. But one of the enemies of intimacy is impersonality. It might be salutary to refer to the discussion on p. 255, about impersonality of the work place. There is no doubt that having opportunity to talk with someone, to express one's feelings, is a safeguard, not only against loneliness and isolation, but against weaving, out of one's defence mechanisms, a blanket to suffocate all feelings. Counselling offers the sort of support that avoids smothering feelings.

Throughout this book it has been stressed that the level of counselling recommended does not equate with the 'in-depth' counselling or psychotherapy that some other professionals are able to offer as a necessary and integral part of rehabilitation. People who suffer from depression of the most severe, incapacitating sort, would need a rehabilitation programme assessed, planned, implemented and monitored by professionals experienced in psychiatry. It has been stressed, repeatedly, that although depression has been covered in some detail, this is not a treatise on depressive neurosis. It has been presented as a necessary part of caring for anyone who is ill and who, as a result of illness or accident, runs the risk of developing depression. As such, the aim of counselling, as recommended here, is supportive and preventive.

In the discussion on anxiety, on pages 235–8, attention was drawn to the coping strategies which people use. Many of these strategies are equally relevant to coping with depression. If support enhances a person's ability to cope with anxiety, it is doubly necessary in coping with depression, particularly when one remembers that self-doubt, hopelessness and isolation are cardinal features of depression. Specific therapies are legion, and many of them could be applied with good results to the treatment of depression. But it rests with every one of us to develop and use therapeutic approaches appropriate for us and for the particular area in which we work.

If this is not a treatise on depressive neurosis, neither is it a comprehensive study of therapies. On page 33, and at various places throughout the book, the importance of relationships has been stressed. When all else fails, when theories fall flat and when techniques fail to satisfy, all the therapist has left are her relationship skills. It is surely upon these, and through these, that theories become fact and techniques become reality. Paykel bears this out when he says, '. . . unless an immediate and intense rapport is established at the beginning of the treatment [although here he is referring to treating depression, what he says could apply with equal force to any treatment], the likelihood of having a successful therapy is considerably reduced.'[24] Beck[5] has described depressed people as 'losers'. If he is correct, one of the aims of the counselling relationship is to make them feel like 'winners'. Cognitive and behaviour therapy approaches, in which graded tasks are set, tackled and accomplished, have much to offer in the way of 'winning'. Physical therapists are well aware of the importance of graded tasks in boosting a patient's confidence. The change in self-esteem that comes with even small successes is essential if the person is to step out of his depression. Maintaining self-esteem is vital, if the ill or disabled person is to stop himself sliding into depression.

This may sound easy. But, as with all counselling, working with those who are depressed is not always easy or successful. Rowe[47] quotes the case of a woman who, because of the negative way she had constructed her life and her relationships, proved to be totally unsuitable for exploratory therapy. Some people, it seems, need to be 'poorly'. In a curious way it makes them feel 'good'. Rowe says that this is the construct of the martyr. Such people resist giving up their suffering. What they gain from being 'ill' is more than they would gain from being well. Thus, counselling — of even the most intense sort — may not always work. Moving out of Limbo — with its implication of being there through no fault of our own — would mean that we could no longer regard ourselves as helpless victims of circumstances imposed upon us by others.

Summary

This chapter has not been a treatise on depressive neurosis and its treatment. There has been no discussion of the classification of depression with its 'endogenous' and 'exogenous', its 'unipolar' and 'bipolar' typologies. Kendall[48] puts the case quite strongly when he says, 'It is clear . . . that there is no consensus of opinion about how depressions should be classified, or any body of agreed findings capable of providing the framework of a consensus.' I have attempted to paint a picture of depression, not present a psychiatric illness.

Indeed, it has been suggested that there is no such thing as mental illness. Szasz[49] is the best-known exponent of this view. What he says is challenging. Perhaps the contents of this chapter have been equally challenging — albeit in a different way. That is the second topic which I chose not to discuss.

Suicide is the third. One reason why it is not included, is that it is too vast and complex a topic to do justice to in such a chapter. Another reason it has not been included is that it would have taken the whole discussion too far into depression as a psychiatric illness, and too far away from depression linked to illness and disability. There is a very useful section on suicide in Davison and Neale.[26]

The one theme that repeats itself throughout this chapter is the isolation felt by depressed people, cut off, as they are, from emotional contact. In a sense, the depressed person pre-empts and pre-experiences his own death — the final isolation. The relationship between therapist and client is crucial in maintaining contact, and thereby reducing the risk of isolation. Human contact has a calming effect on the cardiovascular system of a person under stress.[50] Thus it is quite feasible that our very presence achieves as much, or more, than our words of counsel, however profound. What we do when we counsel is to offer ourselves in a relationship that makes no demands for itself. When we reach out to make emotional contact with depressed people, we break through the invisible barrier that keeps them isolated. This emotional contact builds a bridge. Across this bridge they may walk away from their Limbo.

Notes

1. *Encyclopaedia Britannica*.
2. Lader, M.H. (1981) *Focus on Depression*, Bencard, Great West Rd, Middlesex.
3. Herrington, R.N. (1982) *Anxiety and Depression*, Update Publications Ltd, London.
4. Arieti, S. and Bemporad, J. (1980) *Severe and Mild Depression*, Tavistock, London/Methuen Inc., New York.
5. Beck, A.T. (1976) *Cognitive Therapy and the Emotional Disorders*, International Universities Press, New York.
6. Bowlby, J. (1980) *Attachment and Loss*, The Hogarth Press, London.
7. World Health Organisation (1983) Depressive disorders in different cultures, Using WHO Schedule for a Standardised Assessment of Depressive Disorders (WHO/SADD) 5th edition.
8. Harrow, M., Colbert, J., Detre, T. and Bakeman, R. (1966) 'Symptomatology and subjective experiences in current depressive states', *Archives of General Psychiatry, 14*, pp. 203–12.
9. Rowe, D. (1978) *The Experience of Depression*, John Wiley and Sons, New York.
10. Haber, J., Leach, A.M., Schudy, S.M. and Sideleau, B.F. (eds) (1982) *Comprehensive Psychiatric Nursing*, McGraw-Hill, New York.
11. Becker, J. (1979) 'Vulnerable self-esteem as a predisposing factor in depressive disorders', in Depue, R. (ed) *The Psychopathology of Depressive Disorders: Implications for the Effects of Stress*, Academic Press, New York.
12. Coopersmith, S. (1967) *The Antecedents of Self-esteem*, W.H. Freeman, San Francisco.
13. Stewart, W. (1979) *Health Service Counselling*, Pitman Medical, Tunbridge Wells.
14. Epstein, S. (1976) 'Anxiety arousal and the self-concept', in Sarason, I.G. and Spielberger, C.D. (eds) *Stress and Anxiety*, Volume 3, Hemisphere, Washington.
15. Parkes, C.M. and Weiss, R.S. (1983) *Recovery from Bereavement*, Basic Books, New York.
16. Brown, G.W. and Harris, T. (1978) *Social Origins of Depression*, Tavistock, London.
17. Beaumont, G. (1983) 'Depression and suicide in general practice', *Psychiatry in Practice — a Symposium Supplement*, symposium held at University Hospital South Manchester 19 Jan., Medical News Tribune Group.
18. MacDonald, A. (1982) *Portrait of Depression*, Mind Publications, Leeds.
19. Hartmann, E.L. (1980) 'Sleep' in Freedman, A.M., Kaplan, H.I. and Sadock, B.J. (eds) *Textbook of Comprehensive Psychiatry*, 3rd ed. Williams and Wilkins, Baltimore.
20. Bibring, E. (1953) 'The mechanism of depression', in Greenacre, P. *Affective Disorders*, International Universities Press, New York.
21. Goldberg, D. and Huxley, P. (1980) *Mental Illness in the Community*, Tavistock, London.
22. Watts, C.A.H. (1965) *Depressive Disorders in the Community*, John Wright, Bristol.
23. Shephard, M., Cooper, B., Brown, A.C. and Kalton, G. (1981) *Psychiatric Illness in General Practice*, 2nd ed. Oxford University Press, Oxford and New York.
24. Paykel, E.S. (1982) *Handbook of Affective Disorders*, Churchill Livingstone, Edinburgh/Guildford Press, New York.
25. Seligman, M.E. (1973) 'Fall into helplessness', *Psychology Today, 7*, pp. 43–8.
26. Davison, G.C. and Neale, J.M. (1982) *Abnormal Psychology* (3rd ed), John Wiley, New York.
27. Kennedy, E. (1977) *On Becoming a Counsellor*, Gill and MacMillan, Dublin.
28. Rowe, D. (1983) *Depression: The Way Out of Your Prison*, Routledge and Kegan Paul, London and Boston.
29. Bidzinska, E. (1984) 'Stress factors in affective disorders', *British Journal of Psychiatry, 144*, pp. 161–6.

30. Paykel, E.S., Myers, K., Dienelt, M.N., Klerman, G.L., Lidenthal, J.J. and Pepper, M.P. (1969) 'Life events and depression: a controlled study', *Archives of General Psychiatry, 21*, pp. 753–61.

31. Dorner, S. (1975) 'The relationship of physical handicap to stress in families with an adolescent with Spina Bifida', *Developmental Medicine and Child Neurology, 17*, pp. 765–6.

32. Ben-Sira, Z. (1983) 'Loss, stress and readjustment: the structure of coping with bereavement and disability', *Social Science and Medicine, 17, 21*, pp. 1619–32.

33. Howells, J.G. (1978) (ed) *Modern Perspectives in the Psychiatric Aspects of Surgery*, Macmillan Press, London.

34. Torrie, A. (1971) 'Like a bird with a broken wing', *World Medicine*, 7 April, p. 36.

35. Wassner, A. (1982) 'The impact of mutilating surgery or trauma on body-image', *International Nursing Review, 29 (3)*, pp. 86–90.

36. Bond, M.R. (1978) 'Psychological and psychiatric aspects of pain', in Howells, *Modern Perspectives.*

37. Depue, R. (1979) *The Psychobiology of Depressive Disorders*, Academic Press, New York.

38. Poss, S. (1981) *Towards Death with Dignity*, Allen and Unwin, London.

39. Parkes, C.M. (1965) 'Bereavement and mental illness', *British Medical Psychology, 38*, pp. 13–26.

40. Clayton, P.J., Desmarais, L. and Winokur, G. (1968) 'A study of normal bereavement', *American Journal of Psychiatry, 125 (2)*, pp. 168–78.

41. Rees, W.D. and Lutkins, S.G. (1967) 'Mortality of bereavement', *British Medical Journal*, 7 Oct, pp. 13–16.

42. Ballard, R. (1977) 'Coping with the unthinkable', *Concern* (the Journal of the National Children's Bureau), *No. 23, Spring*, pp. 21–4.

43. Stubbins, J. (ed) (1977) *Social and Psychological Aspects of Disability*, University Park Press, Baltimore.

44. Hamilton, M. (1967) 'Development of a rating scale for primary depressive illness', *British Journal of Social and Clinical Psychology, 6*, pp. 278–96.

45. Zung, W.W.K. (1965) 'A self rating depression scale', *Archives of General Psychiatry, 12*, pp. 63–70.

46. Beck, A.T., Ward, C.H., Mendelson, M., Mock, J. and Erbaugh, J. (1961) 'An inventory for measuring depression', *Archives of General Psychiatry, 4*, pp. 561–71.

47. Rowe, D. (1971) 'Poor prognosis in a case of depression as predicted by the repertory grid', *British Journal of Psychiatry, 118*, pp. 297–300.

48. Kendall, R.E. (1976) 'The classification of depressions: a review of contemporary confusion', *British Journal of Psychiatry, 129*, pp. 15–28.

49. Szasz, T.S. (1960) 'The myth of mental illness', *American Psychologist, 15*, pp. 113–18, or book of the same title (1961) Secker & Warburg.

50. Lynch, J.J. (1977) *The Broken Heart*, Basic Books Inc., New York.

For readers who want to study a personal account of someone suffering from depression the works of Kafka are recommended.

1. Kafka, F. (1971) 'The Complete Stories'.

2. Kafka, F. (1973) 'Letters to his Father'.

Both published by Stocken, New York.

13 CHRONIC ILLNESS — MULTIPLE SCLEROSIS

> We who are handicappped need confidence and friendliness as well as, if not more than, medical treatment. It is not only our muscles and limbs which bother us — sometimes it is our minds as well. A child with a crooked mouth and twisted hands can very quickly and easily develop a set of very crooked and twisted attitudes both towards himself and life in general, unless he is helped to an understanding of them. Life becomes to him just a reflection of his own 'crookedness', his own emotional pain.[1]

Introduction

On the first page of this book a passage was quoted from a speech made in the House of Commons by Alfred Morris. Part of what he said bears repeating '. . . if years cannot be added to the lives of the chronically sick, at least life can be added to their years . . .'[2] These two quotes — by Christy Brown (above) and by Alfred Morris — support each other. There are many people with chronic illness who spend a miserable existence; imprisoned, disabled and handicapped by their illness and kept imprisoned by the attitudes of society toward them, by the lack of adequate facilities to enable them to live as normal a life as their illness would permit. On the other hand, there are many, many others who do enjoy relative freedom of movement, who do participate in social and community activities, who do have jobs to go to and from which they earn a living. What emerges from a study of chronic illness, is that the degree of handicap is not always directly proportional to the severity, or chronicity, of the condition. As we have observed in previous chapters, and particularly in the last one, how a person copes with illness very often *is* directly proportional to the support he receives: the confidence, friendliness and understanding mentioned by Christy Brown.

In chapter 7, another chronic illness — rheumatoid arthritis — was considered. There the discussion focused more on pain than on the disease giving rise to the pain. This chapter will focus on multiple sclerosis (MS) as a chronic disease that brings in its wake many physical, psychological and social problems. It is also an illness that brings together many of the topics which have already been considered in preceding chapters.

Although the focus is on MS, the aim is to use this illness to consider some of the elements that are common to many disabling conditions. This approach is in keeping with the other chapters where less emphasis has been placed on the condition as a medical entity than on the associated physical, psychological and social problems. What must always be considered is, what does this illness mean:

To this person?
In these circumstances?
At this time of life?
With these relatives? (or lack of them)
In this environment?

It has been suggested that '. . . multiple sclerosis provides a paradigm for chronic diseases and all their accompanying problems of adjustment.'[3]

Chronic Illness

Chronic illness is defined as all impairments or deviations from normal which have one or more of the following characteristics:

1. It is permanent.
2. It leaves residual disability.
3. It is non-reversible.
4. It requires special training of the patient for rehabilitation.
5. It is likely to require a long period of supervision, observation or care.[4]

Chronic illness may also seriously affect the person's life style and bring changes in economic, social and inter-personal circumstances.[5] There is a further possibility. The treatment pattern itself often alters the person's life style. People who are unable to adapt their life style, so that treatment becomes a wheel within wheels, often find the whole idea of treatment too difficult to handle.

Dependency

People with chronic illness have to adjust to the 'sick role', a role which has overtones of increasing dependence. Dependency upon 'professionals' is often easier to accept than dependency upon relatives for whom responsibility is increased. Conflict results. The person now becomes a 'patient' and is forced to become more dependent in many areas of his life *but not in all*; at the same time, he is likely to resent and resist his gradual loss of independence. Coupled with this is the social devaluation felt by people with long term illness. This contrasts with what happens in an acute illness, where the patient expects to recover. The person with chronic illness cannot have a realistic expectation of recovery. The expectation is of getting worse.

'Reciprocal dependency' — where there is give and take — is easier to accept than one-sided dependency. Some aspects of dependency were discussed in chapter 10. That discussion — which concentrated on the impact which increased dependency has on the carers — prepared the way for a consideration of the other side of the coin; the impact on the person suffering from illness or disability. In the section, 'Finding meaning in the caring role' (p. 219), Equity Theory was discussed.[6] I would suggest that this theory has equal meaning for the person struggling to find meaning in the new 'sick role'. If the carer needs to find meaning *in the new relationship*, so does the person affected by the illness. The theory suggests that if equity cannot be established, the carer will find the strain intolerable. Breakdown of the relationship will result. This being so, if the ill person cannot establish equity, this will contribute to breakdown. While it may be possible for the carer to 'opt out' and physically leave the ill person, the ill person cannot do this. Yet the psychological stress may be so severe that he opts out by withdrawing from all emotional contact — with his carer or anyone else. A person with a chronic illness may be helped to a better adjustment by being given an opportunity to express how he feels. Counselling affords such an opportunity.

Multiple Sclerosis

This brief excursion into chronic illness and dependency prepares the way for a more detailed examination of MS. Multiple sclerosis has been defined as

> a progressive disease of unknown origin which affects the central nervous system, causing varying degrees of paralysis, impaired vision, slurred speech and bladder and bowel weakness. It is one of the most common cause of crippling in adults. More women are affected than men, in the proportion of three to two. A characteristic of the disease, despite its progressive nature, is periods of remission of the symptoms

The picture painted by this definition, and indeed by most others, is bleak and depressing. It gives little hope. But is there any hope, when one is stricken by a disease, the cause of which is unknown, the course totally unpredictable, with no known cure, which is progressive in its deterioration? On the face of it, no. Yet, in spite of so many negatives, many people with MS live full lives. Others, it is true, do become incapacitated and spend years in a state of total dependence. The only thing that is certain about MS, is its unpredictability. The uncertainty is present from the onset.

The Doctor's Dilemma

'Tell me, Doctor, what is wrong with me?' A natural question posed by Simon, aged 22 years, visiting his doctor. 'About a month ago I stumbled at work. Felt as if my leg had given way. Then a few days later I had pins and needles in the same leg. And I'm so tired lately. Not like me at all. Oh yes, my eyes feel a bit funny; things don't look quite the same.' Presented like this, in this chapter, the natural deduction is 'MS'. But all is not always so obvious.

Incidence

The first of many problems associated with MS is its incidence. A doctor who practises in the South of England, where the incidence rate is around the national average of 50 per 100,000 of population[8] is unlikely to have any more than one or two of his 2000 patients suffering from MS. Indeed, Professor D.L. McLellan (personal communication) suggests that in the South of England the incidence is at least 80 per 100,000, and probably nearer the 120 per 100,000, so that a general practitioner will expect three or so patients with the disease in a practice. The escalating figures are probably caused by improved diagnostic techniques and better epidemiological methods. In contrast, a GP in Shetland or Orkney will have many more patients with MS; 129 per 100,000 of population. As many as 300 per 100,000 have been reported in Shetland.[9] Although the incidence in Great Britain is twice the world average,[9] the numbers *per doctor's practice* are not high. This view is substantiated in, 'Even in those parts of the world where MS is most frequent, it is unlikely that more than one person in 20,000 experiences a clinical onset of the disease each year.'[10] But, as with most conditions, greater exposure means that the doctor is generally more alert. Thus a doctor in Shetland would be more likely to put Simon's symptoms together than a medical colleague elsewhere in the country. The geographical distribution worldwide has been plotted[10] with clearly identified high and low risk zones shown. But in spite of the tremendous research interest shown in MS, its origins remain an enigma.

Multiple sclerosis is '. . . one of the main disorders of the Central Nervous System and its consequences can lead to the disruption of normal functioning of many other parts of the body.'[8] That statement is supported by a study carried out of five residential institutions.[11] Of the 147 residents, 34 (23 per cent) had MS; the highest number for any single illness. If this figure of 23 per cent is nationally representative of those 'in care', then a very high proportion of the estimated 50,000 MS sufferers in Britain are cared for at home by a spouse or other close relative.[12] The inference is that although MS can and does lead to disruption of normal functioning of many parts of the body,[8] most people with MS are not rendered so disabled that they require institutional care, or if they are, their carers are carrying great burdens of responsibility. Campling,[7] although not referring specifically to MS, estimates that '. . . over 84 per cent of all disabled women in GB live at home'. This is particularly relevant when one remembers that more women than men are affected by MS. It is also a misconception that MS always leads to an unproductive life, with the person confined to a wheelchair. In one American study[13] the researchers found that 66 per cent of the patients were ambulatory 25 years after the onset of MS. In another study, of 92 patients with MS, 30 per cent were still working 18.4 years after the onset.[14] The finding of '25 years' is supported by McAlpine.[10] He also says,

> Factors which are associated with a high risk of early disability and premature death are as follows:
>
> (a) slow progression of symptoms from the onset;
> (b) incomplete or poor recovery from the initial attack or from early relapses;
> (c) frequent relapses;
> (d) persistence of pyramidal or cerebellar signs or of sphincter disturbances in the early stages of the disease.

While it is true that MS is a disease that incapacitates some people and ties them to a wheelchair, or confines them to bed, to be looked after, either in hospital or by devoted relatives, others do not progress quite so dramatically down the downhill path to chronic disability and helplessness.

The Clinical Picture

The fact that not all people with MS have the same symptoms, nor the same severity of symptoms, should not disguise the other fact that MS may be devastating in its effect. Since it is predominantly the white matter of the brain and spinal cord that is affected, early disturbances are likely to involve sight, movement and sensation. The cranial nerves may also be affected.[10] Although in many cases these early symptoms disappear, to return only once, in other instances there is steady deterioration.[10]

To Tell or Not to Tell

The typical GP — who sees only one new case of MS every four to five years — would be very unwilling to make a diagnosis of MS. This is understandable, for there are no reliable diagnostic tests available. Accurate diagnosis is vital. But 'When symptoms are intermittent, are as vague as stumbling or slurred speech, and are found in young adults, they do not provide an easy framework for either medical or self-identification.'[5] Sambrook[15] makes the point that the most important indicator of diagnosis is a history of a relapsing and remitting illness with evidence of lesions in the central nervous system. But even then, a positive diagnosis is doubtful. The reluctance some doctors feel about confronting the possibility of MS may be put down to their pessimistic view of the prognosis.[16,17] It is doubtful if any GP would, on his own, make a diagnosis of MS but there is abundant evidence that had GPs — and the specialists to whom the patients were referred — really listened to what the patients were telling them, diagnoses could have been made much earlier than they were. Researchers in one study reported, '. . . the diagnosis of MS was seldom easily or rapidly reached. It took an average of 5½ years for the individual to be correctly diagnosed.'[18] This was a study of 60 people who had suffered from MS for an average of 14 years. A different viewpoint is put forward in another study of 57 patients, resident in a Danish MS nursing home.

> It has been frequently postulated that the medical profession is unwilling to inform patients of a serious illness. Therefore, it seems surprising that 56 per cent of the patients had been informed about their diagnoses less than one year after they had been made with more or less certainty by the medical profession.[19]

It seems, then, that not all doctors put off telling the truth, however difficult they may find it.

Uncertainty would appear to be the major reason why doctors are unwilling to tell patients that they have MS and it is possibly the reason why euphemisms such as 'inflammation of the spine';[17] 'demyelinating condition'; 'inflammatory condition' or 'ideopathic neuritis' are used.[3]

The Patient's Dilemma

Euphemisms may not be actually dangerous; prevarications and misdiagnoses are. Stewart and Sullivan[18] report that 75 per cent of patients in their study were given '. . . unacceptable and inaccurate diagnoses'. The most common types of diagnoses given were: neurological diseases; muscle, bone and joint diseases; eye infection; bursitis; inner ear infection; neuritis; myasthenia gravis; muscular dystrophy and arthritis. Psychosomatic misdiagnoses were also made: nervousness, anxiety, depression and stress. Treatments — based on the wrong diagnoses — ranged from tranquillisers, cortisone-like drugs, pain pills and antidepressants to physical therapy, traction, psychotherapy, vitamins and minerals and even surgery.

Part of the patient's dilemma is, what to believe. His body and his psyche, tell him one thing — there *is* something wrong. The information given the patient by the doctor very often conflicts with his own 'gut reaction'. What, or whom, should he believe? People have expectations of doctors: they believe that they know about all diseases and that they can cure them. If a person is told, 'It's all in the mind; go home and take some Valium', he will believe the doctor — at least for a time, until his psyche says, 'Listen to me!' Many patients try self-diagnosis. Sometimes they are correct but then they have the job of convincing a sceptical doctor. While some self-diagnoses are correct, others are wildly inaccurate. If doctors misdiagnose MS, people with less experience are surely more prone to error. Self-diagnosis can be stressful, particularly if the patient is convinced that he has cancer — quite a common fear.

Another aspect of 'not knowing' is that the person, although feeling unwell, is denied being able to adopt the 'sick role'. A person who is not given a label on which to hang his sickness, runs the risk of being misunderstood by the rest of society. Families and people at work soon begin to wonder if the 'sickness' is not some hypochondriacal manipulation. So, in a way, the person without a diagnosis, or one whom the diagnosis does not fit, is in 'no man's land' — sick, yet not sick. The uncertainty of not knowing, or feeling that the diagnosis is not right, places him under great stress and undermines self-confidence. There is doubtful merit in delaying making the diagnosis known so as to allow more time for data to be collected. But doctors who delay may be guilty of ignoring the personal and social implications of delay.[18]

Some physicians believe that the patient needs protection from the truth. 'They argue that the doctor's first duty is the relief of suffering and that to tell the truth could cause unnecessary anguish rather than be conducive to peace of mind.'[20] But many people who have MS say the exact opposite; knowing the truth although painful, gives them something positive to get to grips with. In any case, the relief of physical suffering which ignores the emotional suffering, caused by uncertainty, is bound to be counter-productive. Knowing that one has MS removes the paralysing fear of other, more terrible, diseases, a point put most graphically by John Brown from New Zealand. At the age of 24, John was diagnosed as having a 'suspected tumour' on his spine. Five years later the correct diagnosis was made. The knowledge that he had a definable condition released an energy that enabled him to work for improved facilities for other people with MS.[21] The view that patients are relieved to know the truth is put very clearly thus, 'Even though it is a matter of a chronic disease with a capricious but usually progressive course with increasing disablement, many patients seem able to accept the truth as an alternative to total and persisting uncertainty and experience a feeling of strength . . .'[19]

The 'strength' referred to, is that which enables a person to be able to plan his life, to be free from the strain of uncertainty, to avoid spending money uselessly, to be able to take care of himself physically, and to remove the fear that he might be neurotic.[22] The person's response to being told that he has MS is influenced by: the severity of the symptoms; how he perceives his illness; his inner strengths; his emotional state and the coping strategies he has already developed; his family's emotional state and how they perceive, and react to, the illness; and the supporting services in the environment.

To summarise the foregoing discussion. Multiple sclerosis is a neurological disease of unknown origin with no known cure. Its course is progressive and characterised by remissions and relapses. Due to the vagueness of the presenting symptoms, many patients are not diagnosed early enough; others are misdiagnosed. Some doctors are loath to tell the patient he has MS, even when the diagnosis is virtually certain. Others tell the patient in such a way that all sensitivity is removed. One male patient of 25, newly married, having been in hospital for several days for investigations, was told by the neurologist, 'You have multiple sclerosis, but there's no need to worry. Go home and read about it.' Luckily, not all are as insensitive as this.

[One] GP's reaction, to a consultant neurologist's confirmation of the diagnosis of MS, was to share the letter with her [the patient] and to say, 'I don't really know much about MS; let's find out what we can together.' Similarly another doctor, when dealing with complications of MS, said to his patient, 'You're the expert; tell me what you know about this problem and I'll do my best to help'.[20]

Matthews says, 'When I am certain of the diagnosis I always tell the patient . . . Moreover, it is distasteful to suspect that your doctor is telling lies and scarcely encouraging to believe that he has no idea what is wrong with you.'[9] People who suffer from MS have to make massive readjustments if they are to cope. The majority do want to know what is wrong with them. Knowing the truth removes some of the uncertainty: uncertainty is an uneasy bedfellow with peace. Knowing that one has MS allows one to concentrate on inner resources on working toward true acceptance built upon understanding, not resignation forced upon one by uncertainty and false hopes constantly dashed. Acceptance, not resignation, allows the person to develop successful strategies to cope with the physical, emotional and social problems that acccompany multiple sclerosis.

Categories of Multiple Sclerosis

The following three categories of MS are adapted from the work of Fritsch.[23]

1. Cerebrospinal Types. These have the highest incidence rate with: defective vision; blindness; trigeminal neuralgia; Bell's paralysis; focal, or in some cases major, epileptic seizures; various forms of spastic paresis of the extremities; disturbed function of bowel and bladder as well as recurrent psychological problems.
2. Spinal Types. Paraplegia; or tetraplegia; early bladder and bowel incontinence; loss of libido and sexual potency; lancinating pain; trophic ulceration.
3. Cerebral Types. Normal bowel and bladder functions; increased libido and sexual potency; deficient peripheral motor functioning.

In types 1 and 3, after many years of suffering, there is likely to be increased euphoria, loss of drive and interest; and a Korsakoff-like picture has been noted.

Fritsch concludes her paper with these words, 'Never measure the success [of rehabilitation] by the tape-measure or the stop-watch, for the treatment of neurological diseases always takes much time and requires even more patience, both on the part of the therapist and on the part of the patient.' This is sound advice indeed; the same advice applies to counselling in rehabilitation.

In the formidable catalogue of symptoms presented above, there is not much space devoted to mental, emotional or social difficulties of people suffering from MS. In order to find a way through what appears to be a jungle of symptoms, from many sources — some not quoted here — they have been re-formed into the following four groupings (Figure 13.1).

Figure 13.1: Signs and Symptoms of Multiple Sclerosis

Physical	Emotional	Mental	Social
Fatigue Motor — paresis — spasms — spasticity — tremors Sensory — loss — pain Ulcers — decubital — trophic Urinary and bowel Visual	Aggression Anxiety Apathy Depression Euphoria Irritability Mood swings Self-concept changes	Disorientation Intellectual — attention — concentration — conceptual thinking — memory — speech — personality change Stress	Employment Finance Housing Mobility Relationships Role change

As with all 'classifications' some items could be included in more than one list. It is worth stressing the inter-relatedness of some of the items here listed. Although the symptoms have been neatly divided into four categories, a symptom from any section is likely to extend its influence into the other three, just as in life.

Physical Dysfunctions

The physical symptoms of MS, listed on the previous page, are the most common. One study (of 92 patients) showed the following incidence of symptoms:[14]

Spasticity	70%	Sensitivity [sensory]	24%
Ataxia	29%	Vision	9%
Bladder/bowel	29%	Psychomental	11%

Some of the disabilities resulting from MS are what Burnfield calls 'visible handicaps'.[16] Other disabilities are 'invisible' and remain so throughout the person's life. Though not wishing to minimise the more obvious symptoms, the discussion here will focus on three invisible disabilities: fatigue, excretory and sexual functions.

Fatigue. Fatigue is a common sign in the early stages of MS. Patricia Wright was working as a district nurse when, '. . . I found that after a couple of turns [on the pedals of her bicycle] my left leg went all weak and wobbly, leaving the work to its mate.'[25] Burnfield said, 'It's curious. One day is fine. I can walk the dogs across the field, and get back without too much difficulty. Another day I can get back only with difficulty. I then have to lie down for an hour or so before I can go on again.'[25] The capricious nature of fatigue is characteristic of the disease that gives rise to it. Everyone has experienced fatigue, particularly following strenuous exercise. The fatigue of MS seems not to be only something that involves muscles but sensory nerves as well.

> Fatigue of motor nerves can cause weakness, a tired heavy feeling of muscles, inco-ordination and shakiness. Fatigue of sensory nerves, which help us to see, to hear, to taste, to smell and enable us to distinguish how objects feel, can cause problems in one or more of these senses.[26]

Fatigue of MS comes on far quicker than 'ordinary' fatigue and often follows even mild exercise or taking a bath that is simply a few degrees hotter than is comfortable for the body. Indeed, the 'hot bath test' is proving to be a sensitive aid to diagnosing MS.[26]

Although fatigue is a physical sign, it may create problems in the emotional, mental and social areas of life — employment, relationships, depression, moodiness and fear of being 'neurotic'. Over-fatigue is to be avoided as it causes worsening of the other symptoms and may lead to relapse. It is by no means certain that fatigue does cause relapse, but chronic fatigue is cause enough for feeling unwell.[9]

Burnfield says that it is essential to keep fit by a balanced programme of daily exercise, *within the individual's capabilities*, and with plenty of rest. He recommends Yoga, calisthenics and swimming.[26] The 'Rest Exercise Programme', as taught by Ritche Russell[27] and advocated by Cross[17] is based on a *gradual* building up of stamina by 20 minute periods of vigorous exercise — '. . . anything appropriate for the particular patient and should demand maximal effort in a short time, after which the heart rate is increased and the patient is dyspnoeic.'[17] Exercise is followed by rest periods of 20 minutes. Such exercise programmes are best supervised by physiotherapists. Progress may be slowed by the patient's feeling of overwhelming fatigue which results from the slightest activity. This '. . . physical exhaustion and lack of exercise tolerance can be a very limiting factor to any rehabilitation programme.'[28] Rehabilitation therapists who disregard the fatigue element may, as so many other people do, put the patient's slow progress down to lack of motivation, apathy, or some such psychological manifestation.

Excretory. Almost two thirds of people with established MS have a combination of urgency of micturition (60 per cent), hesitancy (33 per cent) and incontinence (10 per cent). Almost 80 per cent have some form of bladder disturbance.[29] Urinary incontinence may add to sexual difficulties as well as social and vocational limitations.[30] Constipation, with impacted faeces, is the most common bowel dysfunction.

Bladder dysfunction may be eased by regular voiding, treatment of constipation, prompt treatment of infections and by avoiding excessive fluid intake at certain times of the day.[29] Bowel dysfunction may be avoided by high roughage diet and regular evacuation. The emotional overtones of bladder and bowel dysfunction may be more serious than the physical dysfunctions themselves.

Patricia Wright says, '. . . most of us suffering incontinence feel ashamed of admitting it'.[24] Incontinence renders apparent what is not visible. 'However careful I am, I'm always aware of a smell. It must put people off.' Frequency and urgency also create difficulties. Long car trips — on motorways, or even in rural areas where toilets are sparse — are problematic. Invitations may be turned down for fear of being embarrassed or causing embarrassment. 'How do you explain to someone, that although it was only five minutes ago, you want to go again?' Excretory dysfunction can be a potent isolator.

The psychological significance of incontinence is worthy of mention. Whatever the child-rearing method, control of bladder and bowel are significant achievements to be rewarded with praise. Throughout life the excretory functions are usually carried out in relative privacy. Thus when disability interferes with excretion, and particularly when there is incontinence, the person has to adjust to an enforced return to an infantile stage of behaviour; a stage when there was little or no control over bladder and bowel. If control was linked to praise, lack of control often incurred mother's displeasure. The early feelings of struggling to gain control, of sometimes succeeding and sometimes not, may be long since forgotten. But the feelings, and the associated behaviour, are stored in the unconscious, ready to resurface when they are given the right cues. This regression, to past feeling and behaviour, is usually temporary, lasting ony until the person adjusts to the disability that has led to it.

Sexual. Sexual dysfunction often accompanies MS and may be present in the early stages of the disease. Erection may be difficult, although it is by no means certain that this is always due to neurological damage. The psychological stress may be a contributory factor. 'Not infrequently a failure to obtain satisfactory erection results from disturbance of the sensation in the penis.'[29] In one study[31] all the eight male respondents had partial or total impotence. The author points out that impotence may '. . . vary from minor difficulties in establishing and maintaining an erection, through disturbances of sensation and ejaculation, to absolute failure'.

The main problems of women who have MS are: loss of arousal and orgasm; diminished libido; spasticity; reduced lubrication; anxiety about bladder control. Urinary catheters can prove an embarrassing nuisance to both sexes. Though the sexual difficulties of women are less obvious than those of men, and may be less threatening, to a woman who has enjoyed a satisfying sex life, any of the difficulties mentioned may become real problems.

Sexual difficulties may put the marriage under great strain. As Wright says,

> It can be the last straw for loving marriage partners to find that the illness of one means that their sex life is either impossible or indescribably difficult. Pain, inability to attain certain positions, loss of sensation, all these can put added strain on a marriage which is already under stress.[24]

One of the strains is conflict. Campling puts it thus, 'It is not easy for the disabled woman to be both patient and sexual partner in a relationship which now involves both, or for her husband to fulfil the role of nurse and lover.'[7] The emotional switch is very subtle. The nurse (as an example of a 'carer') employs touch in a very special way and for specific purposes, and she is permitted very intimate contact only by maintaining emotional distance from the patient. Part of the 'contract' (although not made explicit) is that the patient is dependent on the nurse. Another part of the contract is that a sexual relationship is taboo. A related point is that 'being nursed' is reminiscent of the child/parent relationship. For most people, it would be as taboo to make love to one's nurse as to one's father or mother, for in both acts there would be overtones of incest. Thus, when one's spouse takes on nursing functions, a curious relationship-shift takes place as the roles become polarised into 'nurse' and 'patient'. When this polarisation is fixed, sexual relationships are sure to founder. Both partners are caught in a double bind from which it is difficult to escape without psychological assistance.

Children. 'Should we have children?' 'Is MS inherited?' These questions are understandable when it is remembered that the majority of people contract the disease while still young enough to want a family. McAlpine[10] puts the risk for a first degree relative at least 5 times that for a member of the general population. MS, although familial is not inherited.[8,32] and may reflect common exposure to a similar environmental factor, rather than a genetically determined aetiology.[8] The 'environment factor' theory is disputed by Sadovnick and Macleod[33] who studied 416 patients and their 7,945 relatives. These researchers concluded their study by saying,

> Although the risks are low, relatives of MS patients have a greater risk of developing the disease than the general population. Since this is true of second- and third-degree relatives as well as first-degree relatives the increased risk cannot be explained solely by environmental factors.[33]

The main thrust of their argument is that a genetic component in MS does exist although, as they admit, there is no clear Mendelian pattern.

Whether or not couples, after carefully considering the risk, do decide to have children, they may well be worried about the effect on the woman if she is the affected partner. There is an increased risk of relapse within the first months following the birth of a child[10;29;31] but in the long term, the condition of these women does not appear to be different from single women or married women without children. The main contraindication to having children is the severity of the patient's disability. It does seem sensible to suggest that a woman waits for about two years after a diagnosis of MS has been made. She may not wish, or feel able, to take on a family should the course of her MS be a rapid one.[31] But if she does, every measure should be taken to ensure that fatigue is reduced as much as possible.

Emotional Dysfunction

Both anxiety and depression have been discussed previously, so, other than a brief mention, they will not be dealt with here. Anxiety is more common in the early stages of MS,[29] and depression was found in 25 per cent of 108 MS patients studied.[34] Matthews[9] on the other hand, considers the incidence of depression in people with MS to be no more common than in the rest of the population. Although depression may be present in MS, there is no general agreement whether it is caused by actual brain damage, or if it is reaction to the disease. It would be fully understandable if depression was a reactive state, when one considers the number, and the degree, of changes to which the person is forced to adjust. Rehabilitation therapists who understand depression are able to help in the adjustment process of the patient and his relatives.

The discussion in this section will focus on euphoria and changes in self-concept.

Euphoria. Euphoria — a state of exaggerated well-being and cheery good humour — has been quoted by many people as a symptom of MS.[35] Various figures have been given for its incidence. Two extremes are 7 per cent[19] and 26 per cent.[34] This would suggest that, as with most other symptoms associated with MS, there is no certainty that euphoria will be present or that it will prove to be a disabling emotion.

Burnfield[16] says that euphoria may mask depression. With this in mind, it is important to distinguish between the impression the person gives of his mood and how he actually feels. Surridge[34] makes an interesting observation. He found that an exaggerated sense of well-being was more often present in the initial stages of interview than later. He concludes that the later mood was more truly representative. He also suggests that euphoria is associated with the more seriously disabled who also showed intellectual deterioration. He also pointed to a link between euphoria and denial of disability. He sums up his discussion on euphoria in this way, 'These findings would all argue that euphoria is a pathological phenomenon, the direct result of damage to the central nervous system.'

The definition of euphoria given above has been extended to '. . . a marked sense of well-being out of proportion to their physical condition.'[36] A cautionary note is sounded. In some people, particularly the young, who are not severely disabled from MS, '. . . the patient's denial of difficulties and apparent need to present a good front may lead physicians to believe they perceive euphoria.'[37] What has been mistaken for euphoria may be true integration — '. . . a response to a fuller appreciation of life, an appreciation gained by living intimately with the unknown and the threatening.'[38] It is doubtful if patients who are minimally disabled do experience feelings 'out of proportion to their physical condition'. The denial they express '. . . seems to be an adaptive coping mechanism rather than the pathological state implied by Sugar and Nadell.'[37] This seems to substantiate Surridge's findings already referred to.

The comments about denial have implications for rehabilitation. Denial and acceptance are incompatible. Acceptance is necessary for adjustment. If euphoria is linked with denial, the person will be unable to consider rehabilitation as a realistic aim. If euphoria is present in people who are seriously disabled, then it is likely that there is also intellectual deterioration.

Self-concept Changes. One of the points about euphoria is that it could be a compensation for a loss of well-being and a change in self-concept. A person's ideal of self is influenced by being able to look after himself, to be independent, to be able to do — within limits — what he wants to do. Enforced changes in these are likely to produce a diminished sense of well-being and, therefore, of self. Dependence on other people, for the person with MS, may cause emotional distress, coupled with physical distress caused by the disease. The resultant loss of well-being is often quite marked. The person's view of himself changes; his view of the world changes; the world's view of him changes. These feelings of loss are very real. Burnfield[16] has likened the process — of establishing a new identity — to bereavement; a process that may last a long time. He adds, 'If the experience of loss is not expressed, bottled-up feelings may cause serious problems later, such as depression and relationship difficulties.' Opportunities to explore feelings will only be given if other people accept that disability may attack one's inner being — the self. Accepting this, however, is not enough; we need to recognise when a person with MS is *expressing* such feelings.

Having MS demands a restructuring of the self-concept which involves personal identity (who am I?); life's course (where am I going?); relationships (who is going with me?); values (what is my worth?); and expectations (what are my needs?). Self-concept is constantly undergoing change anyway, influenced by circumstances and relationships. This being so, none of us is static and as we get older we are forced (if growing old is to be achieved with grace and dignity) to accommodate gradually to declining bodily functions. The accommodation enforced upon a person with MS is governed by the age at onset, the progress of the disease and its severity.

The person's view of himself in the present is, to a great extent, coloured by the lens of the future, as he sees himself becoming a helpless, devalued person, unacceptable in the eyes of the person or people to whom he most looks for support.[39] If this is so, then significant people (and these will include 'professional carers') have a tremendous responsibility to do everything possible to enhance the self-image of the person who has MS. This is not done by words alone and often not by words at all. Words that are uttered in an attempt to reassure, words that spring from an unaccepting attitude, will wound the sensitive 'self' still further; or at best will be perceived as empty and meaningless and will have the effect of deflating the person's self-worth.

The authors of one study, of coping strategies linked to self-concept,[38] concluded:

1. The longer people have the disease, the more the self-concept improves.
2. Improvement in self-concept is influenced negatively by the restriction in activity.
3. 'Religion', as a coping strategy, is related to a better self-concept.

Points 1 and 2 seem to contradict the commonsense notion of what the case might be. Indeed, these two points have been challenged. Using a broader and better array of personality and health status measures, the authors concluded that, '. . . greater physical disability is associated with decrements in personal efficiency and well-being, adaptive autonomy, self-reliance, social confidence and actual social contacts.'[40] It seems, from their study, that severity, rather than duration of illness, is the factor that most influences self-concept. Increased self-confidence and social contact are directly related to those who have the least physical dysfunction. Physical dysfunction was defined in terms of ambulation, mobility, body care and movement. Another finding in the same study was that marriage did not '. . . appear to serve as a buffer in preserving a sense of well-being in the face of both physical disability and life stress.' The discrepancy between these two studies[38,40] highlights one difficulty in research findings; the two groups, although studying the same illness, used different dependent variables. Because they were looking for different things, perhaps it is not surprising that their results were different. Nevertheless, what they did find is an important contribution to our understanding of MS. But the question, how the person's personality influences the course of the illness and how the illness is coped with, remains unanswered.

Mental Dysfunction

In this section the discussion will focus on personality and personality changes resulting from MS.

Personality. The notion that a person may have a physical disability but remain untouched in all other respects, is an appealing idea which is advocated by some people.[11] There are people with disabilities, no doubt, who would agree with this statement: others would admit to personality changes as a result of having MS. This begs the question, is there one type of person who copes better than another with a chronic disease such as MS? The answer to this is as complex as the question.

On p. 160 the subject of personality was related to stress. Six personality factors of people who cope well with stress were listed. On page 256, nine factors which appear to predispose people to depressive breakdown are given. Stubbins[41] says that the authoritarian personality (the person who perceives everything in black or white terms; is intolerant of ambiguity, contradiction and pluralism) is vulnerable to the threat of disability. This is particularly pertinent to MS sufferers, where the whole progress of their disease is beset with uncertainty. MS often commences at an age before the various characteristics have become fused together as 'personality'. In this instance the person is likely to respond with denial of any distress or difficulty[37] — a point already referred to.

Lloyd says, '. . . people with obsessional traits tend to find illness particularly stressful if there is doubt about the diagnosis, treatment or prognosis.'[42] Again this is relevant to people with MS. This short discussion on personality types and MS is summed up in,

> the vulnerable personality calls for watchfulness: the happy-go-lucky person tends to fare best, whereas someone who has coped badly with minor problems, or the obsessional, controlled type of person may need special help — as do those who have no supporting relationship in their lives.[43]

What must not be inferred from this discussion, however, is that there is one personality type who will cope better than another with a chronic condition such as MS. In trying to assess a person's possible adjustment potential, it is essential to take a multi-factoral approach, such as is recommended on page 266. 'What does this illness mean?'

Personality Changes. Three personality changes, identified by Surridge, are relevant to rehabilitation: memory loss (46 per cent of cases); conceptual thinking impairment (42 per cent of cases); circumstantial talk or wandering off the point (35 per cent of cases).[34]

'When these deficits were marked, confabulation, perseveration, excessive fatiguability and speech disturbances of a dysphasic nature also occurred frequently.'[34] These findings are supported in another study of 43 patients who showed disturbances in short-term memory, learning and delayed recall.[44] Verbal and non-verbal memory were equally affected. Those researchers suggested that memory disturbances might begin early in the history of the disease.

Changes in intellectual functioning are attributed to 'frontal lobe syndrome',[45] and this fact is related to findings that 54.7 per cent of people with MS, with a mean age of 40.62 years, and a mean duration of illness of 10.31 years, suffer '. . . cognitive impairment, as demonstrated on a task of abstract conceptualization'.[46] People in whom memory, conceptual thinking and attention are impaired, are not likely to have a high ability to learn new tasks, to organise or to carry them through. Problem-solving will come with difficulty. Impairment of self-control, with rigidity of attitudes, and inability to adapt to new situations may well be in evidence.[37] Lincoln[45] also suggests that MS patients who have intellectual deficits, give unrealistic reports of how they manage their activities of daily living. While this is undoubtedly linked to their short-term memory loss, it could also be due to their lack of insight, which is another feature of frontal lobe syndrome.[47] Intellectual changes, of the kind here described, make rehabilitation problematic. Counselling, as a part of rehabilitation, because of its cognitive element, may also be difficult. In such instances, counselling may have to be kept very simple. To be able to operate at a simple, feeling level, may not come easily to some therapists who are accustomed to working at a high level of conceptual thought.

Social Dysfunction

In this section the discussion will focus on role change, some aspects of which have already been touched on in previous sections of this chapter. The discussion will cross the boundaries between physical, emotional and mental dysfunctions. This is inevitable, for it is impossible to consider such a topic as role change without the discussion impinging on all aspects of a person's life.

Healthy — Disabled. The person who says, 'I was well now I am ill' is expressing a dramatic change of role. The 'well' person has expectations and obligations that are completely turned on their head when he is ill. Some of these expectations and obligations are:

1. Responsibility for actions. The ill person is deemed to have no control over, or responsibility for, his illness.
2. Independence. The ill person is permitted to be dependent on others, albeit for a limited time.
3. Social obligations to provide for himself and his dependents. The ill person is excused his obligations — examples are, employment, sick pay and social security benefits.

4. Maintenance of health. The ill person is expected to get well as quickly as possible; this involves seeking competent help to get well.
5. To be productive. The ill person is permitted to be a passenger for a limited period of time.

When a person, because of chronic illness, disability or handicap, does not 'get well', sights (his and other people's) have to be readjusted. Some people do not accept the 'sick role' and fight violently against it. Accepting the diminished activities, that accompany the sick role, means relinquishing so many things that reinforce feelings of worth. Some of these will now be considered.

Employed — Unemployed. Occupation means a great deal to most people. Not only is it a means of income — and, therefore, of survival — it is a valuable source of social contact. Working at home is, for many women, just as important as going out to work. Inability to perform household tasks, or when they take far longer than they used to, causes concern. While many people with MS do continue working, many have to adapt to greatly reduced activity which finally makes work difficult.

The Breadwinner — Dependant. 'Often the price of family harmony seems to be an acceptance of a dependent or subordinate role for the disabled woman.'[7] That person was speaking of the dependent role of women, particularly those whose income was a major contribution to the family budget. They are likely to be feel guilty and devalued, because they can no longer contribute as before. Where the person with MS has been the major wage earner, the loss is serious indeed, with overtones of 'idleness', 'sponger', 'shirker' and so on. Many people disabled from MS speak of being a burden.

Marriage Under Threat. Attention has already been drawn to the sexual differences that MS may cause, in the subtle role change from lover to patient and lover to nurse. Some spouses find great difficulty in looking after the physical needs of their spouse.[29] I would suggest that this difficulty has its roots in fear; fear that such attention will get in the way of the love relationship, and so alter that relationship as to make love-making impossible. Wherever one marriage partner is affected by MS, and needs physical care, the husband and wife roles need to be redefined; yet in the redefining lies great stress. This stress puts the marriage at risk. Wright[24] says, 'For of all diseases MS holds the record as the highest marriage-breaker of all.' This statement (not supported by facts) may seem to be too sweeping. It is borne out, to some extent, in Canada where 40 per cent of marriages, where one partner has MS, end in divorce.[32] Burnfield,[16] who agrees that MS does put strain on a marriage, says that it may be used as a scapegoat to take the blame for a relationship which is already strained to breaking point. This view is upheld in a study of 36 disabled women.[48] In those marriages which survive the stresses associated with disability, '. . . some bond of love has been maintained and . . . each partner is directly dependent upon the other for satisfaction of love needs.' MS does put marriages under stress, particularly when the partners do not discuss their feelings. Helping both partners to be aware of the other's feelings would be a valuable counselling input by the rehabilitation therapist.

Coping. Some coping strategies are mentioned earlier.[5,38] The evidence seems convincing that successful coping — with any disabling condition — depends on how well one has coped in the past, coupled with effective and appropriate support. In a study of 22 married couples, where one partner had MS, Miles[49] concluded that such couples have to develop new ways of interacting with people around them. They no longer interact as equals; they feel inferior. Miles used two concepts: 'normalisation' — 'I am not different' and 'dissatisfaction' — 'I am different and inferior'. People who used normalisation maintained contact with healthy people. Those who used disassociation withdrew from involvement with the healthy, not risking being treated as different and inferior persons because of their illness.

One of the elements in successful coping is support from relatives, friends, and groups of various kinds. A curious finding of this study was that 77 per cent of those who were members of the MS society used 'disassociation' as a means of coping. For many of them, their only social contacts were with other MS sufferers or their spouses. It seems that these people had immersed themselves in the 'sick role' so totally as to exclude anyone who was not similarly ill.

Where a couple lived, or chose to move to, after a diagnosis of MS was made, is relevant. A high proportion of those who lived in housing estates used disassociation — 82 per cent;. they had moved *after* a diagnosis of MS was made. But it was not clear if the spouse, or the person with MS, initiated the move to another locality. If the spouse did initiate the move, it could indicate the spouse's difficulty in coping. It was clear, however, that spouses are very caught up in the particular coping strategy; they seemed totally 'at one'. It was also clear that the role of caring for a chronically sick person is an experience for which most people are not prepared. Trying to cope with all this, and possibly living in a locality which they consider hostile, without family ties, was too much for them. Disassociation was their choice of strategy.

People who feel 'different', inferior and stigmatised are likely to seek out those who, by virtue of having a similar condition, do understand. That is when belonging to a local MS group can provide support and so mediate against further disruption and possibly total breakdown.

Summary

There are very definitive statements of fact in this chapter; much of the discussion opens up topics and floats ideas. Indeed, it may be that the whole chapter seems inconclusive. That is precisely the nature of the illness under consideration. If anything emerges with stark clarity, it is that MS is a disease of great uncertainty. It demyelinates not only the nerve sheaths, causing physical disability, but every other fibre of its victim's life, causing emotional, mental and social disability. It is the illness that rightly qualifies as 'the paradigm for all chronic illness'.

The discussion, through free-ranging, has attempted to answer the questions: what does this illness mean:

To this person?
In these circumstances?
At this time of life?
With these relatives? (or lack of them)
In this environment?

But in trying to discover answers, more questions were raised, to which answers were not possible. The uncertainty and ambiguity surrounding MS is similar to that encountered whenever counselling takes place. Very often the person doing the counselling feels impatient and frustrated that there seems so little he can actually do. Responsibility for change is the client's. In MS, great changes are forced upon the client; changes which may be so rapid that adaptation lags far behind. In such a situation, counselling is a rearguard action, the aim of which is to salvage as much as possible from the wreckage that many clients feel their lives to be. Where the progress of the disease is slow, the client has more opportunity to adapt; yet the eternity of certain uncertainty proves too much for some people, whose coping strategies prove inadequate. Withdrawal from social relations and marriage breakdown are two examples of how destructive any chronic illness may be.

The formidable list of symptoms associated with MS gives the impression of inevitable and total incapacitation, hopelessness and uselessness. That some people do feel this, cannot be denied; others still manage for years to live lives which they feel are useful and productive.

Many people with MS have learned the most valuable lesson, that of living a day at a time. These are those who have reached the stage of 'integration',[38] not resignation — acceptance. To reach this stage of integration, the majority of people would need psychological help — of the type suggested in this book. Some may receive it from relatives and friends; others, by force of circumstances, unless they receive help from professional carers, will not receive it at all. Resignation is unlikely to have the insight to say, 'a day at a time', but rather 'where have my days gone?' To offer rehabilitation to a person suffering from MS, without offering counselling as an integral part, is like throwing to a drowning man a life-raft with a puncture in it.

Notes

1. Brown, C. (1972) *My Left Foot*, Secker and Warburg, London. And re-published (1972) as *The Childhood Story of Christy Brown*, Pan Books.

2. Morris, A. (1970) *Chronically Sick and Disabled Persons Bill*, United Kingdom.

3. Marsh, G.G., Ellison, G.W. and Strite, C. (1983) 'Psychological and vocational rehabilitation approaches to M.S.', *Annual Review of Rehabilitation, 3*, pp. 242–67.

4. Strauss, A.L. (1975) *Chronic Illness and the Quality of Life*, Mosby, St Louis.

5. Brooks, N.A. and Matson, R.R. (1982) 'Social-psychological adjustment to Multiple Sclerosis: a longitudinal study', *Social Science and Medicine, 16*, pp. 2129–35.

6. Walster, E., Berscheid, E. and Walster, W. (1976) 'New directions in Equity research', in *Advances in Experimental Psychology, 9*, Berkowitz, L. (ed.), Academic Press, New York.

7. Campling, J. (1979) *Better Lives for Disabled Women*, Virago Ltd, London.

8. Office of Health Economics (1975) *Multiple Sclerosis.*

9. Matthews, B. (1979) *M.S.: The Facts*, Oxford University Press, Oxford and New York.

10. McAlpine, D., Lumsden, C.E. and Acheson, E.D. (1965) *Multiple Sclerosis: A Reappraisal*, Livingstone Ltd., Edinburgh.

11. Miller, E.J. and Gwynne, G.V. (1972) *A Life Apart*, Tavistock Publishing Ltd., London.

12. Cannon, J. (1983) *M.S. and the Problem of Dependency*, Southampton University 4th year Medical Student Project, Book No. 83 — 102970.

13. Kurtzke, J.F. (1965) 'Further notes on disability evaluation in MS with scales modifications', *Neurology, 15*, p. 661.

14. Poser, S., Bauer, H.J., Ritter, G., Friedrich, H., Beland, H. and Denecke, P. (1981) 'Rehabilitation for patients with M.S.?', *Journal of Neurology, 224*, pp. 283–90.

15. Sambrook, M.A. (1975) 'Medical management of M.S.', *Physiotherapy, 61*, pp. 2–4.

16. Burnfield, A. and Burnfield, P. (1978) 'Common psychological problems in M.S.', *British Medical Journal*, 6 May, pp. 1193–4.

17. Cross, V. (1980) 'M.S.: the physiotherapist's approach', *Journal of Community Nursing, 3, 8*, pp. 22–6.

18. Stewart, D.C. and Sullivan, T.J. (1982) 'Illness behaviour and the sick role in chronic disease: the case of Multiple Sclerosis', *Social Science and Medicine, 16*, pp. 1397–1404.

19. Christensen, D. and Clausen, J. (1977) 'Social remedial measures for Multiple Sclerosis patients in Denmark', *Acta Neurologica Scandinavica, 55 (5)*, pp. 394–406.

20. Burnfield, A. (1984) 'Doctor-patient dilemmas in Multiple Sclerosis', *Journal of Medical Ethics, 1*, pp. 21–6.

21. Brown, J. (1984) 'One man's experience with M.S.', in Simon, A.F. *Multiple Sclerosis: Psychological and Social Aspects*, William Heinemann Medical Books, London.

22. Wright, B.A. (1960) *Physical Disability — A Psychological Approach*, Harper and Row, New York.

23. Fritsch, M. (1972) 'Possibilities in the medical treatment and rehabilitation of severely handicapped patients suffering from Multiple Sclerosis', *Proceedings* of the 12th World Congress of Rehab. International, pp. 473–6.

24. Wright, P. (1978) 'At home with MS . . . a patient's view', *Journal of Community Nursing, 1, 10*, pp. 16–28.

25. Burnfield, A. A personal conversation.

26. Burnfield, A. (1983) 'Coping with fatigue in MS takes understanding and planning', *MS Canada*, July.

27. Ritchie, Russell, W. (1976) *Multiple Sclerosis*, Pergamon Press, Oxford.

28. Nosworthy, S.J. (1976) 'Physiotherapy', in 'A Symposium on Multiple Sclerosis', *Nursing Mirror*, 5 August, pp. 45–57.

29. McLellan, D.L. (1981) 'A neurologist's view of MS', *Newsletter* of the Wessex Neurological Rehabilitation Group.

30. Kelly-Hayes, M. (1980) 'Guidelines for rehabilitation of Multiple Sclerosis patients', *Nursing Clinics of North America, 15, 2*, pp. 245–56.

31. Burnfield, P. (1979) 'Sexual problems and MS', *British Journal of Sexual Medicine*, July, pp. 33–7.

32. Multiple Sclerosis Society of Canada (1984) MS: *Model 2. A Personal and Family Focus*, Toronto, Ontario M55 1N5.

33. Sadovnick, A.D. and Macleod, M.J. (1981) 'The familial nature of Multiple Sclerosis: empiric recurrence risks for first, second-, and third-degree relatives of patients', *Neurology, 31*, pp 1039–41.

34. Surridge, D. (1969) 'An investigation into some psychiatric aspects of Multiple Sclerosis', *British Journal of Psychiatry, 115*, pp. 749–64.

35. Whitlock, A. (1980) 'Emotional disorders in Multiple Sclerosis', in Simon, *Multiple Sclerosis*.

36. Sugar, C. and Nadell, R. (1943) 'Mental symptoms in Multiple Sclerosis', *Journal of Nervous and Mental Disorders, 98*, pp. 267–80.

37. Peyser, J.M., Edwards, K.R. and Poser, C.M. (1980) 'Psychological profiles in patients with Multiple Sclerosis', *Archives of Neurology, 37*, pp. 437–40.

38. Matson, R.R. and Brooks, N.A. (1977) 'Adjustment to Multiple Sclerosis: an exploratory study', *Social Science and Medicine, 11*, pp. 245–50.

39. Bolding, H. (1960) 'Psychotherapeutic aspects in the management of patients with Multiple Sclerosis', *Diseases of the Nervous System, 21*, pp. 24–86.

40. Zeldon, P.B. and Pavlou, M. (1984) 'Physical disability, life stress and psychological adjustment in Multiple Sclerosis', *Journal of Nervous and Mental Disorders, 172, 2*, pp. 80–4

41. Stubbins, J. (ed) (1977) *Social and Psychological Aspects of Disability*, University Park Press, Baltimore.

42. Lloyd, G.G. (1977) 'Psychological reactions to physical illness', *British Journal of Hospital Medicine*, October, pp. 352–8.

43. Editorial, *British Medical Journal*, 23 September 1978, p. 847.

44. Grant, I., McDonald, W.T., Trimble, M.B. and Smith, E. (1984) 'Deficient learning and memory in early and middle phases of Multiple Sclerosis', *Journal of Neurology, Neurosurgery and Psychiatry, 47*, pp. 250–5.

45. Lincoln, N.B. (1981) 'Discrepancies between capabilities and performance of activities of daily living in Multiple Sclerosis patients', *International Rehabilitation Medicine, 3*, pp. 84–8.

46. Peyser, J.M., Edwards, K.R., Poser, C.M. and Filskov, S.B. (1980) 'Cognitive functioning in patients with Multiple Sclerosis', *Archives of Neurology, 37*, pp. 577–9.

47. Vowells, L.M. and Gates, G.R. 'Neuropsychological findings', in Simon, *Multiple Sclerosis*.

48. Skipper, J.K., Fink, S.L. and Hallenbeck, P.N. (1968) 'Physical disability among married women: problems in the husband-wife relationship', in Stubbins, *Social and Psychological Aspects*.

49. Miles, A. (1978) 'Some psycho-social consequences of Multiple Sclerosis: problems of social interaction and group identity', *British Journal of Medical Psychology, 52*, pp. 321–31.

Recommended Reading

Burnfield, A. *Multiple Sclerosis: a Personal Exploration* (Souvenir Press Ltd, London, 1985).

Glastonbury, G., Cantrell, T. and Dawson, J. *Prisoners of Handicap* (University of Southampton, 1983).

14 TOWARDS INDEPENDENT LIVING: SEPARATION OR RECONCILIATION

> A body is not a single organ, but many. Suppose the foot should say, 'Because I am not a hand, I do not belong to the body', it does belong to the body none the less. Suppose the ear were to say, 'Because I am not an eye, I do not belong to the body', it does still belong to the body. If the body were all ear, how could it smell? But, in fact, God appointed each limb and organ to its own place in the body, as he chose. If the whole were one single organ, there would not be a body at all; in fact, however, there are many different organs, but one body. The eye cannot say to the hand, 'I do not need you', nor the hand to the feet 'I do not need you', . . . If one organ suffers, they all suffer together. If one flourishes, they all rejoice together.
>
> (The New English Bible. 1 Corinthians 12: 14–26)

Introduction

In this final chapter we shall consider the place in society of the person with disability. We have already considered the dramatic change of role from 'healthy' to 'disabled' and the problems that disablement often brings, as the person and the significant people in his life struggle to make sense of what has happened. They have to establish new identities for themselves. Part of those new identities involve the remainder of society. For every person who becomes disabled, society is forced to establish for *itself*, a new identity. Many people with disabilities find this struggle too great, and give up. If society is to function effectively, and that means the disabled too, there needs to be far greater understanding and acceptance of every single person, as someone without whom the rest of us cannot function to our full potential.

The 'Body' Concept

The analogy of society as a human body is apt, when one thinks of 'all parts working together'. The human body is complex in its composition, construction and function. But the perfect functioning of the body depends upon all parts working together in balance and harmony. Any disturbance in one part of the body, and 'dis-harmony', will affect the whole body; the body will feel 'out of sorts' and will misfunction. When we consider the body, we think of its various systems, every single one functionally perfect, yet unable to exist independently of any of the others. If every system of the body was a personality in its own right, would they each claim pre-eminence? Would each battle for supremacy and seek to adopt a dominant position over the others? No one system could isolate itself from the others, by adopting a 'superior' attitude. Nor could one system, or a number of them 'gang' up on another and isolate it. No one system may, because it feels 'more important', 'more needed', demand more attention than any other. When every system is inter-dependent, no one is less, nor more, important than any other. For it to be otherwise, would impose intolerable stress on the body and chaos would result. This is what happens in illness.

Illness is not caused by one part of the body 'deciding' that it will assume dominance; neither is illness caused by one system being isolated by all other parts. Yet in a sense, at that time, the affected part *is* demanding more attention from every other part; the other parts respond in sympathy. Their own needs become subservient to the needs of the affected part. Witness the reaction of the hand when the leg is injured; the natural response is to hold, or rub, the affected part and so to soothe away the pain. When disease strikes the body, defending white blood cells rush to devour the intruders. All parts work together.

This analogy, taken from the Biblical quotation that heads this chapter, was used, by St. Paul, to demonstrate the inter-dependence of every member of the Christian church, where each may have had a different function. These functions were generally thought of as gifts or talents which, if not used, caused the rest of the Christian fellowship to function imperfectly. Paul was exhorting his readers to work together, in the same way as the body does, for the good of the whole.

Body-image and Society

Society's view of itself is similar to the view a person has of his own body. This is the body-image, which in turn is part of the self-concept. I would like to propose that society has a 'collective body-image'. The inner picture that society has of itself is as complex as the picture the individual has of himself. Reference to chapter 6 shows that the individual has an 'ideal self' and a 'personal self'. A significant point is that the body-image is constantly changing — at least for the majority of people who realistically accept changes. A dramatic change in body-image results from chronic illness and disability.

The self-image, that society has internalised, corresponds to the idealised image which the individual holds of himself. The discrepancy between society's idealised image and the realistic image, is great. This is because there are many individuals and groups of people who 'spoil' that image. People with chronic illness and disability form such a group. Individuals who retain a 'healthy' and realistic body-image, are those who have accommodated changes. Societies who reject disabled people — striving desperately to retain an unchanged body-image — are not 'healthy'. A pathological example of such 'disassociation' was Nazi Germany's attempt to exterminate the Jews. The 'healthiest' societies are those who accommodate people who are 'different'. Disability makes people different.

Most people would regard, as pathological, the person who, not liking the shape of it, cuts off his nose. In much the same way, parents who 'disown' their son, because he does not match up to their ideals, are regarded with suspicion by other people. Yet, on a larger scale, society does this to those who are disabled. It cuts them off and disowns them, because they do not match up to an ideal; they spoil the image. The person who cuts off his nose mutilates himself, yes, but he also does irreparable harm to his body-image. Though his intention was to improve his looks, he has disfigured himself, thereby creating a massive scar in his body-image. His ideal self is pushed further away. The parents who disown their son have carved a hole in their family body-image, a hole that no other person can fill and which, if it is not filled by the son, will never shrink. When society cuts disabled people off and disowns them, it mutilates and creates holes that cannot be filled. The result is a spoiled body-image. Society has achieved, by its actions, what it hoped to avoid — a spoiled identity, a spoiled self-concept. A society which acts like this toward disabled people is not whole, and never will be until it incorporates those whom it has cut off and isolated — those whom it regards as not 'normal'. Individuals, if they are to remain emotionally healthy, have to accept themselves as they are — warts and all. Society must do likewise.

The Concept Applied

The man who, as the result of a stroke, is left with the legacy of a weakened arm, may do one of two things. He may totally ignore the arm. 'It is no longer mine' and end up crippled; or he can tenderly love it back to a degree of usefulness. The one approach is 'separation', the other is 'reconciliation'. Separation implies incompleteness; reconciliation, wholeness. The man needs to discover what his arm can do and what it cannot. He may regret that it can no longer function alone; that it has to be aided by his good arm, but he adjusts to its limitations. He — and the rest of his body — adjusts to his arm's limited function. But they, all the body members — become reconciled to what is, in effect, a 'new body'. In like manner, society is given two choices to deal with those who are disabled — separation or reconciliation.

Society, at its peril, says, 'We don't need you. Go away, we cannot stand the sight of you. Look! we have provided you with this beautiful place, where you can be happy with people who are like yourself. You can be sheltered there, protected, fed, watered and groomed. We are a caring society.' But this is separation, not reconciliation. Is this not the hand saying to the foot, 'I have no need of you?' This is not all parts working together for the good of the whole.

Give and Take

The weakened arm could say (had it a voice) 'I am weak, no good and useless. I want to be looked after. It is my right.' The other members of the body could then rightly say, 'We will help you, but we cannot do everything for you. There are certain things that you, and only you, can do. If you do not do them, either they will not be done at all, or they will be done badly because we were not designed like you. Without you we are incomplete.' Some people become so immersed in their disability and self-pity that they expect — as their right — that other people will function for them. But these are a minority. Many more desperately want not to be separated from society, but to be reconciled to it, to be restored to active partnership, to function once more as a hand, foot, eye, or tongue. Reconciliation accepts that the function may not be quite as vigorous as before but even reduced function has a definite place.

Separation may be easier for society to bear than reconciliation. The one approach is statutory and fiscal; the other is hard work and is emotionally demanding. In the process of reconciliation, many of the feelings within society are thrown into sharp relief against the backcloth of chronic illness and disability. For it is as the person with disability struggles back to a degree of independence that society's attitudes toward disability are questioned. If we are to be reconciled with people who have disabilities, we need, like the body, to establish a new identity in which the reconciled person has a definite place and is able to function as an integrated 'member' *in spite of limitations*.

The foregoing discussion does not imply that society should do all the giving: reconciliation is a relationship of give and take. We all have rights, privileges, needs and wants. But hand in hand with these go responsibilities, obligations and duties. None of us, and this includes the person with a disability, may expect to exercise the first group without accepting the second. To do so is synonymous with the hand saying to the foot, 'I am more important than you'. The more that people with disabilities are reconciled to society — truly reconciled, accepted and helped to function as valuable, wanted and needed members — the less they will need to regard themselves as 'special' and expect (and sometimes demand) what may be denied to other members of society who are not disabled.

In the first chapter we considered certain constraints upon rehabilitation. None of us could be so complacent as to suggest that enough resources are devoted to people with disabilities, but a great deal has been, and is being, achieved. While it is absolutely right and proper for people with disability to let their voices be heard, they may, if not careful, become so dominant a voice that other groups — other parts of the body, also struggling to be reconciled — do not receive a fair share of scarce resources.

None of us goes through life without struggle; it would scarcely be to our benefit if we did. But when considering people with disability, one does sometimes wonder if impediments are deliberately put there (or not taken away) to ensure that life is made as difficult as possible. It would be too strong to condemn this attitude as 'sadistic', but it is certainly an attitude of indifference. Indifference is the offspring of ignorance. Much has been accomplished in the past 25 years to make known the feelings of many people who are disadvantaged, not only by illness and disability, but by bad housing, poverty and hunger. Perhaps at no other time in the world's history has the impact of suffering of whole communities engendered such response in the way of aid. The impact which suffering millions has made on many people, has been made possible by rapid spread of information by radio and newspapers but more startlingly, by television. In much the same way illness, of all kinds, has been brought into people's sitting rooms — *whether they want to know about it or not*. This may produce favourable results, and people respond by wanting to know more, thereby increasing their understanding of other people. Sometimes, however, people react in much the same way as when confronted with the sight of starving, dying people in Africa — they switch their emotional receiver off even though the television set is left receiving. Some people are so overwhelmed by suffering — *over which they have no influence* — that their only safeguard is to 'switch off'. In a sense, this re-echoes the 'learned helplessness' model of coping, referred to in chapter 11.

Publicity, then, for chronic illness and disability, may be constructive, but it can also be so stunning in the way it is presented as to be counter-productive. People who respond to the suffering of others by turning away, cannot be protected from chance encounters with people who are disabled, any more than the person who is disabled can, or should, be shielded from possible contact with people who would shun him because of his disability. That's life! But if provision for people with chronic illness and disability is to be improved, more people — of the sort who are prepared to do something to change the system — need to be better informed.

When society becomes better informed, and when the majority of people accept illness and disability as a part of a 'healthy' and 'whole' society, then, and only then will reconciliation and not separation operate. Then, and only then will Alfred Morris's hopes (stated on page 1), which hitherto have been little more than images drifting in the wind, take on solid form and become reality. That reality is a society where quality has been added to years and disabled people are truly members of, and working together as, one body.

NAME INDEX

SUBJECT INDEX